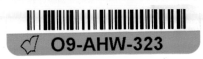

Your Career in

Cardiovascular Technology

Roberta C. Weiss, LVN, Ed.D.

Allied Health Curriculum Specialist
Vocational Education Teacher and Trainer

Your
Career
in

Cardiovascular Technology

W.B. Saunders Company
A Division of Harcourt Brace & Company
Philadelphia London Toronto
Montreal Sydney Tokyo

W.B. SAUNDERS COMPANY

A Division of Harcourt Brace & Company

The Curtis Center
Independence Square West
Philadelphia, Pennsylvania 19106

Library of Congress Cataloging–in–Publication Data

Weiss, Roberta C.
    Your career in cardiovascular technology / Roberta C. Weiss.—
1st ed.
        p.   cm.
    ISBN 0–7216–6074–6
    1. Cardiovascular system—Diseases—Diagnosis.   2. Medical
technology—Vocational guidance.   3. Cardiology—Vocational
guidance.   I. Title.
    [DNLM: 1. Heart Function Tests.   2. Diagnosis, Laboratory.
3. Respiratory Therapy.   4. Allied Health Personnel.   WG 141 W432y
1996]
RC670.W45   1996
616.1′023—dc20
DNLM/DLC   95–17718

YOUR CAREER IN CARDIOVASCULAR TECHNOLOGY   ISBN 0–7216–6074–6

Printed in the United States of America

Last digit is the print number: 9   8   7   6   5   4   3   2   1

This book is very lovingly dedicated
to my dear friend, Betsy Raulerson,

who taught me the importance of discipline
and the meaning of "unconditional friendship."

Preface

With all of the technological breakthroughs, the ever-changing and increasing costs in medical care, and the constant need to fill new positions in all health-related disciplines, the delivery of health care as we once knew it no longer exists. Instead, we are rushing to meet the demands of a society that, because its members live longer, is in greater need of care by health care professionals trained in a number of occupations within the same educational discipline. According to the United States Department of Labor, health care will continue to be one of the fastest-growing industries in our economy. By the year 2005, employment in health-related occupations is projected to grow from 8.9 million in 1994 to 12.8 million. Of those many millions of jobs, the majority of employers agree that those individuals trained in more than one occupation will have the greatest opportunity to fill them.

Your Career in Cardiovascular Technology is a textbook based on the concept of training a professional in more than one occupation within the same health care discipline. It is written in simple, yet comprehensive language, and is accompanied by photographs and basic illustrations to provide the reader with a well-rounded introduction to the principles and techniques involved in the various allied health occupations in the field of cardiovascular technology.

Although this author and educator firmly believes that there are many adequate textbooks currently in use that provide information for the person interested either in advanced techniques in cardiovascular technology or in a specific area of interest, no other text exists that covers more than one occupation in that field.

The text consists of 36 chapters and covers concepts and hands-on skills and techniques involved in the study of basic health careers opportunities, scientific principles and medical terminology, electrocardiography, echocardiography, laboratory assisting, respiratory therapy assisting, and administrative and job-seeking skills for the cardiovascular worker. To assist readers in their understanding of the subject matter, each chapter is accompanied by performance objectives and a list of terms and abbreviations at the beginning of each chapter, and a short summary of the material at the end of each chapter. In addition, to assist both the student and the instructor, the text is accompanied by a *Teacher's Resource Package,* which covers such concepts as teaching methodologies and strategies, resources and references, clinical and classroom activities, and an in-depth glossary of medical terms used in the study of cardiovascular technology.

Roberta C. Weiss, LVN, Ed.D.
North Hollywood, California

Acknowledgments

———————
———————
———————

———————

———————

I would like to extend my deepest gratitude and appreciation to all those who have assisted me in the preparation and development of this textbook, including: the members of the staff at Huntington Memorial Hospital, Pasadena, CA, who caringly gave of their time, energy, and expertise in the preparation of this text; the individual patients undergoing cardiovascular treatments and procedures in Huntington Memorial Hospital's cardiology department, respiratory therapy department, clinical laboratory department, and central supply department who gave of their time and provided that "personal touch" by allowing their photographs to be taken.

Thanks to my very dear friend and colleague, Ms. Marla Keeth, LVN, Coordinator of the Health Careers Academy at Blair High School, Pasadena Unified School District/Los Angeles County Regional Occupational Programs for her assistance and continued sustenance in providing time for her health career students to be photographed and to work with actual patients for the preparation of this textbook.

The highly professional health careers students enrolled in Blair High School's Health Careers Academy provided their time, expertise, and participation while being photographed; Debbie Ogilvie, Career School Sales Representative for W.B. Saunders Company, gave her time and energy in bringing me and my "new" concept to the right people at Saunders.

And finally, thanks to Lisa Biello, Vice-President and Editor-in-Chief for Health-Related Professions for W.B. Saunders Company, who was willing to take a chance on something that had never been done, and who has provided me with many hours of guidance and inspiration throughout the development of this project.

Contents

————
————
————

————

————

Introduction to Health Careers

Chapter 1

Career Opportunities in Cardiovascular Technology

Performance Objectives

Upon completion of this chapter, you will be able to:

1. Discuss career opportunities available in cardiovascular technology.
2. Describe the training required by various levels of health care providers in the field of cardiovascular technology.
3. Distinguish among divisions within health care facilities.
4. Discuss some of the personal characteristics and technical skills required of a cardiovascular technology worker.
5. Identify several potential duties of the cardiovascular technology worker.
6. List potential employers of cardiovascular technology workers.

Terms and Abbreviations

AAMA abbreviation for the American Association of Medical Assistants, Inc., a national association for medical assistants and medical assistant students that provides medical assisting instructions.

CMA abbreviation for Certified Medical Assistant, which is a certification earned through examination and after appropriate training or work experience as a medical assistant in certain institutions.

Diagnostic services services within a medical facility that deal with identifying pathological conditions or diseases.

Environmental services services within a medical facility that provide properly furnished facilities for safe use by patients and staff.

General services services within a medical facility that include admitting, feeding, and medicating patients and preserving records concerning both patients and medical personnel.

HMO abbreviation for Health Maintenance Organization, which is an organization comprising various medical professionals and services to which a patient can have access.

Medical record a document that includes a patient's evaluation, testing, and treatment received during his or her health care.

Patient care services services within a medical facility that manage the activities of daily living for patients.

Therapeutic services services within a medical facility that treat pathological conditions and diseases.

We give periods of time descriptive names in order to indicate something important about that particular time. For example, when we speak of the "stone age," we are referring to a time when humans had stone tools and simple survival skills. Now commentators are saying that we live in the "information age." Computers and electronic technology make global transfer of data instantaneous. Thus workers in the health care industry must be versed in information systems for recording, storing, and retrieving data related to the health and wellness of those entrusted to their care. In addition to the various clinical skills required of the cardiovascular worker, health care providers involved in the field of cardiovascular technology must also be able to use various types of machines, equipment, and computers and information systems, since some of their responsibilities also require basic interpretation of data.

History of Cardiovascular Medical Services

Early in the twentieth century, the clinical or hands-on aspects of a medical practice were quite simple. A doctor performed all the procedures, clinical tests, and treatments on his or her own, or, in some cases, had only one assistant who worked in all aspects of the practice. More recently, clinical health care providers, in particular those associated with the administration of cardiovascular procedures, have become a necessity in almost all health care facilities and in most private medical practices and clinics. As a result of the great changes made in health care technologies and the ever-increasing role of the cardiovascular health care provider, the individual who has been trained in more than one of the cardiovascular disciplines and medical services continues to gain more and more authority, along with increased responsibility. There are now exciting possibilities for both variety and specialization in the workplace.

Careers in cardiovascular technology can be found in many facets of the health care industry, such as small and large hospitals, multispecialty clinics and out-patient centers, urgent care centers, private medical offices, private and nonprofit laboratories, clinical trials companies, and health insurance companies. These positions can also be found in skilled nursing facilities, board and care homes, and retirement hotels. Ambitious members of the cardiovascular team may also choose to work for private health care registries, government agencies, and in some cases, their own businesses.

All members of the cardiovascular team are concerned with providing care and treatment to patients in need of their services. This includes caring for patients suffering from disorders of the heart, lungs, and cardiovascular system. The procedures which you, as a cardiovascular worker, will provide to patients can range from something as basic as taking and recording a patient's blood pressure, temperature, pulse, and respiration, to performing an echocardiographic or electrocardiographic study on a patient who recently suffered a heart attack. In addition to the skills that you will have to possess in order to work with patients with cardiovascular and other medical conditions, you will also have to become knowledgeable and skilled in working with other members of the health care team. You will have to learn how to gain access to records about a patient's health and treatment, and at the same time learn what you can and cannot do with those records. Since there are many occupations involved in the field of cardiovascular technology, for our purposes, in this chapter we will deal specifically with those careers available to the allied health worker who wishes to specialize in one or more aspects of cardiovascular technology.

Training and Education

No matter what aspect of cardiovascular technology services you choose to work in, the fact that you have selected an occupation in the health care industry says a lot about you and your interest in helping others. Unfortunately, however, not all people are cut out to work in an area in which many of the patients who you encounter are quite sick, comatose, or in some cases even terminally ill. Only you will be able to make that decision.

If you are to be successful in your position, it is important that you not only possess certain educational and technical skills, but also the personal qualifications necessary to work well with others. In addition to being a compassionate person, you must also be dependable and punctual. You must be flexible and organized. You should be able to work well under pressure and take pride in both yourself and the job you are doing. And above all, you must like working with people, and when doing so, you must be able to be tactful, be able to accept criticism, and be able to follow rules and detailed instructions.

Most allied health cardiovascular positions do not require national licensing or certification. However, all occupations under the cardiovascular umbrella do require someone who is able to follow and understand directions and instructions. Therefore, most employers of cardiovascular technologists require their workers to have a minimum of a high school diploma or its equivalent. It goes without saying that to be successful in the field of cardiovascular technology, you should also have received some advanced technical training in the field. This generally includes both classroom training and many hours of hands-on operation of the medical equipment used in this profession. It also includes some computer training and training in basic office machines, medical terminology, and a basic understanding of anatomy and physiology. Most workers receive this training as part of an overall education program in a vocational or adult school, community college, or regional occupational program.

Cardiovascular Technology Careers and Employment Opportunities

Health care facilities and private medical practices use many different titles for their cardiovascular workers. Doctors' offices and clinics often hire *clinical medical assistants*, *laboratory assistants*, and *ECG technicians* to perform many of the cardiovascular procedures. Larger health care institutions often have job titles such as *echocardiographic* and *clinical sonography technicians*, *respiratory therapy* and *pulmonary function assistants*, *phlebotomists*, *laboratory assistants*, *medical technologists*, *ECG technicians*, and *cardiac catheterization* and *cardiology monitor technicians*. No matter what your job title may be, there are certain necessary tasks that are common to all of these jobs, including taking and recording vital signs; proper use of medical asepsis and body mechanics; understanding and being able to use the proper medical terminology and medical abbreviations as part of your charting; being able to determine the differences between the anatomical and physiological functions of patients; and having an understanding of such concepts as medical law and ethics, confidentiality, and preserving patient's rights.

During the normal day, the cardiovascular worker comes into contact with a wide variety of people. In addition to dealing with the many variations of patients and their individual problems and personalities, you will also interact with members of the nursing staff, doctors and pharmacists, laboratory and radiology technicians, supervisors, housekeepers, hospital volunteers, and many other people who both work as members of the hospital staff, as well as visitors seeking understanding and answers about their loved ones. You must always be prepared to communicate with surgeons, who may use very technical terms, as well as patients, some of whom may speak very little English. Such diversity creates a work environment filled with frustrating and rewarding challenges (Figure 1-1).

Employment Opportunities

Over the past several decades, employment opportunities for cardiovascular medical services workers have expanded far beyond the one-person clinical or medical assistant who was only responsible for assisting the doctor and completing such basic tasks as answering the telephone. Where a physician's office once offered the only jobs for someone interested in the field, today the options are much more extensive.

Medical care has never been more expensive or competitive. Insurance companies are not willing to pay for unnecessary procedures. Many different institutions are competing with one another for providing patient services. In today's economy, the health care institution, as well as the private medical practice, must run in a cost-efficient manner if it is to survive. Because of the escalating costs of health care and the great demand put on health care providers in today's ever-changing, highly technological health care world, there has become an increased need to train people in more than one occupation within the same medical discipline.

Ten years ago, it was acceptable to hire one person to complete only one task. The employee, for example, who was hired to work as an ECG technician, only worked as an ECG technician. Today, however, that same person might be expected to work in the respiratory therapy department as a pulmonary function assistant, or in the clinical laboratory as a laboratory assistant or phlebotomist.

Today there are many different types of health care facilities and institutions that can be very rewarding places of employment for the cardiovascular worker. These include general acute care hospitals, where patients are hospitalized for a short period of time, anywhere from a day to a few weeks; specialized hospitals, which have facilities that provide care for specific problems, such as respiratory care hospitals or facilities for chronic diseases; long-term-care facilities, also known as convalescent hospitals, which concentrate on providing care to the elderly; and outpatient clinics, which generally house several doctors with varied specialties combining their practice. Other types of facilities that are available for employment of the cardiovascular services worker include private physicians' practices, rehabilitation centers, health maintenance organizations, and home health care and cardiovascular care agencies.

In addition to working in a health care facility, the cardiovascular worker may also seek employment within university medical schools, research centers, pharmaceutical and medical supply companies, laboratories, insurance companies, and in some cases, even freelance self-employment.

Hospital Organization and Medical Specialties

If you choose to work in the hospital environment, as a member of the cardiovascular team, it is very important for you to understand how today's medical facilities function. These facilities must be well organized, with a "chain of command" that informs each

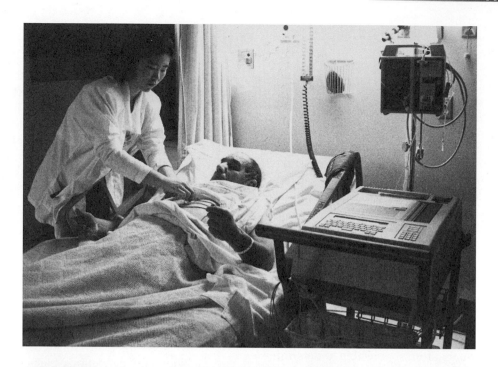

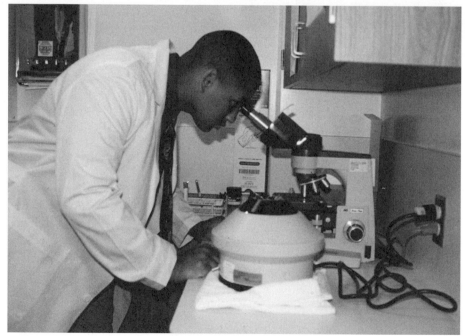

Figure 1-1
The cardiovascular technology worker.

employee as to who his or her immediate supervisor is. Such organization provides an efficient way for the facility to fulfill its mission and purpose.

An example of a hospital organization chart is shown in Table 1-1. As you can see, each service has specialized departments. These departments are determined by the type of service they provide.

Medical Specialties

If you are working in the hospital or clinic environment, more than likely you will come into contact with many different medical specialties. A medical specialist is a physician who devotes himself or herself to a single branch of medical knowledge. You

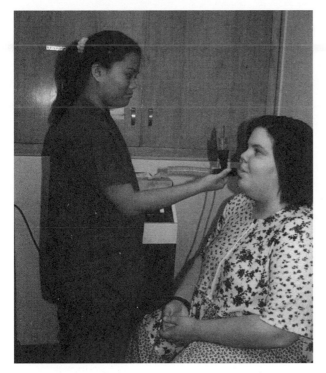
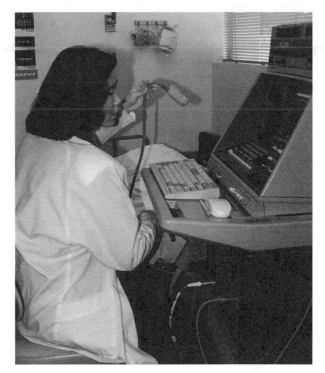

Figure 1-1
Continued.

may find yourself working in an area that deals often with one branch of medicine, such as cardiology or hematology. Table 1-2 provides a listing of the definitions of most of the present-day medical specialties and what the physician practicing those specialties is called.

Summary

In this chapter, we discussed the rapidly changing field of cardiovascular technology and the various occupations comprising this very demanding, yet highly rewarding branch of medicine. We deter-

Table 1-1
Organizational Chart of a Health Care Facility

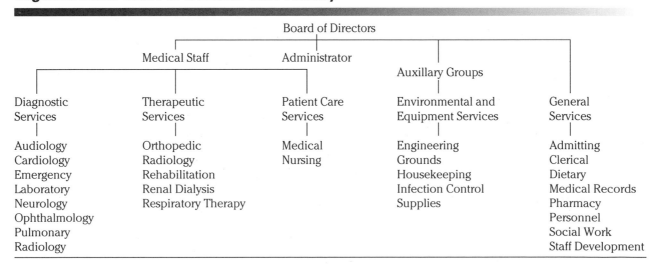

Board of Directors				
Medical Staff	Administrator		Auxillary Groups	
Diagnostic Services	Therapeutic Services	Patient Care Services	Environmental and Equipment Services	General Services
Audiology	Orthopedic	Medical	Engineering	Admitting
Cardiology	Radiology	Nursing	Grounds	Clerical
Emergency	Rehabilitation		Housekeeping	Dietary
Laboratory	Renal Dialysis		Infection Control	Medical Records
Neurology	Respiratory Therapy		Supplies	Pharmacy
Ophthalmology				Personnel
Pulmonary				Social Work
Radiology				Staff Development

Table 1-2
Medical Specialties

Specialty	Name of Physician	Description of Specialty
Allergies	Allergist	Diagnoses and treats reactions resulting from sensitivity to foods, pollens, dust, medicine, or other substances
Anesthesiology	Anesthesiologist	Administers various forms of anesthesia in surgery or to diagnose causes of loss of feeling or sensation
Cardiology	Cardiologist	Diagnoses and treats diseases of the heart
Dermatology	Dermatologist	Diagnoses and treats diseases of the skin
Endocrinology	Endocrinologist	Diagnoses and treats diseases of the endocrine system and the hormones produced by the ductless glands
Family Practice	Family Practitioner	Diagnoses and treats diseases by medical and surgical methods for all members of the family
Gastroenterology	Gastroenterologist	Diagnoses and treats diseases of the digestive system
Gynecology	Gynecologist	Diagnoses and treats disorders of the female reproductive system
Internal Medicine	Internist	Diagnoses and treats diseases of adults
Neurology	Neurologist	Diagnoses and treats diseases of the nervous system and brain
Obstetrics	Obstetrician	Cares for women during pregnancy, childbirth, and the interval immediately following
Oncology	Oncologist	Diagnoses and treats cancer
Ophthalmology	Ophthalmologist	Diagnoses and treats disorders of the eye and prescribes glasses
Orthopedics	Orthopedist	Diagnoses and treats disorders of the muscular and skeletal systems
Otolaryngology	Otolaryngologist	Diagnoses and treats disorders of the eyes, ears, nose, and throat
Pathology	Pathologist	Studies and interprets changes in organs, tissues, cells, and changes in the body's chemistry to aid in diagnosing disease and determining the type of treatment that may be necessary
Pediatrics	Pediatrician	Deals with the prevention, diagnosis, and treatment of children's disease
Proctology	Proctologist	Diagnoses and treats diseases of the rectum
Psychiatry	Psychiatrist	Diagnoses and treats mental disorders
Radiology	Radiologist	Uses radiant energy, including x-rays, radium, and cobalt, in the diagnosis of diseases
Urology	Urologist	Diagnoses and treats diseases of the kidneys, bladder, ureters, and urethra and of the male reproductive system

mined that there were many varied career opportunities available to graduates of this field, both in private and public health care agencies and institutions, as well as in other industries, such as insurance and preventive health and health care maintenance. We also talked about some of the personal characteristics and technical skills that are necessary in order to be successful as a professional member of the cardiovascular team, as well as defining the basic level of training for these occupations. Finally, we defined the various types of medical specialties and the name of each of the medical specialists involved in the various branches of medicine, noting that all of these were available to the cardiovascular technology worker as a means to employment.

Review Questions

1. What is the name of the services provided for patients within a health care facility that is responsible for treating pathological conditions and diseases?

2. What is the name of the services provided for patients within a health care facility that is responsible for managing the activities of daily living for patients?

3. What is the name of the services provided for patients within a health care facility that is responsible for properly furnishing the facility for safe use by all patients and staff?

4. What is the name of the services provided for patients within a health care facility that is responsible for admitting, feeding, and medicating patients and preserving records that concern both patients and medical personnel?

5. A(n) _____ is an organization that comprises various medical professionals and services to which a patient can subscribe.

6. Give at least three examples of departments that would be found under diagnostic services:

   a. _____

   b. _____

   c. _____

7. Give at least two examples of an auxiliary group working within a health care facility:

   a. _____

   b. _____

8. Under what services would the *pharmacy* be found within a health care facility?

9. Under what services would *staff nurses* be found within a health care facility?

10. Under what services would the *respiratory therapy department* be found within a health care facility?

Health, Wellness, and Illness

Performance Objectives

Upon completion of this chapter, you will be able to:

1. Define health, wellness, illness, and disease and briefly explain their relationship.
2. Briefly discuss nontraditional views of health and illness.
3. Identify and briefly discuss health beliefs and behaviors.
4. Identify and briefly discuss the five basic stages of illness.
5. Identify and briefly discuss the 11 sequential stages of illness.
6. Describe what is meant by sick role behavior.
7. Explain the effects of illness on family members.
8. Discuss the effects of hospitalization.
9. Identify patterns and trends that influence health and illness.

Terms and Abbreviations

Compliance   the extent to which a person's behavior coincides with the health care provider's recommendations.

Disease   an alteration in the body's functions that results in a reduction of capacities or a shortening of the normal lifespan.

Health   the state of complete physical, mental, and social well-being, and not merely the basis of disease or infirmity.

Health status   the state of an individual at a given time.

Illness   a highly personal state in which the individual feels unhealthy or ill.

Model   an abstract outline or a theoretical depiction of a complex phenomenon; also *paradigm*.

Morbidity   pertains to illness; the morbidity rate is the ratio of sick to well people in a given population.

Wellness   the active process through which an individual becomes aware of and makes choices that lead to a more successful existence.

Health is an ever-changing, evolving concept, which is basic to the study of medicine, and as it relates to us, to the study of cardiovascular technology. For centuries, the concept of disease was the yardstick by which all health was measured, and it wasn't until as late as the 19th century that health care providers began to deal with the causes of diseases. More recently, there has been an increased emphasis on health.

There is no general consensus regarding the definition of health. There is, however, knowledge as to how one can attain a certain level of health, but health itself cannot be measured. According to the World Health Organization (WHO), *health* can be defined as a state of complete physical, mental, and social well-being, and not merely as the absence of disease or infirmity. Because this definition was proposed in the late forties, when thousands of soldiers were returning home from World War II with serious injuries and traumas, many health care providers of the time thought this definition to be impractical. Today, however, some view it as a possible goal for all people, while others consider complete well-being unobtainable.

Because health is a complex concept, much research has been done in an attempt to measure it. Out of this research, specific models or paradigms have been developed to explain health and, in some instances, its relationship to illness. The five models of health care delivery that are most widely accepted include the *clinical* model, the *ecological* model, the *role performance* model, the *adaptive* model, and the *eudaimonistic* model.

Models of Health Care Delivery

Clinical Model

The clinical model is the narrowest of the health care delivery models. According to this model, people are viewed as physiological systems with individual and related functions. Health is used as a concept to identify the absences of signs and symptoms of disease or injury.

In the clinical model, disease is seen as the opposite of health and health as a relatively passive state of freedom from illness. The extreme of health, according to this model, is the absence of any signs or symptoms of disease, and the presence of such signs or symptoms is an indication of illness. Today, the focus of many medical practices is to relieve the signs and symptoms of disease and thus eliminate the malfunction and pain of patients. When the signs and symptoms of the disease are no longer present, the physician considers that individual's health as being restored.

Ecological Model

The ecological model of health care delivery is based upon the relationship of all humans to their internal and external environments. The model covers three concepts (Figure 2-1): the *host*, which is a person or group of people who may or may not be at risk of acquiring an illness or a disease; an *agent*, which can be any factor within either the internal or the external environment that, by its presence or absence, can lead to illness or disease; and the *environment*, either internal or external, which may or may not predispose the person to the development of a disease or illness.

Role Performance Model

The role performance model of health care delivery adds the social and psychological implications and standards to the concept of health. In this model,

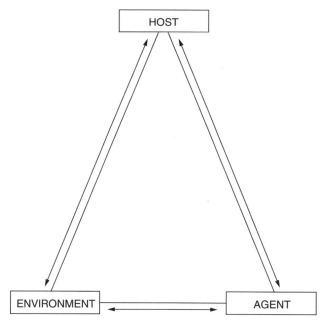

Figure 2-1
Ecological model of health care delivery.

health is defined in terms of the person's ability to fulfill his or her role in society, that is, to be able to perform work. According to this model, people who can fulfill their roles are considered healthy even if they appear clinically ill. The emphasis of the delivery of health care, in this model, is placed upon a person's capacity rather than his or her committment to roles and tasks.

Adaptive Model

The focus of this adaptive model of health care delivery is adaptation. Diseases are seen as a failure in the person's ability to adapt, and the treatment is seen as an ability to restore the person to a state in which he or she can cope with illness or disease.

Eudaimonistic Model

The eudaimonistic model of health care delivery incorporates the most comprehensive view of health. Health, according to this model, is seen as an actualization or realization of a person's total potential, and the highest aspiration of an individual is his or her fulfillment and complete development. Illness is seen as a condition or situation that prevents self-actualization.

Developing a Personal Definition of Health

As you begin your journey into a career as a provider of health care, you will soon realize that health is a highly individual perception. Meanings and descriptions of health vary considerably, and an individual's personal definition of health may not necessarily agree with that of other health care professionals.

There are several factors that influence one's personal definition of health. These include the developmental status of that person, social and cultural influences, previous experiences, and personal expectations.

Wellness, Disease, and Illness

The concept of wellness has received increasing attention in recent years. Some people believe that wellness and health are one and the same, whereas others believe that the two differ. In one respect, wellness is very similar to self-actualization as defined by the eudaimonistic model of health care delivery. It, like good health, can only exist as a relatively passive state of freedom from illness in which the individual is at peace with his or her environment.

Wellness can also be defined as an active process through which an individual becomes aware of choices that can lead to a more successful existence. These choices are influenced by the person's self-concept, his or her culture, and the environment. Wellness, therefore, is seen through a continuum whose extremes are total wellness and premature death (Figure 2-2).

Disease and Illness

Disease is a medical term that is used to describe any alteration in a person's body functions that results in a reduction of his or her capacities or a shortening of the normal lifespan. The goal of physicians has always been eliminating or decreasing the disease process. Primitive people thought that disease was caused by outside forces or spirits. Later on, however, this belief was replaced by the single-cause the-

ory. Increasingly, a number of factors are considered to interact in causing disease and a person's response to a given treatment.

Illness, while it may or may not be related to disease, differs from disease, in that it is defined as a highly personal state in which a person feels unhealthy or ill. Someone who feels pain or nausea tends to modify his or her behavior in some way and thus may consider himself or herself ill. An individual could have a disease, for example, a growth in the intestine, and not feel ill. According to researchers in the theory of illness and disease, for a person to feel ill, the physician must be able to determine if that person meets three distinct criteria. First, there must be a presence of symptoms, such as an elevated temperature or pain. Second, the person affected by the illness must be able to describe his or her state, for example, good, bad, or sick. And third, the ability to carry out daily activities, such as a job or schoolwork, must have had to been affected.

Relationship of Health, Illness, and Disease

Health and Illness

One's state of health or illness can be considered either as points along one continuum, as related but separate entities, or as completely separate entities. A continuum of well-being, or health, can be viewed as a grid or graduated scale, in which peak wellness is at one end and death is at the other. Such a continuum accommodates a wide range of normal health, which reflects the fact that no one ever attains perfect health, and not everyone becomes sick.

Illness and Disease

Traditionally, health care providers have dealt with diseases at a subsystem level. Subsystems are those aspects of the human body that are subsumed

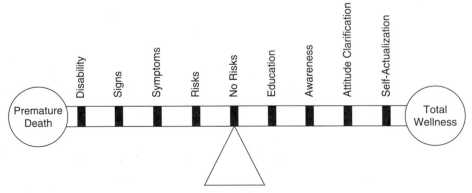

Figure 2-2
Continuum between total wellness and premature death.

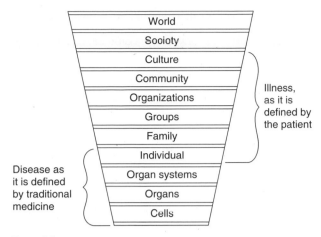

Figure 2-3
Systems hierarchy differentiating illness from disease.

in the larger system of the whole body. A subsystem, for example, may be a cell, an organ, or an organ system. Only recently have medical practitioners started looking at the person as a whole being. Health care providers, such as cardiovascular technicians, by contrast, have traditionally viewed the person as an entity, meaning that they have viewed the patient from a holistic point of view. Cardiovascular providers today base their scope of practice on the multiple-causation theory of health problems or illness. For example, unemployment, pollution, lifestyle, and stressful events may all contribute to illness. In effect, these can all be considered subsystem problems, that is, problems that stem from systems in which the patient is a subsystem (Figure 2-3). Therefore, the concept of illness must include all aspects of the total person as well as the biological and genetic factors that contribute to disease. Illness, then, is influenced by a person's family, his or her social network, the environment, and culture.

Understanding the Concept of Holistic Health

The concept of *holistic health* is based upon the belief that the whole is more than the sum of its parts. When using a holistic health approach to health care, you must consider the event's affecting the whole person. Illness is viewed as an opportunity for growth;

health is a dynamic state of being that moves back and forth along a continuum. The extremes of the continuum are highest health potential and death; good health, normal health, mild illness, illness or poor health, and critical illness are points along the continuum (Figure 2-4).

In the holistic health model of health care delivery, wellness is seen as an ever-changing growth toward self-actualization. It considers the person's needs, abilities, and disabilities. A critical assumption in holistic health is that the perception of health is an individual decision, encouraging self-responsibility and self-control. Health can exist in the presence of illness. For example, a man who is feeling pain in his heart may perceive himself as being near or at the point of highest health potential along the continuum if he feels he is functioning to his highest potential relative to his pain.

Health Beliefs and Behaviors

The *health status*, or state, of a person is the health of that person at a given time. In its general meaning, the term may refer to anxiety, depression, or acute illness, and thus describes the individual as a whole. Health status can also describe such specifics as a person's vital signs, such as a pulse rate and a body temperature. The *health beliefs* of an individual are those concepts pertaining to his or her health that that individual believes to be true. Such beliefs may or may not be founded on fact.

Health behaviors are defined as those actions that a person takes in order to understand his or her state of health, maintain an optimal state of health, prevent illness and injury, and reach his or her maximum physical and mental potential. Behaviors such as eating wisely, exercising, paying attention to signs of illness, following treatment advice, and avoiding known health hazards such as smoking are all examples. The ability to relax, achieve emotional maturity, lead a productive life, and give way to self-expression also affect one's state of health.

Influences Affecting State of Health

There are many variables that affect or influence one's state of health. Some of these are internal fac-

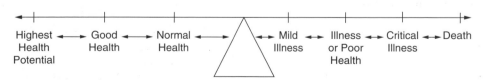

Figure 2-4
Health-illness continuum representing the holistic health model.

tors, such as the person's genetic makeup, and others are external, such as the person's culture and physical environment.

Of the many internal and external factors influencing how one achieves his or her state of health, there are 13 that have a direct effect on the person. These include the person's genetic makeup, race, and culture; the sex, age, and developmental level of the person; the mind-body relationship, meaning how that person allows his or her emotional responses to affect his or her body function; the lifestyle, physical environment, occupation, and standard of living the person enjoys; family makeup and support network; self-concept; and the geographic area in which the person resides.

Factors Influencing Health Behavior

In addition to those factors that influence one's state of health, there are other factors that also influence one's health behavior. Culture and family influences are two examples. People can usually control their health behaviors and can choose healthy or unhealthy activities. In contrast, people have little or no choice over their genetic makeup, age, sex, physical environments, culture, or area of residence.

Individual behavior is based upon one's own perceptions and modifying factors that influence one's own life.

Individual perceptions generally include:

- The importance of health to the person.
- Perceived control over one's own life.
- Any perceived threat of a specific illness.
- Perceived susceptibility toward a specific illness or disease.
- Perceived seriousness of a specific illness or disease.
- Perceived benefits of preventive action toward a specific illness or disease.
- Perceived value of early detection.

Individual factors that generally modify a person's perceptions generally include:

- Demographic variables such as age, sex, and race.
- Interpersonal variables, such as concern of significant others, family patterns of health care, and interactions with health care professionals.
- Situational variables, such as the cultural acceptance of specific health-related behaviors.

Stages of Illness

Throughout the evolution of medicine and health care, various scientists and researchers have described the various stages of illness. The stages of ill-

ness are generally classified according to *basic*, or physical, stages and *sequential* stages.

Basic Stages of Illness

There are five basic stages to illness. The first stage is the transition during which most people come to believe something is wrong with them. We refer to this as the *symptom experience* stage. The stage at which a patient accepts his or her illness is called the *acceptance of the sick role*. At this time, the patient has decided that his or her symptoms or concerns are sufficiently severe to suggest that they are sick.

Medical care contact is the third basic stage of illness. During this stage, the patient seeks the advice of a health care provider, either on his or her own initiative, or at the urging of a significant other. When people go through this stage, they are usually seeking three types of information: validation of a real illness, explanation of the symptoms in understandable terms, and reassurance that they will be alright or a prediction of the likely outcome.

During the fourth basic stage of illness, known as the *dependent patient role* stage, the patient has already gone through the process of having his or her illness validated by the health care professional. The person now sees himself or herself as a patient, dependent on the professional for help. Oftentimes during this stage, the person becomes reluctant to accept a professional's recommendation.

The final basic stage of illness is the *recovery* or *rehabilitation* stage. During this stage, the patient learns to give up the sick role and return to former roles and functions. For people suffering from acute illnesses, the time as an ill person is generally short, and recovery is usually rapid. Thus, they find it relatively easy to return to their former life-style.

Sequential Stages of Illness

There are 11 sequential, or consecutive, stages of illness. Many of these stages vary in duration, and some may occur simultaneously. They usually include the following:

- *Symptoms experience.* During this time the patient begins to experience actual symptoms, such as pain; he or she may also become more aware that there may be a problem and begins to respond with fear or anxiety, while at the same time, often giving the symptoms a label and a meaning.
- *Self-treatment.* During this time, the patient often tries to treat himself or herself, especially if it is believed that the symptoms are not serious.

· *Communication to significant others.* During this time, the patient will begin to communicate and confide their symptoms to support persons, significant others, or health care providers.

· *Assessment of symptoms.* During this time, the assessment of the patient's symptoms may be made by the patient, support persons, or a health care professional.

· *Assumption of the sick role.* At this point, the person has accepted his or her illness, has been declared sick, and has accepted the role of being a sick person.

· *Expression of concern.* During this stage, support persons and friends begin to offer the patient sympathy and express concern; some people may even recommend practitioners to their sick friend.

· *Assessment of probable efficacy of treatment or appropriateness of treatment.* During this time, the person may begin to assess the variety of treatments available; a number of variables may affect this assessment, including previous experience and availability of information.

· *Selection of a treatment plan.* During this time, a treatment plan may be selected with or without the advice of a health care professional; such factors as cost, time, knowledge, and effects are often involved during the selection process.

· *Implementation of treatment.* During this stage, the patient allows the health care practitioner to implement the prescribed treatment.

· *Evaluation of the effects of treatment.* During this stage, the patient begins to see and accept the possible outcomes of his or her treatment, including a full recovery with a change in treatment, recovery with some disability, and no recovery; at this time, the patient may also choose to exercise his or her right to completely reject or terminate all treatment.

· *Recovery and rehabilitation.* During this final stage, the patient begins to make his or her return to usual social roles.

Sick Role Behavior

Sick role behavior concerns activities that are undertaken by those who consider themselves ill for the purpose of getting well. Such behavior usually includes four aspects: the patient's inability to be held responsible for his or her condition; allowing the patient to be excused from certain social roles and tasks; encouraging the patient to try to get well as quickly as possible; and assisting both the patient and his or her family members in seeking competent health care and treatment.

Effects of Illness on Family Members

A person's illness often affects the family or significant others. The effect and its extent depend chiefly on three factors: which member of the family is ill, the seriousness of the illness and length of recovery, and the cultural and social customs of the family.

Changes that most frequently occur in a family include role changes, task reassignments, increased stress arising from anxiety about the outcome of the illness for the patient and conflict about unaccustomed responsibilities, financial problems, loneliness as a result of separation and pending loss, and change in social customs.

Each family member may be affected differently, depending, for example, on whether a grandparent, the father of a nuclear family, or a teenager is ill. Each of these people plays a different role in the family, and each supports the family in different ways. Parents of young children, for example, have greater family responsibilities than parents of grown children.

The degree of change that family members experience is often related to their dependence on the sick person. For example, when a child is ill, there are few changes other than added responsibilities directly related to the child's illness. When the mother is ill, however, many changes are often necessary because other family members must assume her functions.

Effects of Hospitalization

Normal patterns of behavior generally change with illness; with hospitalization, however, the change can be even greater. Hospitalization usually disrupts a person's privacy, autonomy, life-style, roles, and economics.

When a person enters a hospital or other health care institution, the greatest loss comes in the patient's privacy. *Privacy* is often described as a comfortable feeling reflecting a deserved degree of social retreat. It is a personal, internal state that cannot and should not be imposed upon without an agreement by the person seeking the privacy, and its boundaries are considered to be highly individual. People need varying degrees of privacy and establish their boundaries accordingly. When these boundaries are crossed, they feel invaded. Hospital personnel sometimes show little concern for their patients' privacy. Patients are asked to provide information that often they consider private; they may share a room with a stranger; and their health is frequently discussed with many health care providers.

A person's *autonomy* deals with those activities

that allow a person to be independent and self-directed. People vary in their sense of autonomy; some are accustomed to functioning independently in most of their life activities, while others are accustomed to direction from others. Hospitalized patients frequently give up much of their autonomy. Decisions about meals, hygienic practices, and sleeping habits are frequently made for them. The loss of individuality is difficult to accept, often leading to feelings of dehumanization.

Hospitalization often makes a drastic change in a person's life-style and social role. Many hospitals determine when people wake up and when they should go to sleep. Food in a hospital is usually mass produced, and individual differences in taste are not always accommodated. Hospitalization not only affects a person's life-style; it frequently affects their life roles. A woman or man may no longer be capable of earning wages; a single parent may be unable to fulfill his or her normal parental responsibilities. Such changes not only affect the patient's physical and emotional well-being, but just as important, hospitalization can often place a genuine financial burden on patients and their families. Even though many people have health insurance, it may not reimburse all costs; in addition, many patients lose wages while they are hospitalized.

As a health care provider, you can become aware of costs sustained by the patient, and by doing so, can provide care and treatment that is as economical and safe as possible. For example, you can use only the minimum supplies necessary for providing a patient's breathing treatment. You can also support activities that promote health and that return patients to their normal activities as soon as possible.

Patterns and Trends in Health and Illness

The health of most Americans is steadily improving. This is primarily because of early preventive efforts based on new knowledge obtained through research; improvements in sanitation, housing, nutrition, and immunization essential to disease prevention; and individual members of society taking measures to promote health and prevent disease. There are other health risks that people take upon themselves that make them more susceptible to illness and disease. These factors include *cigarette smoking, alcohol and drug abuse, injuries* sustained from automobile and other types of accidents, and *occupational risks* suffered as a result of not following safety standards in the workplace. All of these risks present challenges to the health care worker, especially members of the cardiovascular team, whose goal is to promote and

provide the patient with care and treatment relative to his or her cardiovascular system.

Measuring Trends in Health Care Delivery

Evidence of change in health status of the population is measured in various ways. Measurements are made of longevity or life expectancy; the way people feel about their health; mortality rates and causes; morbidity rates and causes; the type of health behaviors people practice; and the amount and kind of health services used.

Longevity

In 1960, life expectancy at birth was about 70 years of age. By 1983, it reached almost 75 years. Differences exist among races and between males and females. In 1982, for example, the life expectancy for a caucasian male was 71.5 years of age. For a caucasian female, it was 78.8 years of age. For an African-American male, it was 64.9 years, while it was 73.5 years for an African-American female.

How People Feel about Their Health

The way a person feels about his or her health is one way in which a person's health status can be ascertained. Over the past several years, people of all ages have generally held the same perception of their health status. In 1981, for example, when most people were asked how they felt about their state of health as compared to other people of the same age, approximately 87.3 percent said they felt good or excellent. What was most interesting, is that about 70 percent of people who stated they felt good or excellent were elderly persons.

Summary

In this chapter, we discussed the concepts of health, wellness, illness, and disease, and explained their relationship to one another. We also talked briefly about nontraditional views of health and illness, as well as health beliefs and behaviors, the basic and sequential stages of illness, what is meant by sick role behavior, and the effects of illness on both the patient and family members. Finally, we discussed the effects of hospitalization and the role it plays in caring for an ill person, as well as identified various patterns and trends that influence both health and illness.

Review Questions

1. Briefly define the meaning of *disease*.

2. Briefly define the meaning of *health*.

3. Briefly define the meaning of *wellness*.

4. Briefly define the meaning of *illness*.

5. The _____ rate is the ratio of sick to well people in a given population.

6. The term _____ pertains to the extent to which a person's behavior coincides with health care providers.

7. What model of health care delivery is based upon the relationship of all humans to their internal and external environments?

   a. eudaimonistic

   b. adaptive

   c. ecological

8. What model of health care delivery incorporates the most comprehensive view of health?

   a. eudaimonistic

   b. adaptive

   c. ecological

9. What model of health care delivery sees disease as a failure in the person's ability to adapt?

   a. eudaimonistic

   b. adaptive

   c. ecological

10. Health _____ are defined as those actions that a person takes in order to understand his or her state of health and prevent illness or injury.

Medical Law and Ethics

Performance Objectives

Upon completion of this chapter, you will be able to:

1. Delineate the difference between medical law and medical ethics.
2. Discuss the Code of Ethics that members of the cardiovascular team are morally bound to follow.
3. Identify at least four examples of ethical behavior for the cardiovascular professional.
4. Discuss the Patient's Bill of Rights.
5. Discuss the purpose of licensing medical personnel.
6. Explain the Rule of Personal Liability.
7. Briefly discuss the Good Samaritan Act.
8. Demonstrate an understanding of specific patient consent forms.
9. Discuss the legal implications of a patient's medical record.

Terms and Abbreviations

Battery pertains to any unlawful touching of another person without his or her consent, regardless of resultant injury.

Civil law differentiated from criminal law in that it enforces private rights and liabilities.

Defamation pertains to any attack on a person's reputation; called *libel* when the written word is used, and *slander* when the spoken word is used.

Duty of care a lawful obligation that protects the patient by requiring the health care worker to provide safe care to the patient.

Ethics moral standards and principles.

Good Samaritan Act a law, differing in various states, that protects a health care worker from a malpractice suit when coming to the aid of a person in an emergency situation.

Informed consent pertaining to the act of informing the patient of the risks and alternatives to a medical procedure; the patient is asked to sign a consent form, acknowledging the assumed risks.

Malpractice literally meaning "bad practice" by a professional; any care below an expected standard that results in injury.

Medical Practice Acts statutes dealing with licensing of medical personnel.

Negligence failing to perform or to do something for a patient that another person of the same training and position would do under the same or ordinary circumstances.

Patient's Bill of Rights a document produced and adopted by the American Hospital Association which states what a patient has the right to expect during his or her medical treatment.

Privileged information information given by a patient to a medical care provider that cannot be disclosed without the consent of the patient.

Reasonable care the health care professional is protected by law if it is proven that he or she acted reasonably compared to fellow workers.

Rule of Personal Liability all health care workers are held responsible for their own conduct.

The laws and ethical codes of conduct for the medical profession must be understood by all members of the cardiovascular technology team. These laws and ethics codes protect all members of the medical profession, as well as the patient.

Medical ethics has been important to medical practice as far back as 400 B.C., when Hippocrates wrote the Hippocratic Oath, a document that first developed the standards of medical conduct and ethics. Today, many individual health care professional associations have adopted their own codes of ethics in order to govern their health care workers. Laboratory assistants, ECG and echocardiography technicians, and respiratory therapy assistants all have ethical codes that provide guidelines for professional behavior.

The practice of medicine today exists within a framework of laws. Such laws vary from state to state, so it is important to know your state's laws governing the cardiovascular technologist, as well as federal and any other local statutes.

Understanding Medical Ethics and Medical Law

Medical ethics are concerned with whether a health care provider's actions are right or wrong. *Ethical behavior* represents the ideal conduct for a certain group. Each group of health care professionals who require a license to function in their position have drafted and adopted a specific code of ethics. These ethics are based upon moral principles and practices. If accused of unethical behavior by a medical worker's professional association, you can be issued a warning or expelled from the association.

Medical law is concerned with the legal conduct of the members of the medical profession. There are federal, state, and local laws that must be followed, and violation of such laws may subject the offender to civil or criminal prosecution. Professional licenses can be taken away, fines can be levied, and prison sentences can be imposed. Often, the line between what is unethical and what is illegal can be unclear. If you, as a member of the health care delivery system, decided, for example, you were going to be rude to a patient, that is unethical behavior. But if you decided to inform the patient's neighbor of his or her disease, that is illegal behavior. In addition, you can also be sued by a patient for *defamation*, which is considered an attack on a person's reputation. This is called *libel* when the defamation is written, and *slander* when spoken.

Another example of the difference between un-ethical and illegal behavior concerns the viewing of a friend's chart in a part of the hospital where you do not work. If you read it out of curiosity, that is unethical. If you talk about it, that is illegal. If an action is illegal, it is always unethical. However, it can be unethical without being illegal. Remember, ethics represents the highest standards of behavior.

Ethical Behavior

As a member of the cardiovascular team, you are responsible for displaying ethical behavior at all times. This means maintaining the highest level of ethical conduct. To accomplish such a task, you should always:

- Respect the rights of all patients to have opinions, life-styles, and beliefs that are different from your own.
- Remember that everything seen, heard, or read about a patient is considered confidential and does not leave the jobsite.
- Be conscientious in doing your work, doing the best you can at all times.
- Be ready to be of service to patients and coworkers at any time of the workday.
- Let the patient know that it is a privilege for you to assist him or her.
- Follow closely the specific rules of ethical conduct prescribed by your employer.

The Patient and the Health Care Worker

The Patient's Bill of Rights

Awareness of the patient's rights is the responsibility of all members of the health care team. Because this is such a vital aspect of providing care and treatment to the patient, the American Hospital Association (AHA) felt it was necessary to establish a document that identified what patients could expect from the individuals who cared for them. As a result, the *Patient's Bill of Rights* was adopted. The intent of the document is to make both members of the health care system and patients aware of what the patient has a right to expect. According to the AHA, the patient has a right to:

- Considerate and respectful care.
- Obtain from their physician complete current information concerning their diagnosis, treatment, and prognosis, in terms that they can be reasonably expected to understand.

- Informed consent, which should include knowledge of the proposed procedure, along with its risks and probable duration of incapacitation; in addition, the patient has a right to information regarding medically significant alternatives.
- Refuse treatment to the extent permitted by law and to be informed of the medical consequences of such action.
- Have case discussion, consultation, examination, and treatment conducted discretely, and have those not directly involved in the patient's care be granted permission by the patient for their presence.
- Expect that all communication and records pertaining to his or her care be treated in a confidential manner.
- Expect the hospital to make a reasonable response to request for services, and the hospital must provide evaluation, service, and referrals as may be indicated by the urgency of the case.
- Obtain information as to any relationship of the hospital to other health care and educational institutions, insofar as his or her care is concerned, and the relationship among individuals, by name, who are treating the patient.
- Be advised if the hospital proposes to engage in or perform human experimentation affecting his or her care or treatment, and the right to refuse to participate in such research projects.
- Expect reasonable continuity of care.
- Examine and receive an explanation of the bill regardless of the source of payment.
- Know what hospital rules and regulations apply to his or her conduct as a patient.

Licensing of Health Care Workers

The medical profession and many of the individual health care professions are legally regulated throughout the United States by the issuing of licenses and certificates. All 50 states require the licensing of hospitals. The statutes dealing with licensing and certification of individual health care professionals are commonly referred to as *medical practice acts*.

Licenses can be revoked or suspended when a medical professional has been found guilty of having violated various statutes. Grounds for losing a medical license include serious crimes such as murder, rape, and arson. Crimes of "moral turpitude," such as tax crimes, minor sexual offenses, and false statements while applying for a license, can also be grounds for loss of the license. Other crimes that may cause the worker to have his or her license suspended or revoked include incapacity because of insanity, excessive use of alcohol, or drug addiction.

Protection Under the Law

In the health care environment, both the patient and the health care worker must be assured protection under the law. For the patient, this means being assured of safe care. For the health care professional, it means being protected from irresponsible lawsuits.

The patient is protected by a process known as *duty of care*. This entitles the patient to safe care by making it mandatory that he or she be treated by meeting the common or average standards of practice expected in the community under similar circumstances. The duty of care also provides that the patient be treated with *reasonable care*, that is, protection of the health care professional by law if it can be proven that he or she acted reasonably as compared to fellow workers of the same or similar training in a situation of the same nature. If it is proven that the health care worker failed to meet such a standard and harm comes to the patient as a result, negligence may be proven.

Negligence is the failure to give reasonable care or the giving of unreasonable care. The patient is harmed because the health professional did something wrong or failed to do something that he or she should have done under the circumstances.

The Good Samaritan Law and Medical Malpractice

The *Good Samaritan law* is a law that addresses the problem of medical malpractice suits for a physician or any trained health care professional who comes upon an accident scene and attempts to render aid to the victim. The law, which has been enacted in all 50 states, encourages members of health care professions to offer treatment without fearing the possibility of a malpractice suit. Laws throughout the country do differ, so it is wise to check the law in your own state in order to determine what professional liability may exist during an emergency situation.

Malpractice, unfortunately, is a term that is familiar to all of us, because of the large number of lawsuits being filed and settled throughout the country. For the medical worker, it seems that the higher the educational level and requirements of the worker, the greater is the likelihood that they may be responsible for their actions.

When used in the medical professions, malpractice refers to any misconduct or lack of skill that results in the patient's injury. A patient who thinks that his or her physician has been negligent in diagnosing and treating an illness or accident can file a medical malpractice claim. Most claims are generally made against physicians; however, any employee working in the health care environment can be named in a malpractice lawsuit. Most insurance companies who issue medical malpractice policies on physicians take into account that the policy will also cover the physician's employees, but medical office or hospital employees may also wish to purchase their own insurance policy, which is usually quite inexpensive.

Physicians are liable for the actions of their employees while the employee is on duty. For example, suppose a laboratory assistant accepts a specimen from each of two patients and then mislabels them. Subsequently, one patient is told that his specimen is normal and the other is told she has an infection. The patient who has been told that everything was alright develops an infection that could have been prevented if antibiotics had been administered. In this case, the doctor could be sued for the negligence of the employee who mislabeled the specimens.

In health care, under the *rule of personal liability*, all individuals are held responsible for their own personal conduct. In a medical malpractice suit, such as the example, previously described, both the physician and the laboratory assistant could be held jointly liable for medical malpractice.

You can also be held jointly responsible if you work for a doctor who is involved in an illegal act and you are aware of the crime but fail to report it. Physicians must also report crimes that they learn about when practicing medicine, such as a shooting, child or elder abuse, or rape. As a health care professional, you can also be held jointly responsible with the physician if you fail to report such crimes. In some cases, protecting patient confidentiality and the patient's right to complete privacy of their records does not apply. Births, deaths, communicable diseases, and crimes are all examples of times when the physician is bound by law to report what has occurred. If you fail to report these types of cases, you may also be held liable.

In some instances, the law is very specific regarding confidentiality and reporting of information. In cases dealing with acquired immunodeficiency syndrome (AIDS), for example, there are laws and regulations that take into account the confidential nature of the patient's illness. However, these regulations are constantly changing; therefore, it is important that you keep current as to the laws and regulations of the state in which you are working regarding confidentiality and patient's records in treating this disease.

Obtaining Patient Consent

When a doctor makes a diagnosis and recommends a specific mode of treatment, the patient has the responsibility to decide whether or not to accept such diagnosis and treatment. The physician has the responsibility of informing the patient in words that he or she can understand as to the risks of and alternatives to any suggested procedure. The patient has the responsibility of deciding whether or not to accept all the explained risks. Once it is ascertained that the physician has properly explained the procedure and the patient fully understands it and the risks, a consent form must be signed by the patient, indicating that he or she fully accepts the risk of the procedure. The process is called *informed consent*. As part of your responsibilities as a cardiovascular care worker, you may be asked to prepare the consent form (Figure 3-1) for any type of procedure, whether it is to be performed in the office or in the hospital. Consents are also required before an experimental procedure or prior to any other unusual procedure taking place. Consent forms are also used prior to the administration of any experimental drugs or medication.

In cases where the patient may have difficulty understanding or speaking the English language, the consent form must be translated or prepared in the patient's native language. A patient who has not been properly informed through the "informed consent" process can sue the physician for medical malpractice.

Specific guidelines have been established in regard to the details and the signing of the consent form. These include the following:

- Always make sure that the patient fully understands the consent form and realizes what he or she has signed; patients who are mentally handicapped should be given an explanation that can be understood completely, with as few confusing terms as possible.
- The patient must never be forced to sign the consent form, and must not be allowed to sign it under the influence of alcohol or drugs.
- All signatures must be witnessed, dated, and signed in ink, with the full legal names used.
- Any patient over 18 years of age may sign his or her own consent unless the patient is incompetent and has a guardian, or there is an emergency, in which case, two physicians must sign the consent form.
- Married minors may sign their own consent forms for treatment.
- Unmarried minors must have a consent form signed by one parent or legal guardian; however, consent of both parents is usually suggested; a stepparent may not sign a consent form.
- An emancipated minor, who is under the age of 18 and who has been declared by a court of law to be legally responsible for himself or herself, may sign his or her own consent form.

Patient or someone acting for the patient agrees to the following terms of hospital admission.

1) **MEDICAL TREATMENT:** Patient will be treated by his/her attending doctor or specialists. Patient authorizes Hospital to perform services ordered by the doctors. Special consent forms may be needed. Many doctors and assistants (such as those providing x-rays, lab tests, and anesthesiology) may not be Hospital employees and are responsible for their own treatment activities.

2) **GENERAL DUTY NURSING:** Hospital provides only general nursing care. If the patient needs special or private nursing, it must be arranged by the patient or by the doctor treating the patient.

3) **MONEY AND VALUABLES:** The Hospital has a safe in which to keep money or valuables. It will not be responsible for any loss or damage to items not deposited in the safe. The Hospital will not be responsible for loss or damage to items such as glasses, dentures, hearing aids and contact lenses.

4) **TEACHING PROGRAMS:** The Hospital participates in programs for training of health care personnel. Some services may be provided to the patient by persons in training under the supervision and instruction of doctors or hospital employees. These persons may also observe care given to the patient by doctors and hospital employees. Photos or video tapes may be made of surgical procedures.

5) **RELEASE OF INFORMATION:** The Hospital may disclose all or any part of the patient's medical and/or financial records (INCLUDING INFORMATION REGARDING ALCOHOL OR DRUG ABUSE), to the following:

   a. **Third Party Payors:** Any person or corporation, or their designee, which is or may be liable under a contract to the hospital, the patient, a family member, or employer of the patient, for payment of all or part of the hospital's charges, including but not limited to, insurance companies, utilization review organizations, workman's compensation payors, hospital or medical service companies, welfare funds, governmental agencies or the patient's employer;

   b. **Medical Audit:** The Hospital conducts a program of medical audit and the patient's medical information may be reviewed and released by employees, members of the medical staff or other authorized persons to appropriate agencies as part of this program.

   c. **Medical Research:** Information may be released for use in medical studies and medical research.

   d. **Other Health Care Providers:** Information may be released to other health care providers in order to provide continued patient care.

   I understand that the authorization granted in items 5. a, b, c and d may be revoked by me at any time, except to the extent to which action has been taken in reliance upon it. The authorization will stay in effect as long as the need for information in items 5. a, b, c and d exist.

I have read and understand this Admissions Agreement, have received a copy and I am the patient, the parent of a minor child or the court appointed guardian for the patient and am authorized to act on the patient's behalf to sign this Agreement.

Harriet Culver   _Bertha C. Young_
WITNESS   PATIENT   PARENT OF MINOR CHILD   COURT APPOINTED GUARDIAN
(PLEASE CIRCLE THE CORRECT TITLE)

October 6, 19XX 1:00 p.m
DATE

MEDICAL POWER OF ATTORNEY A.R.S. §14-5501: I appoint _____ as my agent to act in all matters relating to my health care, including full power to give or refuse consent to all medical, surgical and hospital care. This power of attorney shall be effective upon my disability or incapacity or when there is uncertainty whether I am dead or alive and shall have the same effect as if I were alive, competent, and able to act for myself.

_____   _____
WITNESS   PATIENT

FINANCIAL AGREEMENT

I agree that in return for the services provided to the patient, I will pay the account of the patient, and/or prior to discharge make financial arrangements satisfactory to the hospital for payment. If the account is sent to an attorney for collection, I agree to pay reasonable attorney's fees and collection expenses. The amount of the attorney's fee shall be established by the Court and not by a Jury in any court action. A delinquent account may be charged interest at the legal rate.

If any signer is entitled to hospital benefits of any type whatsoever under any policy of insurance insuring patient, or any other party liable to patient, the benefits are hereby assigned to hospital for application on patient's bill. However, IT IS UNDERSTOOD THAT THE UNDERSIGNED AND PATIENT ARE PRIMARILY RESPONSIBLE FOR PAYMENT OF PATIENT'S BILL.

IN GRANTING ADMISISON OR RENDERING TREATMENT, THE HOSPITAL IS RELYING ON MY AGREEMENT TO PAY THE ACCOUNT, EMERGENCY CARE WILL BE PROVIDED WITHOUT REGARD TO THE ABILITY TO PAY.

Bertha C. Young
PATIENT
Harriet Culver   _____
WITNESS   OTHER PARTY AGREEING TO PAY
October 6 19XX
DATE   RELATIONSHIP TO PATIENT

09-1542 1-84

Figure 3-1
Consent form. (Reprinted with permission from LaFleur, M. W. and Starr, W. K. *Health Unit Coordinating*. Philadelphia, W. B. Saunders, 1986, p 483.)

- Because any break in the skin may be considered an operation, a consent form must be signed in order to avoid liability for battery.
- Telephone consents are valid in an emergency situation, provided that the telephoned consent is witnessed by two people and is immediately followed by a written confirmation.
- A consent is valid for a reasonable time after signing, as long as there is no change in the anticipated procedure.

Patient Medical Records and the Law

A patient's medical record is a legal document and as such is the property of the physician if the patient is an outpatient, and the property of the hospital if the patient has been hospitalized. It is extremely important that these records be as accurate, complete, up to date, and as neat as possible, in order to protect members of the medical staff from any future litigation, as well as evidence of truth if there is a lawsuit or court case regarding the patient's care or treatment. Although all patient's records are considered confidential, any or all parts of it may be summoned and used during a court action. Therefore, most hospitals and private medical practices make it a standard practice to obtain a signed "release of information" form from the patient when they are first seen or admitted into the hospital.

If you are required to write in the patient's medical records, always remember to use only permanent ink, and *never* erase an entry. If an error has been made, simply cross the error out, using only one line, initial it, and rewrite the correct entry above or next to the original entry. No documentation written in pencil or with erasures is acceptable, and any record with either of these can be automatically rejected as legal evidence.

Summary

In this chapter, we discussed some of the very important concepts dealing with medical law and ethics, including the differences between each, as well as what constitutes medical negligence and medical malpractice. We also talked about ethical behavior on the part of the administrative medical services worker, as well as the role of the Patient's Bill of Rights and what the patient has the right to expect from those health care professionals caring for him or her. In addition, we talked about the need to license medical personnel, as well as the purpose of the rule of personal liability and Good Samaritan acts. Finally, we talked about patient consent forms and defined the legal implications of the patient's medical record.

Review Questions

1. A patient's _____ is a document that states what a patient has the right to expect during his or her medical treatment.

2. Briefly define the *Good Samaritan Act.*

3. _____ pertains to any attack on a person's reputation.

   a. ethics

   b. negligence

   c. defamation

4. _____ pertains to any member of the health care delivery system failing to perform or to do something for a patient that another person of the same training and position would do under the same or ordinary circumstances.

   a. negligence

   b. defamation

   c. malpractice

5. _____ pertains to any care which is provided to a patient which is below an expected standard and which can result in injury.

   a. negligence

   b. defamation

   c. malpractice

6. Briefly define what is meant by *duty of care.*

7. When the written word is used to defame someone, it is called _____; when the spoken word is used to defame someone, it is called _____.

8. Briefly explain the concept of *medical ethics.*

9. Give at least two examples of ethical behavior:

   a. _____

   b. _____

Health and Safety in the Cardiovascular Environment

Performance Objectives

Upon completion of this chapter, you will be able to:

1. Identify factors associated with making some people more susceptible to infection than others.
2. Explain the difference between medical and surgical asepsis.
3. Describe and be able to demonstrate how to perform correct handwashing techniques.
4. Explain the relationship between good body alignment and practicing good body mechanics.
5. Identify specific types of activities that will ensure a safe environment for both patients and members of the cardiovascular health care team.
6. Identify potential emergency situations and how to respond to them.
7. Discuss the skills necessary for providing privacy for patients seen in the hospital and in the cardiovascular department.
8. Discuss methods for maintaining treatment rooms within the cardiovascular department.

Terms and Abbreviations

Alignment having parts in their proper relationship to one another.

Asepsis the absence of disease-producing organisms.

Bacteria one-celled microorganisms that are capable of causing fermentation, decay, and, in some cases, disease.

Bacteriology the study of bacteria.

Balance keeping an object in a steady position, or stable.

Base of support the area on which an object rests; when the body is upright, the feet form the base of support of the body.

Body mechanics the efficient use of the body during activity.

Center of gravity the point at which the mass of the body is centered.

Infection process that occurs when pathogens attack a person and produce signs and symptoms of an illness.

Line of gravity the imaginary vertical line that passes through the center of gravity.

Medical asepsis medical techniques used to reduce the number and prevent the spread of pathogens.

Musculoskeletal system made up of the bones, joints, and muscles of the body.

Nosocomial infection an infection acquired by the patient while being cared for in the hospital.

Pathogen any disease-producing organism.

Posture the position of the body parts in relation to one another.

Susceptible having a very low resistance to disease.

For as many years as people have lived on earth, they have suffered from infectious diseases. For a very long time, however, it was thought that an infection might be part of the actual healing process. No one knew how or why infections were transmitted. Physicians would move from one patient to another, without ever washing their hands or changing their dirty lab coats. And who ever heard of wearing sterile gloves or isolation gowns? It wasn't until as recent as the middle of the nineteenth century that the germ theory of disease was even suggested.

Asepsis and Infection Control

Asepsis is defined as the absence of microorganisms that are capable of causing disease. As it is now practiced, asepsis is based upon the many discoveries of scientists from around the world. One of the greatest of these was Louis Pasteur. Born in France, Pasteur made tremendous strides in the prevention and treatment of disease. It is for all his work that he is considered the founder of the study of bacteriology. In fact, today there are millions of people around the globe who owe their very lives to this man. It was his work that ultimately proved that germs could be spread through the air, but that the spread of such germs could in fact be controlled. In addition, he also proved that these germs could be killed. Because of his knowledge and his work in the study of bacteriology, Pasteur was also one of the very first to practice surgery with the use of antiseptics to prevent infection.

Susceptibility and Infection

Some people tend to be more susceptible to infection than others. One factor is the age of the person. The very young and the very old seem to develop infections easily. This is because a small child does not have the mature immune system that is needed to fight off infections, and the immune system of an elderly person is in decline.

People weakened because of disabilities also seem to be more susceptible than others to infection. One example are patients who suffer from spinal cord injury. They are more susceptible to urinary tract and bladder infections because of their inability to empty the bladder effectively. Another example are patients with multiple sclerosis; they are more susceptible to pneumonia because of impaired lung capacity and muscle paralysis.

People who are well nourished are less suscep-tible to infection than the malnourished. Nutrition plays an important role in the prevention of infection and in recovery from illness. Without proper nourishment, our bodies would not be able to function properly. A good diet, therefore, can provide the substances the body needs to repair itself.

Ingestion of medications can also increase one's incidence of infections. Drugs used in the treatment of leukemia, for example, will decrease the number of white blood cells being manufactured by the body. These cells are part of the body's immune system and are necessary to fight infection.

Patients who have been diagnosed with acquired immune deficiency syndrome, or AIDS, also have a weakened immune system. These patients are very susceptible to all kinds of infections.

The Infection Cycle

Microorganisms move from place to place in a cycle (Figure 4-1). If the cycle is broken, the microorganisms cannot grow, spread, or cause disease. A person with an infection acts as a reservoir for the microorganisms, allowing them to grow and multiply. The infection may be spread by such things as the hands, bed clothes or linens, and equipment. Microorganisms can even be transmitted by a simple cough or a sneeze. The person exposed and receiving the organism is called the *host*. The infectious agent may enter the host via an opening in the skin, mouth, or nose. If the host is unable to fight off the infecting organism, that person will begin to show signs or symptoms of a disease or an infection.

Germs and microorganisms are everywhere. They are in the air, in the soil, in the food and water we consume, and even on other people. The skin is called our first line of defense, and if this is broken, germs and organisms may enter the body. In order for an infection to occur, the environment for the microorganisms to grow and multiply must be just right. This means that food and moisture are needed. Oxygen is also needed, except in those cases where the microorganisms are anaerobic, that is, not requiring oxygen for growth. There are a few bacteria that fall into this category. One common example of an *anaerobic* bacterium is the one that causes tetanus. It generally grows well in a puncture wound because of the absence of oxygen. Bacteria needing oxygen for growth are called *aerobic* bacteria. Normal body temperature is best for most bacteria to grow and multiply. High temperature kills most microorganisms, while low temperatures tend to slow the growth rate. Finally, many bacteria need darkness to grow and

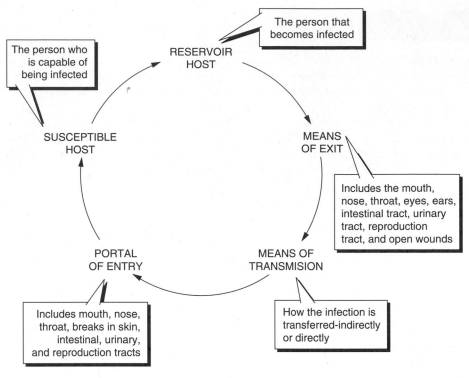

Figure 4-1
The infection cycle.

multiply. When exposed to light, they die. Food, moisture, oxygen, warm temperature, and darkness all encourage the growth of bacteria. In order to break the infection cycle, you must modify at least one of these factors.

Practicing Medical and Surgical Asepsis

The most common means by which organisms are transmitted are the hands, since they carry germs to the mouth, eyes, nose, and to other people. The best way to inhibit this transmission is through the practice of medical and surgical asepsis. *Medical asepsis* is the practice of reducing the numbers and preventing the spread of microorganisms. It is a practice that can be accomplished in a number of ways, such as covering your nose and mouth when you sneeze or cough, washing your hands before you handle food and after you have used the restroom, washing your hands before and after you have treated a patient, wearing a clean uniform or lab coat each day to work, practicing good body hygiene, and keeping dirty items such as linen and equipment separate from clean items in your department.

Surgical asepsis is the practice of eliminating all microorganisms, both pathogenic, or disease-producing, and nonpathogenic. Examples of surgical asepsis include using sterile equipment for giving injections, performing venipuncture, starting IVs, surgery, and

using sterile dressings and bandages to cover open wounds.

One of the most important tasks you will be faced with in health care is to provide the very best possible surroundings for you and the patients intrusted into your care. A clean, dry, well-lit, and airy department will help prevent the growth of pathogens.

One of the easiest and best ways of preventing the spread of bacteria is through using correct *handwashing* techniques. Figure 4-2 shows the correct procedure for handwashing. It is a skill used not only for your protection, but also for those around you—patients, co-workers, and visitors. You will wash your hands before and after doing treatments and at any other time your hands become dirty.

When washing your hands, always remember to use plenty of flowing water, a good germicidal soap, and friction. It is the friction, or strong rubbing movement of both hands against one another, that loosens the bacteria from the skin. The water is directed so that it flows from the wrist down toward the fingers. This carries the suds and dirt down the drain. Never lean against the sink or allow your uniform or lab coat to touch it. After drying your hands with a paper towel, before you discard it in the trash, you must always remember to use the towel to turn off the faucet. After you have finished washing your hands, you may also apply some lotion to them to prevent any chapping and to keep the skin soft.

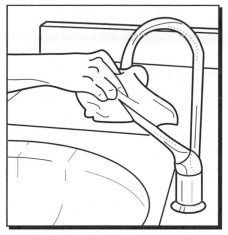

Step 1: Never touch sink with your uniform.

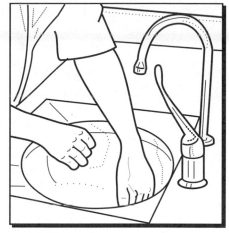

Step 2: Wet hands.

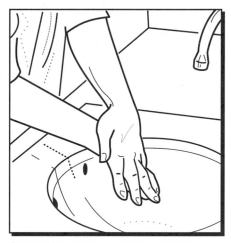

Step 3: Use strong rubbing movements.

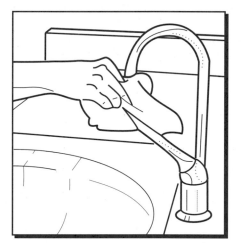

Step 4: Rinse well, with hands lower than wrist.

Figure 4-2
Steps in handwashing to prevent the spread of bacteria.

Medical Asepsis in the Cardiovascular Department

In most large medical facilities, the cardiovascular department is usually self-contained. This makes it easier to keep it clean and thus prevent the growth and spread of bacteria and microorganisms. Tables and equipment should have adequate space between them so that they may be kept spotlessly clean.

All articles that are used in the cardiovascular department must be cleaned after each use. This prevents the spread of pathogens between patients. It also protects your coworkers from the possibility of contracting an infection from a patient. In the past, many hospitals placed articles in the direct sunlight in order to destroy pathogens. Since this is not very practical today, equipment can be soaked in an antiseptic solution or wiped off with a disinfectant.

Antiseptics are used to inhibit and stop the growth of pathogens, yet they are mild enough to be used on the skin. A *disinfectant* is used to stop the growth of the pathogenic organisms, but it is harmful if used directly on the skin. *Sterilization* is a process used to kill all microorganisms. Items that have been sterilized are usually marked or wrapped in special containers in order to maintain their cleanliness until they are to be used.

It is the responsibility of all members of the cardiovascular department to continuously be on guard against the spread of infections. If you start to perform a procedure on a patient and suddenly remember that you failed to wash your hands since working with your last patient, you must immediately stop the procedure and wash your hands. A clinician who observes that medical aseptic techniques are not being followed and does nothing to correct it, is not safe to practice as a member of the health care profession. Nothing should ever be assumed when practicing asepsis.

Following Universal Precautions

In today's medical and health care facilities, all cardiovascular departments must practice universal precautions to prevent the spread of communicable diseases and infections. All patients and staff are considered possible carriers of potentially harmful pathogens. Blood and body fluids carry many pathogens. Body fluids that may be infected include blood, sputum, urine, stool, and drainage from open wounds. In order to decrease the risk of accidental exposure to body fluids, the cardiovascular department will have strict infection control procedures that must be followed by all members of the staff. This is especially true when working with patients who have open wounds. These precautions are for all patients, and they stress *prevention* of exposure and possible infection. As a member of the cardiovascular health care delivery team, you should make yourself aware of the infection control procedures followed by your department and the facility.

Providing for a Healthy and Safe Environment

Health care workers are active people. In the performance of your work, you will use a variety of movements. You may be required to reach, pull, lift, stoop, sit, stand, carry objects, push wheelchairs and stretchers, and stand at the treatment area or a patient's bedside. Your body must be in good physical condition. This means being constantly aware of how to most effectively and efficiently use your muscles. Doing so will prevent injury to yourself as well as your patients.

Practicing Good Body Mechanics

Body mechanics is the efficient use of the body during an activity. Good posture is insurance for health and happiness. *Posture* pertains to the position of your body and the relationship of its individual parts to one another. Once you know your faulty posture habits and have a corrected posture image, you can begin to control alignment. Your movements will be safer and more efficient. You will feel tall, poised, and graceful. You should always remember to practice good posture in your walking, sitting, and working. It will decrease the fatigue you may experience during the day. Figure 4-3 shows the correct alignment of body parts.

The most common complaint of all health care workers is lower back pain. Often this involves lifting a load while twisting around at the waist. It may result in severe muscle strain, or in some cases, even disc herniation or rupture. It is costly in loss of salary and

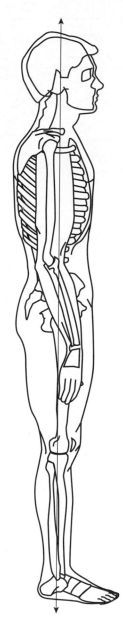

Figure 4-3
Correct postural body alignment.

medical expenses. The important point is that it is preventable.

When the parts of the skeletal system are aligned, balance can be maintained (Figure 4-4). *Balance* is the maintaining of an object in a steady position so that it does not tip or fall. To maintain balance, the body must have a wide base of support. In a standing position, the feet are the base of support. The *center of gravity* is located at the center of the pelvis just below the umbilicus. To maintain balance, the center of gravity must fall within the base of support (between the feet). When the center of gravity falls outside of the base of support, you will lose stability or balance.

In order to use your muscles most efficiently and

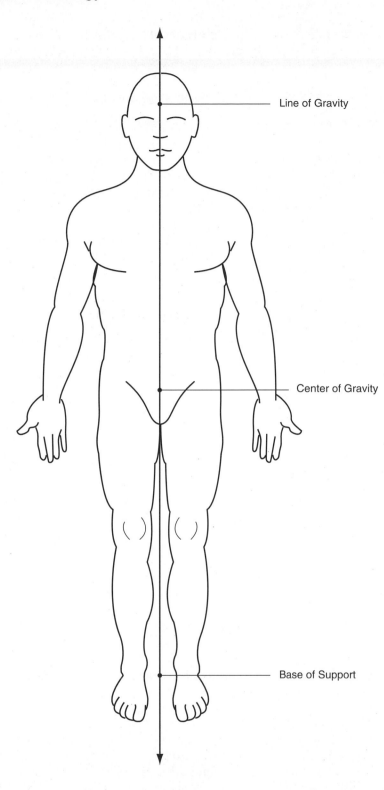

Line of Gravity

Center of Gravity

Figure 4-4
Maintaining balance through body alignment.

Base of Support

prevent the possibility of muscle strain or other injury, there are certain guidelines you can follow when lifting objects or helping patients. These include

- Always remember to size up the load and never lift more than you feel comfortable lifting. When in doubt, get help!

- Always remember to stand with your feet shoulder-width apart or with one foot slightly in front of the other.
- If you have to squat, always remember to bend at your knees, and never at the waist. This will only add more stress to your back.
- Always remember to bring the load close to your body, using a firm grip with both hands.

- When lifting an object, always remember to tighten your abdominal muscles, and then lift the load using your leg muscles.

It's important to remember that even lifting very light loads can result in injury if you do not use proper body mechanics. Using good posture and body mechanics in your everyday work will decrease the amount of energy expended and provide more ease and grace in your movements. The knowledge of proper body mechanics and alignment will help you prevent injury to yourself and to others (Figure 4-5).

Providing a Safe Environment

The makeup of the cardiovascular department is important to the well-being of the patient. The goal is to have a therapeutic or healing environment. Therefore, it is the responsibility of all members of the cardiovascular team continuously to provide for safety, privacy, and order.

You must be constantly alert to provide safe care during every treatment and procedure for each and every patient. A safe environment will help prevent injuries and potential lawsuits. Falls, which are considered to be the leading cause of most lawsuits in the hospital environment, can be prevented by taking a few precautions, including

- Keeping the floor clean and dry and putting things away as soon as you are through using them.
- Cleaning up all spills immediately after they occur.
- Checking with the nursing station before performing a procedure on a patient of whom you are unsure regarding his or her level of consciousness or orientation.
- Giving extra attention to patients with vision or hearing impairments.

Any time you are required to use an electrically operated piece of equipment, you must make sure it is in proper working condition. Make sure there are no frayed wires or faulty plugs. Report equipment problems to your supervisor and move faulty equipment out of patient care areas so that it will not be used accidentally.

Another aspect to providing a safe environment is providing for your patient's privacy. Privacy is the legal right of every patient, and anytime you are required to perform a procedure, you must also provide for the patient's privacy. Always remember to knock before entering a patient's room or a treatment area. If you are performing a procedure that requires the patient to disrobe, always make sure that you only expose the part of the body needed for the pro-

cedure. And if you must perform the procedure in the patient's hospital room, make sure you remember to have the privacy curtain pulled around the patient. Remember, as health care workers, we are accustomed to situations that would be embarrassing to the average person. Always be careful to provide for the privacy of each of your patients.

Finally, another very important aspect of providing for a safe environment has to do with knowing your hospital floor plan regarding exits, locations of fire extinguishers, and how to use them. Make a point of finding out how to report a fire. Many clinics and hospitals have special code words that alert the entire building of fires and emergencies. You should know these codes and be aware of your responsibilities if an emergency does occur in your facility.

Common Emergencies

Part of providing a safe environment means being aware of potential crisis or emergency situations and then responding appropriately. Patients want to feel that you will know what to do if an emergency does occur. Naturally, any emergency should be reported to your supervisor immediately.

A common emergency is *fainting*, which is the temporary loss of consciousness. This occurs quite often and is not considered a serious malady. It is generally associated with illness or emotional stress. The patient shows pallor, sweating, and a slow, weak pulse that later becomes rapid. To treat the patient, first check the pulse, respirations, and blood pressure and make sure the airway is open, elevate the patient's feet, and provide supportive care.

Another common emergency that you may encounter is a *convulsive seizure*. These are disorders of the central nervous system and are characterized by recurrent attacks. They generally involve changes in the patient's level of consciousness, motor activity, or sensory phenomena. The onset is usually sudden and lasts only a brief time. The individual convulses, falls to the floor, and in some cases, may exhibit violent, involuntary contractions of the muscles.

The aim of treatment during a seizure is to prevent the person from injuring himself or herself. Move furniture out of the way, loosen the clothing around the person's neck, and place a pillow or soft roll under the person's head. After the seizure is over, the patient will be sleepy and lethargic. Rest should be encouraged.

Falls, which may lead to contusions, sprains, or dislocations, are another common emergency, and as we have already noted, are one of the leading causes of lawsuits in the hospital environment. A contusion or bruise is an injury to the muscle and soft tissues as a result of a blunt force. Discoloration occurs

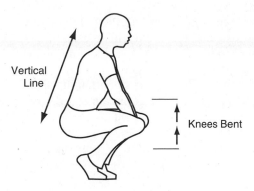

Vertical Line

Knees Bent

A. Lifting Heavy Objects

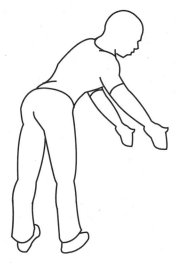

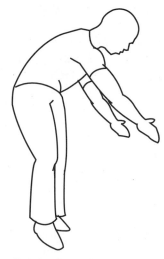

Figure 4-5
Using correct body alignment to prevent injuries.

B. Twisting Incorrectly

Twisting Correctly

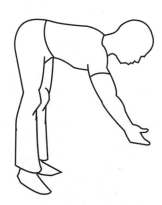

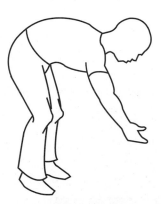

C. Bending Incorrectly

Bending Correctly

when small capillaries break and leak into the tissues. The area is usually quite painful and is generally swollen.

To treat a sprain, gently apply cold compresses or icepacks to the area. This will cause vasoconstric-

tion, which slows the internal bleeding and thus decreases the pain. The injured part should be elevated and wrapped in an elastic bandage for compression and support.

An emergency that could have a deady result is

cardiac arrest. In this very serious crisis situation, there is a sudden stoppage of the heart. The patient loses consciousness, stops breathing, as has no pulse and no heart sounds. Time is the most important factor in resuscitation. You must quickly assess the situation and call for help. A delay of more than 4 to 6 minutes could result in irreversible brain damage. As a member of the cardiovascular team, you must be familiar with standard cardiopulmonary resuscitation (CPR) techniques, and if necessary, begin rescue breathing or CPR immediately.

Maintaining the Treatment Area

By keeping your department neat, you will be doing much toward keeping things running smoothly. You will also find that your own work, as well as everyone else's, is much easier once there is a system for keeping everything in order. As soon as possible, you should learn exactly where different articles and equipment and supplies are kept and always return them to the same place. This keeps the shelves, cabinets, and treatment rooms in a state of readiness. Shelves should be labeled so that everyone will know at a glance where a particular item is located. Tabletops should be kept clear and clean so that there is always workspace. Wastebaskets should be emptied regularly, and the rest of the department should be kept clean and in perfect working order.

Equipment should be checked often and cleaned with the recommended disinfectant after being used. Movable equipment should be placed where it will not tilt or roll. Water should be drained from the autoclave or sterilizer after each use. It is a good idea to check with your supervisor frequently for any ideas or suggestions regarding changes in the normal cleanup routine of the department.

An inventory is important in any department. A good reference file, listing the names, addresses, and telephone numbers of the companies from which supplies and equipment can be ordered, should be kept. Prices and order numbers of supplies and equipment are usually listed with information supplied from the company. Supplies on hand should be checked often so that new supplies can be ordered

before they are needed. Do not order more supplies than will be used in a reasonable length of time. Storage space should be available for anything that is ordered. If you are required to keep the inventory for your department, always make sure that you have your list approved by the department supervisor before you make out a requisition or take an order.

Any equipment needing repairs should be reported to your supervisor as soon as possible. Never try to repair the equipment or take advice from another employee who is not qualified to repair the equipment, because more damage and greater costs may result. Most equipment requires certification as being "safe" before it can be used for patient care.

Medical supplies are very expensive. Therefore, you should only use what is necessary and return reusable supplies to their proper places. In some institutions, supplies are ordered for each individual receiving treatment. This is especially true when ordering medications, dressings, and bandages. Wise use of medical supplies in your department will decrease the cost of the patient's medical care, which will ultimately decrease the costs for the medical facility, thus putting additional monies back into your pocket in the form of increases in salary.

Summary

In this chapter, we discussed the important aspects of cleanliness and safety in the health care environment. We talked about medical and surgical asepsis and infection control procedures, noting the importance of each in the protection of both the patient and the health care worker. We also discussed awareness of posture and maintenance of good body alignment and use of proper body mechanics. We explained the role safety played in the health care environment and discussed some of the more common emergencies that occur in health care settings. Finally, we discussed how to maintain the cardiovascular department and its individual treatment areas properly, noting that it is the responsibility of all members of the department to maintain the department in a state of readiness and order.

Review Questions

1. Briefly define *medical asepsis.*

2. What does the term *alignment* mean?

3. A one-celled microorganism that is capable of causing fermentation, decay, and in some cases, disease, is called

   _____ .

4. What type of infection is acquired by the patient while being cared for in the hospital?

   a. bacteriological

   b. nosocomial

   c. viral

5. _____ pertains to keeping an object in a steady position, or stable.

   a. alignment

   b. center of gravity

   c. balance

6. The point at which an object rests, when the body is upright, is called:

   a. base of support

   b. center of gravity

   c. line of gravity

7. A(n) _____ is a process that occurs when pathogens attack a person and then produce signs and symptoms of an illness.

8. Briefly explain the *infection cycle*.

9. What is the easiest and best way a health care provider can prevent the spread of bacteria?

10. What is the name of the process used to kill all microorganisms?

    a. disinfection

    b. sterilization

    c. sanitization

5

Medical Terminology and the Medical Record

Performance Objectives

Upon completion of this chapter, you will be able to:

1. Identify specific prefixes, suffixes, and root words related to medical terms.
2. List common medical abbreviations used in the health care environment.
3. Identify body structure terms related to position, direction, anatomical planes, posture, and types of movement.
4. Explain the importance and uses of the medical record.
5. Distinguish between subjective, objective, assessment, and plan information on a patient's medical record.

Terms and Abbreviations

Combining form created by the joining of word elements and the combining vowel together.

Combining vowel adding an "o" to a prefix for ease in pronounciation.

Prefix a word element placed at the beginning of a word that, combined with the root, changes or adds to the root word's meaning.

Root the main part of a word, referring to the primary meaning of the word as a whole.

Suffix a word element placed at the end of a root that, combined with the root, changes or adds to the meaning of the word.

Word elements the five word elements that make up the basis of medical terminology: the prefix, suffix, root, combining form, and the combining vowel.

The discussion of medical terminology will help you to understand the many terms commonly used in medicine and in your individual department. The prefixes and suffixes of many medical terms give definite information about the meaning of the term. If you know these prefixes and suffixes, it will be much easier to understand many medical words. A *prefix* is a word fragment placed in front of the basic or root word (Appendix B). A *suffix* is a word fragment added at the end of the basic or root word (Appendix B). The *root word* is the main body of the word, that is, the part that usually gives the meaning to the word (Appendix B).

There are no specific rules governing the pronunciation of medical terms. A medical dictionary will give you some suggestions as to the pronounciation of words. However, in many hospitals and medical facilities, these pronunciations will vary among professionals and individual departments.

Using Medical Abbreviations

Many abbreviations for words and phrases are used in the treatment of patients to save time and space. As a member of the cardiovascular team, you must learn these abbreviations so that you can follow directions and communicate with other health care workers (Appendix A). Since the cardiovascular profession has adopted many abbreviations that are commonly used by health care professionals in writing their notes in the patient's medical record, it is very important that you study and learn these common abbreviations so that you will be able to recognize their meanings easily.

Body Structure and Medical Terminology

The human body can be compared to a smooth-running machine. It has many parts that must work together in order to promote good health, growth, and life itself. The body is a combination of organs and systems supported and protected by a framework of bones known as the skeleton. The muscles working upon the skeleton provide for the movements as we work and play through each day. All of this is then protected by an external covering known as the skin, which is considered the largest of all our body organs. You will need to know the various parts of the body and how to describe them in medical terms.

The human body is divided into five specific *cavities* or compartments: thoracic, abdominal, pelvic, cranial, and spinal (Figure 5-1). Within the thoracic cavity are the lungs, heart, aorta, and the thymus gland. The brain lies within the cranial cavity, and the spine is located within the spinal cavity. The abdominal cavity contains the stomach; liver; gallbladder; small intestine; colon, or large intestine; spleen; and the pancreas. The reproductive organs and the urinary bladder are all located within the pelvic cavity. Various structural units make up the body. Cells, tissues, and organs are organized into individual systems. These systems include the skeletal, muscular, nervous, circulatory, digestive, respiratory, urinary, reproductive, and endocrine.

Anatomical Position

Many terms are used to describe the body and to identify the position, direction, and location of the parts of the body. In addition, these terms are also used to describe various medical characteristics of the body, such as the location of incisions or injuries on the body. In order for the health care professional to be able to read the patient's medical record and thus have a mental picture of the patient's condition, all descriptive terms are based on an accepted standard position. This standard is known as the *anatomical position* (Figure 5-2). In this position, the person is standing erect, facing forward, with the head and trunk aligned, the arms straight by the sides with

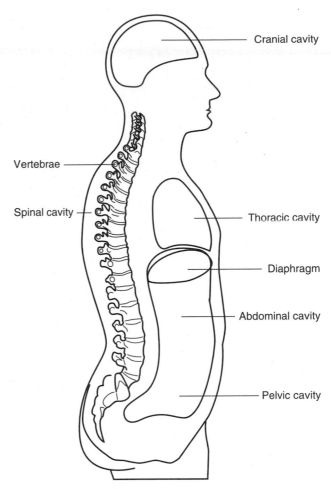

Figure 5-1
Body cavities.

palms facing forward, and the legs straight with the feet together.

Defining Position and Direction

Once you know the definition of the anatomical position, you can begin to use specific terms to describe position, direction, and location. Whereas Figure 5-3 shows the relationship of some of these terms to one another, the following is a list of all of the terms which are used to describe the body's position and direction:

- *Anterior.* Toward the front or in front of; ventral
- *Posterior.* Toward the back or in back of; dorsal
- *Medial.* Nearest the midline
- *Lateral.* Away from the midline or toward the side
- *Internal.* Inward or inside
- *External.* Outward or outside

36

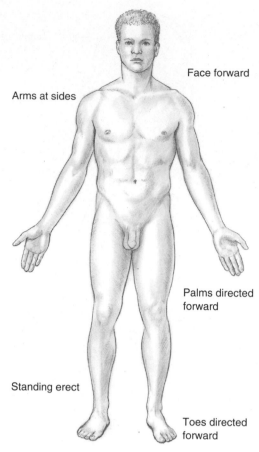

Face forward

Arms at sides

Palms directed
forward

Standing erect

Toes directed
forward

Figure 5-2
**Anatomical position. (Reprinted with permission from
Applegate, E. J. *The Anatomy and Physiology Learning
System*. Philadelphia: W. B. Saunders, 1991, p 14.)**

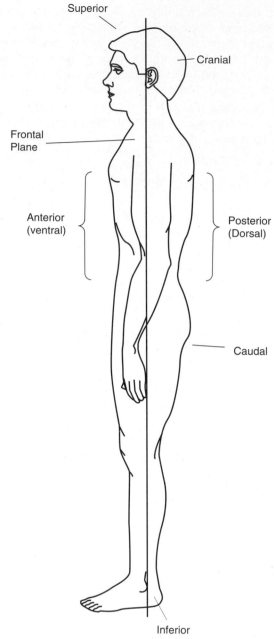

Superior

Cranial

Frontal
Plane

Anterior
(ventral)

Posterior
(Dorsal)

Caudal

Inferior

Figure 5-3
Body positions and directions.

- *Proximal.* Nearest the point of reference
- *Distal.* Farthest away from the point of reference
- *Superior.* Above
- *Inferior.* Below
- *Cranial.* Toward the head
- *Caudal.* Toward the tail

Defining Anatomical Planes

There are specific terms used to describe and identify structures, areas of the body, and certain types of movement of the extremities (Figure 5-4). These include

- *Sagittal.* An imaginary plane that runs parallel to the long axis of the body dividing it into right and left sections
- *Frontal.* An imaginary plane that runs through the side of the body dividing it into anterior (front) and posterior (back) sections

- *Transverse.* An imaginary plane dividing the body into superior (upper) and inferior (lower) sections

Defining Anatomical Postures

There are specific terms used to describe anatomical postures. These include

- *Erect.* Standing position
- *Supine.* Lying down

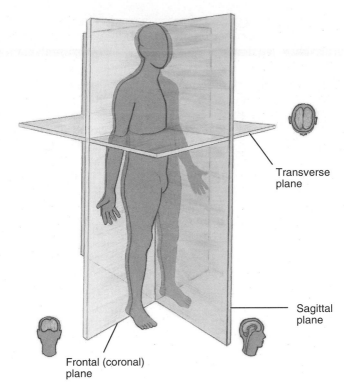

Figure 5-4
**Anatomical planes.
(Reprinted with permission
from Applegate, E. J.** *The
Anatomy and Physiology
Learning System.*
**Philadelphia: W. B. Saunders,
1991, p 14.)**

Transverse
plane

Sagittal
plane

Frontal (coronal)
plane

- *Prone*. Lying flat on the stomach, with the face down
- *Side-lying*. Lying with the body positioned on either the left or right side

Defining Types of Movement

There are specific terms used to describe various types of body movement. These include

- *Flexion*. Bending at a joint
- *Extension*. Straightening at a joint; unbending
- *Abduction*. Moving away from the center of the body
- *Adduction*. Moving toward the center of the body
- *Rotation*. Rolling a part on its own axis, such as the turning of the head
- *Pronation*. Moving the palm from the anatomical position into a position with the palm facing posteriorly or backward
- *Supination*. Moving the palm into the anatomical position facing anteriorly or forward
- *Eversion*. Turning the foot outward
- *Inversion*. Turning the foot inward

It's very important to remember that not all joints can perform all motions. The immovable joints are, of course, incapable of performing any of them. Of the freely moving joints, only the ball-and-socket joints, such as the hip and the shoulder, can perform all motions. The hinge joints, such as those found at the knee and the elbow, are only able to flex and extend.

Understanding the Patient's Medical Record

Memory is oftentimes fleeting and inaccurate. Medical records fill the need by containing accurate and detailed facts. These facts serve as a basis for the study, evaluation, and review of the patient's medical care.

Patient's medical records have been found among the earliest writings of Egyptians and in Hindu literature. Until modern times, however, no effort was made to keep patients' histories in any type of systematic order. These records are of the greatest importance to the physician while the patient is under his or her care. They are also extremely valuable if the patient returns for treatment after several years. For the patient, the record has a historical value, because it is the document that forms his or her case history.

Patients' histories also have great statistical value. For instance, they may be of use to the physician in evaluating a specific type of treatment or to find out the incidence of a particular disease. They may also be used as the basis for a lecture, an article, or a textbook. Further, patients' histories have legal importance. They may be summoned as a legal document and used in a court of law either to uphold the rights of the doctor, if he or she is involved in litigation, or they may be used to confirm the claim of the patient if the doctor is called as a witness.

The medical record is used by health care practitioners to exchange information or as a means of communication. The physician, nurses, and other personnel contribute information to the record. A doctor may change a patient's care if the nurse has observed a change in the patient's condition. Likewise, after reading the notes written by the ECG technician, a nurse may plan specific nursing care that will allow the patient the greatest degree of comfort toward the prevention of any future cardiac symptoms.

There are many different types of printed forms available for keeping medical records. Some hospitals print their own forms. Preprinted forms are useful because they save time. They also assist the recorder in remembering questions he or she will want to ask. They are a way to record accurately the details of the patient's care and treatment.

The physician is always the person who initiates the treatment by checking the appropriate referral blanks or writing directions or "orders" for treatment in a narrative form. The request for a lab test or an electrocardiogram, for example, is then sent to the cardiovascular department or the laboratory, as soon as possible, so that the procedure or lab test can be scheduled and carried out. Usually, the hospitalized patient and the chart are brought to the department from the nursing unit. Information relating to how the testing or procedural goals are being accomplished, and the patient's response to the procedure, is then recorded in the medical record after the test or procedure has been completed.

Charting Notes in the Medical Record

Most large health care facilities and individual medical practices document the patient's care and treatment in the medical record by utilizing a four-point system known as *SOAP notes*. The SOAP abbreviation refers to the four methods in which the patient's care is identified, assessed, and, ultimately, carried out. The *S* stands for *subjective* symptoms that the patient may be presenting, and includes any information the patient says, family remarks made regarding the patient, and any other information stated by other health care providers. The *O* refers to any

objective information, tests, or treatments that may have been provided for the patient, as well as any observations or measurements made by a member of the health care team. The *assessment*, or how well the patient is responding to a given treatment, is abbreviated by the *A*. It includes any professional opinions or goals of a specific type of therapy or treatment made by the health care provider. The *P*, which pertains to the *plan*, is what needs to be done or what will be done for the patient, based on the objective and subjective findings and the assessment.

Not all hospitals or individual departments will use the SOAP note format. Your department may choose to set up its own method of keeping records. Some departments use 5-by-8-inch file cards and record only the visits of the patients. Others may use an 8-by-11-inch file folder that encloses individual progress notes. In any case, the SOAP format is a good way of organizing your written data, no matter what type of forms the department uses.

Writing in the Medical Record

Since the patient's medical record is considered a legal document, it should always be written in ink. The information should be factual and have meaning. Notes must be accurate, without any spelling or grammatical errors. Any errors must be properly corrected by drawing one line through the error, with the person making the correction, writing his or her initials to verify that an error has been made. You must never scratch out mistakes and/or use correction fluids. Remember, too, that all information within the medical record is confidential. This means that the record should not be used for any other reason but as a means of exchanging information between members of the professional medical staff.

Summary

In this chapter, you were introduced to medical terminology and the medical record. In doing so, we determined that a basic knowledge of medical terms will make you better able to assess your patient's condition and thus allow you to read medical reports and records with greater understanding. As you continue to gain experience in the field of cardiovasuclar technology, you will recognize the importance of using proper terms and abbreviations to save time and space when documenting patients' responses to medical treatments.

Review Questions

1. A _____ is always placed at the beginning of a word.

    a. prefix
    b. suffix
    c. root

2. A _____ is always placed at the end of a word.

    a. prefix
    b. suffix
    c. root

3. A _____ is the body or main part of a word.

    a. prefix
    b. suffix
    c. root

4. A(n) _____ _____ always requires an "o" for ease in pronounciation.

    a. combining form
    b. combining vowel

5. What does the term *anterior* mean?

6. What does the term *lateral* mean?

7. Define the following prefixes:

    a. anti _____
    b. erythro _____
    c. leuko _____

8. Define the following suffixes:

    a. ectomy _____
    b. itis _____
    c. ology _____

9. Define the following abbreviations:

    a. ECG _____
    b. CHF _____
    c. H&P _____

10. Define the following abbreviations:

    a. npo _____
    b. tid _____
    c. ac _____

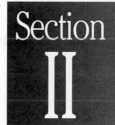

Section

II

Scientific Principles in Cardiovascular Technology

6

Applied Anatomy and Physiology of the Cardiovascular System

Performance Objectives

Upon completion of this chapter, you will be able to:

1. Discuss the functions of blood and the individual formed elements of it.
2. Discuss blood coagulation and identify the role platelets play in the process.
3. Discuss the significance of ABO blood types and briefly tell why the Rh factor is important in some pregnancies and transfusions.
4. Describe the structure of the heart and be able to trace the course of blood as it travels through it.
5. Define pulse and blood pressure.
6. Identify the different types of blood vessels found in the human body and describe the two major circuits formed by the blood vessels.
7. Distinguish between breathing (pulmonary ventilation) and external and internal respiration.
8. Identify the parts of the respiratory system and briefly describe the structure and function of each.
9. Discuss how sound is produced by the vocal cords.
10. Describe and be able to demonstrate the Heimlich maneuver.
11. Explain how air is caused to flow in and out of the lungs.
12. Explain the movement of gases between alveolar walls and the blood and tell how oxygen and carbon dioxide are transported in the blood.
13. Briefly explain how breathing is controlled by the nervous system and chemical stimulation.

Terms and Abbreviations

Agglutination   the clumping together of small particles.

Alveoli   minute, balloonlike sacs in the lung through which oxygen and carbon dioxide are exchanged.

Antibody   protein substance found in blood serum, that has been developed in response to an antigen and that reacts specifically against that antigen.

Anticoagulant   a substance that prevents the coagulation of blood.

Antigen   any substance that stimulates the body to produce antibodies.

Asphyxiation   a condition caused by an insufficient intake of oxygen; suffocation.

Breathing   the mechanical process by which atmospheric air is taken into the lungs and waste air is expelled.

Ciliated   covered with short, bristlelike hairs.

Coagulation   the process of clotting.

Cyanosis   a bluish-gray skin color that is caused by a lack of oxygen in the blood.

Diapedesis   the movement of leukocytes through the unbroken capillary wall.

Electrocardiogram the recording of the electrical activity of the heart.

Embolus a blood clot that has dislodged from its place of origin.

Expiration (exhalation) the process of breathing out.

External respiration the exchange of gases between the lungs and the blood.

Fibrinolysis the mechanism by which blood clots are dissolved.

Hematology the study of the blood.

Hemorrhage pertaining to copious bleeding; undue loss of blood.

Inspiration (inhalation) the process of breathing in.

Intercostal between the ribs.

Internal respiration the exchange of gases between the blood and the body cells.

Lymph clear, watery fluid found in lymphatic vessels.

Matrix intercellular material of a tissue.

Medulla the part of the brain that controls respirations.

Megakaryocyte large bone marrow cell; cells from which platelets develop.

Mitotic pertaining to mitosis or cell division.

Olfactory pertaining to the sense of smell.

Phagocyte a cell that engulfs and destroys bacteria and cellular debris.

Plasma the liquid part of the blood that has been prevented from clotting by the addition of an anticoagulant.

Pleural thin tissue covering the lungs and lining the chest cavity.

Pulmonary pertaining to the lungs.

Respiration the interchange of gases between organisms and the environment; the taking in of oxygen, its use in tissues, and the giving off of carbon dioxide.

Reticuloendothelial a term used for cells scattered throughout the body, such as the liver, spleen, tonsils, lymph nodes, and others, that ingest foreign particles.

Serum the liquid portion of coagulated blood.

Sinus a cavity.

Spirometer a device used to measure the air capacity of the lungs.

Surfactant phospholipid produced by the alveoli that forms a lining that prevents the thin membranes of the alveoli from sticking together.

Thoracic pertaining to the chest region.

Thrombus a blood clot.

When we discuss applied anatomy and physiology of the cardiovascuar system, we are actually talking about five different areas of concentration. These individual components include hematology; the heart; the blood vessels that carry blood to and from the heart and throughout the rest of the body; the lymphatic system, which acts as a transportation system for circulation; and the respiratory system, which provides us with the ability to take in oxygen and rid our body of unwanted gases, such as carbon dioxide.

Hematology and the Functions of Blood

Everyone knows that blood is important to life. Even primitive civilizations were able to correlate blood with health and loss of blood, with death. Modern studies have shown us that blood is as awesome today as the ancients believed. We refer to the study of blood as *hematology*, and scientists who study blood are called *hematologists*.

Blood is a type of connective tissue. The liquid plasma is the matrix of intercellular space of the tissue, while the blood cells are the solid or formed elements. An easy way to visualize the parts of the blood is to allow a tube of whole blood, to which an anticoagulant has been added, to stand until the cells fall to the lower part of the tube. The yellowish, liquid part that remains at the top is the plasma (Figure 6-1).

Blood, which makes up about 8 percent of our total body weight, is a thick, sticky liquid in which cells are suspended. An average person who weighs 150 pounds has about 10 pints of blood. About 92 percent of blood is made up of water, but many important things are either dissolved or suspended in it. Soluble components include three plasma proteins: albumins, which maintain the blood's viscosity; globulins, which are antibodies produced by leukocytes; and fibrinogen, which is necessary for clot formation. Other soluble components of blood include nutrients, such as glucose, lipids, and amino acids, and organic wastes, such as urea, uric acid, ammonia salts, and creatine. Inorganic salts in the plasma maintain a normal pH balance in the blood. Small quantities of oxygen and carbon dioxide are carried in the blood plasma, although larger quantities are carried by the hemoglobin. Regulatory substances, such as enzymes and hormones, are dissolved in the plasma, and thus transported from their source to all parts of the body.

When whole blood is allowed to clot, the liquid that separates from the solid constituents is serum. Serum differs from plasma in that it contains the clotting elements of blood.

One very important function of the blood is transportation. It carries oxygen and nutrients from the digestive and respiratory systems and then delivers them to each cell. It also transports waste products of metabolism from the cells to the excretory organs.

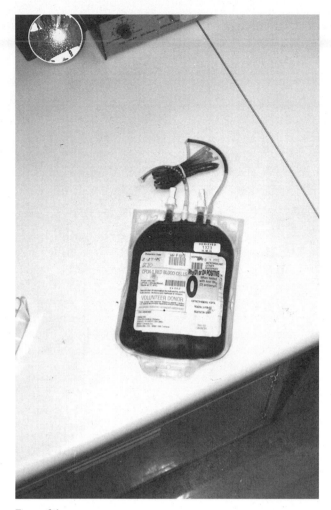

Figure 6-1
Whole blood.

This includes carbon dioxide from the cells to the lungs, and wastes from the cells to the kidneys. It also transports hormones produced by the endocrine glands from their production site to the cells and tissues.

Another important function of blood is to regulate and equalize the body's temperature by distributing heat to all parts of the body. Blood also acts as a defense mechanism, using white blood cells to engulf and destroy pathogens, and thus defend the body against invasion by unwanted bacteria and viruses.

Blood Cells

The formed elements in the blood are the cells. These include the erythrocytes, or red blood cells; the leukocytes, or white blood cells; and the thrombocytes, called platelets. The red blood cells are most numerous, averaging 4.5 million per cubic millimeter in females and 5.5 million per cubic millimeter in

males. In adults, the average total number of red blood cells is about 35 trillion. Of course, such a figure is not important to remember, but it is important to understand that each person has a great many red blood cells.

The total number of red blood cells varies with a person's age and degree of activity. Infants have a higher red blood cell count than children and adults. The number increases with activity and decreases during sleep. The number also increases at higher altitudes. These factors must be taken into account in determining normal numbers of cells.

Red blood cells are produced in the red marrow of bones by specialized cells. There, they go through several stages of development before they mature and are liberated into the circulating blood as they are needed. Unlike most other body cells, mature blood cells do not reproduce by mitotic cell division. Immature erythrocytes have a nucleus, but the nucleus is extruded before they enter the bloodstream. The nucleus is not needed for cell division to occur, and the cellular space is used for the cell's transport activities.

Red blood cells that are immature are spheroid in shape, but once the nucleus has been lost, they become biconcave (Figure 6-2). This shape increases the surface area of the cell while it decreases the amount of space that is needed for each cell. Red blood cells are only about 7 to 7.5 micrometers in diameter. This small size and their shape make it possible for them to move through the intercellular spaces of the capillary walls.

All red blood cells contain hemoglobin, which gives blood its characteristic bright red color. The hemoglobin gives the red blood cell its ability to oxygenate.

Red blood cells can only survive in the circulating blood for an average of 120 days. Then they break apart, and the pieces are engulfed and destroyed by the *reticuloendothelial* cells of the liver and spleen. In the cellular breakdown, iron is released from the hemoglobin, and compounds such as bilirubin are formed. Iron is stored in the liver until it is transported to the bone marrow, where it is used in building more red blood cells. The bilirubin is excreted in the bile.

The function of red blood cells is the transportation of oxygen and carbon dioxide. As the blood passes through the lungs, oxygen combines with hemoglobin and is then transported to all the tissues. In the tissues, oxygen is released. Carbon dioxide from the tissues combines with the globin portion of the hemoglobin molecule and is then taken back to the lungs. There the carbon dioxide is released and excreted by the lungs.

White blood cells, or leukocytes (Figure 6-3), are

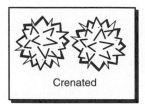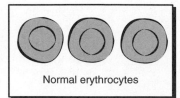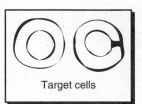

Figure 6-2
Red blood cells (erythrocytes).

classified by the presence or absence of granules in the cytoplasm. Cells that contain such granules are called *granulocytes*; there are three kinds of granulocytes, each named for its reaction in the staining process. The first type, called *neutrophils*, have fine cytoplasmic granules that stain lavender. The nuclei have several lobes, so one name for these cells is *polymorphonuclear leukocytes*, shorted to "polys." *Eosinophils* are another type of granulocyte. They have large cytoplasmic granules that stain red. Their nuclei are bilobed. *Basophils* have large cytoplasmic granules that stain purple. The nuclei of basophiles are usually S-shaped. Granulocytes are formed in the red bone marrow.

Agranulocytes are leukocytes that lack granules in the cytoplasm. They are formed in bone marrow and lymphoid tissue. There are two kinds of agranulocytes, lymphocytes and monocytes. *Lymphocytes* are small and have a large, round central nucleus and a small amount of cytoplasm. *Monocytes* are larger. They also have a large central nucleus, but it is surrounded by a large amount of cytoplasm.

Leukocytes have one main objective: to combat pathogenic organisms that have invaded the body. They are capable of ameboid motion. Thus, they can move between the intercellular spaces of the capillaries into the tissues and migrate to the invading microorganisms where they engulf and destroy them.

This movement through the capillary walls is called *dipedesis. Phagocytosis* is the term used to describe the process by which white blood cells engulf and destroy invading microorganisms. Neutrophils are most active in phagocytosis (Figure 6-4). They also produce the enzyme lysozme (muramidase), which destroys some bacteria.

In studying the blood, a test, called a *differential* white blood cell count, is done in order to determine the percentage of each kind of leukocyte. Of course, these numbers can vary, however, the average percentage of individual groups of white blood cells are as follows:

- *Lymphocytes*: 20 to 25%
- *Monocytes*: 3 to 7%
- *Neutrophils*: 60 to 70%
- *Eosinophils*: 2 to 4%
- *Basophils*: 0 to 2%

The differential is a valuable diagnostic tool because numbers of the various kinds of leukocytes increase or decrease in specific diseases. For example, in any bacterial infection, such as pneumonia, the number of neutrophiles rises. In allergic reactions, the number of eosinophiles increases. Monocytes tend to increase in the presence of some chronic infections.

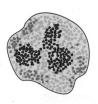

Figure 6-3
White blood cells (leukocytes).

Monocyte

Lymphocyte

Neutrophil

Basophil

Eosinophil

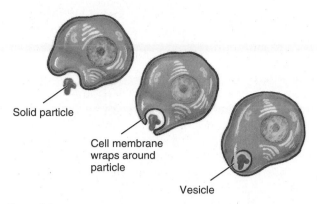

Figure 6-4
Phagocytosis: White blood cell engulfing bacteria. (Reprinted with permission from Applegate, E. J. *The Anatomy and Physiology Learning System.* **Philadelphia: W. B. Saunders, 1991, p 53.)**

Solid particle

Cell membrane wraps around particle

Vesicle

Platelets

Platelets, or *thrombocytes*, are actually fragments of large cells that have been formed in the red bone marrow. These cells break apart, leaving the fragments enclosed in part of the cell membrane to form the platelets. These small cells have no nucleus and are vital to the process of the coagulation of blood. A platelet count is a useful procedure in diagnosing some types of anemia.

During the clotting process, the thrombocytes first disintegrate, releasing thromboplastinogenase. This enzyme causes thromboplastinogen to be transformed to thromboplastin. The thromboplastin in the presence of calcium ions brings about the conversion of prothrombin to thrombin. Fibrinogen in the presence of thrombin is then converted to fibrin, which is made up of fine threads that are insoluble and that form a network that traps red blood cells and forms a clot.

Some hematologists believe that the tiny vessels of the circulatory system are constantly rupturing and that clots immediately form in order to stop the bleeding. Thus, two opposing processes, fibrinolysis, which results in bleeding, and clot formation, which stops the bleeding, go on all the time. Antithrombins are the agents that prevent clotting by inactivating thrombin, thus inhibiting the conversion of fibrinogen to fibrin. Two antithrombins are heparin, found in the liver and basophils, and coumarin compounds, which inhibit the liver's use of vitamin K.

Antigens and Antibodies

There are other important factors in the blood. Among these are the antigens and antibodies that determine our blood type. An *antigen* is a substance that reacts with its specific antibody. Antigens are named for the type of antigen-antibody reaction they may bring about. The antigens on the surface of red blood cells are called *agglutinogens*.

Antibodies are protein substances in the plasma that react with their specific antigen. Thus, agglutinogens, or antigens, will react with agglutinins, or antibodies, in order to bring about agglutination. There are many different kinds of antigen-antibody reactions.

There are two kinds of agglutinogens that may be found in the surface of human red blood cells, called A and B. An individual may have either A or B, or both A and B, or neither A nor B. A person's blood group or type is determined by the presence or absence of these A and B antigens.

If an individual has A agglutinogens on the red blood cells, then he or she will also have corresponding antibodies called anti-B agglutinins in the plasma. Persons with B agglutinogens will have anti-A agglutinins. Those with both A and B agglutinogens will have no agglutinins; and those with neither A nor B agglutinogens, will have both anti-A and anti-B agglutinins. Plasma could never contain antibodies against the antigens on its own red blood cells. If so, the antigen and antibody reaction would bring about the agglutination of the person's own red blood cells. Table 6-1 shows the antigens and antibodies present in the various blood types.

Blood Types and the Rh Factor

Blood types are important in blood transfusion because, if donor blood is of a type containing antigens and/or antibodies of a type different from that of a recipient, the red blood cells will agglutinate and cause severe reactions, or even death. The blood group O has no antigens. It is called the *universal donor* because theoretically the blood would not react with any cells in transfusion. In actuality, patients are almost always transfused with their own blood type. The anti-A and anti-B antibodies in the serum and other factors in the blood could cause an undesirable reaction.

Blood types are hereditary and do not change

Table 6-1
ABO Blood Types

Blood Group	Agglutinogen on Red Blood Cells	Agglutinin in Serum	Cells Agglutinated
A	A	Anti-B	B, AB, O
B	B	Anti-A	A, AB, O
AB	A, B	None	A, B, AB, O
O	None	Anti-A, anti-B	None

during one's lifetime. The pattern of inheritance is predictable. It is possible, by determining blood types, to know whether a given person *could be* the parent of a particular child, but not that he or she *is* the parent. Further research of blood factors may provide definite proof of parentage.

The percentage of a given blood type in various ethnic groups tends to vary. In the United States, 47 percent of the population has Type O blood; 41 percent has Type A; 10 percent has Type B; and only about 4 percent has Type AB.

Another factor that may cause the cells to agglutinate is the *Rh factor*. It gets its name from rhesus monkeys, the only animals in which it is found besides humans. Approximately 85 percent of the population in the United States has this factor. They are said to be Rh-positive. Those who lack the factor are said to be Rh-negative. Rh antigens are on the surface of the red blood cells as well as the A and B antigens. Thus, a person can be Type A, B, AB, or O, and also be Rh-positive or Rh-negative.

The Rh factor is of little importance except in the pregnancy of Rh-negative persons, or if they receive blood transfusions. If an Rh-negative person receives a blood transfusion from an Rh-positive donor, the body is stimulated to produce specific anti-Rh antibodies. These remain in the blood. If the patient receives further transfusions of Rh-positive blood, the Rh antigen on the donor's red blood cells and the Rh antibody in the patient's blood will react, causing the red blood cells to agglutinate, with serious consequences, in some cases even death. To avoid this problem, Rh determinations are done prior to transfusion with whole blood, and Rh-negative patients are given only Rh-negative blood. Therefore, there can be no antigens to stimulate the production of antibodies.

Current thought indicates that if an Rh-negative mother delivers an Rh-positive baby, but has no anti-Rh antibodies, she is given anti-Rh immune globulin during the first 72 hours following the delivery. These antibodies react with the fetal antigens in the mother's blood, if any, so she will not produce anti-Rh antibodies. Then, if a second pregnancy with an Rh-positive fetus occurs, there will be no Rh-positive antibodies present to cause a reaction.

Although Rh factors must be determined in order to provide adequate care of both the mother and the child, the actual numbers involved are quite small.

Structure and Function of the Cardiovascular System

The cardiovascular system is composed of the heart and blood vessels. The heart is the organ that moves blood through the circulatory system and thus to and from each part of the body. It is located in the chest cavity. The top of the heart is at a point between the second and third ribs. The *apex* is located between the fifth and sixth ribs and points to the left. About one-third of the mass of the heart lies to the right of the sternum, or breastbone, and two-thirds lies to the left. The size, and even the shape, of the heart varies. It is a hollow, muscular, cone-shaped organ, about the size of the individual's fist. An average weight for the heart of an adult male is about one pound.

The heart has four chambers. The two upper chambers are called the *atria* or *auricles*. The two lower chambers are called the *ventricles*. The right and left sides are divided by a *septum* and have no communication.

The heart wall is made up of three separate and distinct layers. The outer layer is called the *epicardium*, the middle layer, the *myocardium*, and the inner layer, the *endocardium*. The endocardium is a thin membrane that lines the chambers of the heart, covers the valves, and is continuous with the lining of the major blood vessels that enter the heart. The myocardium is made up of cardiac muscle. The heartbeat is the result of the rhythmic contraction and relaxation of the myocardium. The *pericardium* is a tough, but loose-fitting sac that covers and protects the heart.

There are four valves located within the heart that prevent the backflow of blood. The *semilunar valves* keep the blood from reentering the heart. The *pulmonary semilunar valve* prevents the backflow of blood into the right ventricle as it leaves by way of the pulmonary artery. The *aortic semilunar valve* prevents the backflow of blood from the aorta into the left ventricle. The valve between the right atrium and the right ventricle is called the *tricuspid valve*. It has three flaps or cusps, thus the name "tricuspid." The valve between the left atrium and the left ventricle is the *bicuspid* or *mitral valve*. These two valves are called *auricular-ventricular valves*.

Blood carrying carbon dioxide returns from the body by way of the *superior vena cava* and then enters the right atrium. It leaves the right atrium and falls through the tricuspid valve to the right ventricle. There it passes through the pulmonic or semilunar valve to the *pulmonary artery*, which is the only artery that carries carbon dioxide–laden blood, and then to the lungs. In the lungs, carbon dioxide is given off, and the blood is replenished with oxygen. The *pulmonary veins*, which are the only veins that carry freshly oxygenated blood, return oxygenated blood from the lungs to the heart. There it enters the left atrium and passes through the bicuspid valve into the left ventricle. From there it passes through the aortic semilunar valve to the aorta to be distributed throughout the body (Figure 6-5).

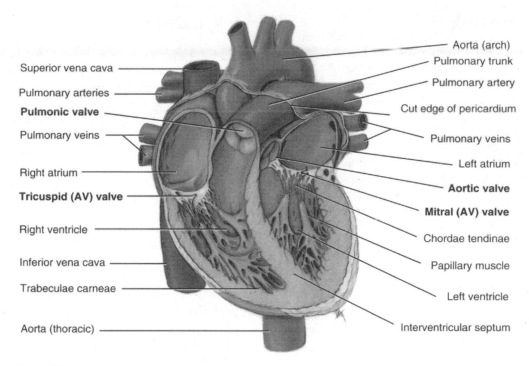

Superior vena cava —
Pulmonary arteries —
Pulmonic valve —
Pulmonary veins —
Right atrium —
Tricuspid (AV) valve —
Right ventricle —
Inferior vena cava —
Trabeculae carneae —
Aorta (thoracic) —

— Aorta (arch)
— Pulmonary trunk
— Pulmonary artery
— Cut edge of pericardium
— Pulmonary veins
— Left atrium
— **Aortic valve**
— **Mitral (AV) valve**
— Chordae tendinae
— Papillary muscle
— Left ventricle
— Interventricular septum

Figure 6-5
The heart. (Reprinted with permission from Applegate, E. J. *The Anatomy and Physiology Learning System.* Philadelphia: W. B. Saunders, 1991, p 248.)

The heart must pump blood to every part of the body in order to meet the metabolic needs of the cells. The atria contract, forcing the blood into the ventricles. At the end of the atrial contraction, the ventricles contract, forcing the blood out of the ventricles. Blood from the right ventricle is then forced into the pulmonary artery and finally to the lungs. Blood from the left ventricle is forced into the aorta.

The heart has a built-in regulating system called the *conduction system* (Figure 6-6). It is composed of cardiac muscle modified to conduct impulses. Heart action is automatic, that is, it is independent of outside impulses to initiate its contractions.

There are three structures that make up the heart's conduction system. The first is called the *sinoatrial* or *SA node*. It is located in the upper wall of the right atrium. It is called the "pacemaker" because it initiates the heartbeat and sets its rate. These impulses initiated by the SA node travel through the muscle fibers of both atria, causing them to contract.

The *atrioventricular* or *AV node*, which is located in the lower part of the right atrial wall, is stimulated next. This impulse is transmitted to the *bundle of His*, which is a group of specialized cardiac muscle fibers that are adapted for conduction of impulses. The bundle of His branches to go down each side of the septum, which divides the right and left ventricles. Each branch divides to form a network called the *Purkinje fibers*. Thus, the walls of the ventricles are supplied with conducting fibers.

As the impulse originates from the SA node, the atria contract almost simultaneously, forcing the

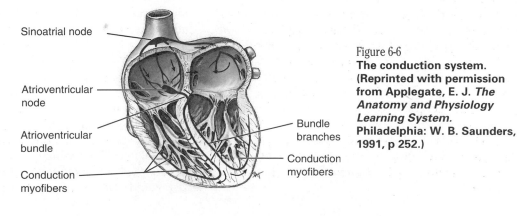

Sinoatrial node —
Atrioventricular node —
Atrioventricular bundle —
Conduction myofibers —
— Bundle branches
— Conduction myofibers

Figure 6-6
The conduction system. (Reprinted with permission from Applegate, E. J. *The Anatomy and Physiology Learning System.* Philadelphia: W. B. Saunders, 1991, p 252.)

blood into the ventricles. The impulse reaches the AV node at about the conclusion of atrial contraction. Then the impulse travels over the bundle of His, which is the connecting link, and causes the ventricles to contract, thus forcing blood from the left ventricle into the aorta, and the right ventricle to the pulmonary artery.

The electrical impulses generated by the heart's conduction system are recorded from the surface of the patient's skin. This record is called an *electrocardiogram*. It is of great clinical significance because it records any variations in the heart muscle's action. Persons skilled in the interpretation of the electrocardiograms can use the recording to help determine disease and follow the patient's progress.

Pulse and Blood Pressure

Pulse is defined as the waves of increased pressure in the arteries as a result of ventricular contraction. Perhaps a better definition is the alternate expansion and recoil of an artery. The *pulse rate* is actually the rate at which the heart beats. It is affected by the patient's body size, muscular activity, emotional disturbance, infections, and endocrine secretions. In general, the smaller the person, the faster the pulse rate. Newborn babies have a pulse rate of 120 to 140, while in normal adults, the rate is about 70 to 82.

The pulse is a useful diagnostic tool in determining disease. One of the most commonly performed procedures in the care of the ill is a determination of vital signs, that is, the temperature, pulse, respiration, and blood pressure. Most often, the pulse rate is counted at the radial artery of the wrist. Sometimes this is not convenient, so other sites may be used, such as the carotid artery of the throat; the temporal artery, located on the side of the head; the popliteal artery, found behind the knee; and the dorsalis pedis artery, located at the ankle.

Blood pressure refers to the pressure the blood exerts on the inside walls of the blood vessels. It is measured in millimeters of mercury (mm Hg). The pressure during the contraction of the heart muscle, or *systole*, is the systolic blood pressure. The pressure during the relaxation of the heart muscle, or *diastole*, is the diastolic blood pressure. Normal blood pressure varies widely. Also, as is the case with the pulse rate, blood pressure varies with a person's age, amount of activity, and emotional disturbance. Blood pressure is recorded as systolic over diastolic pressures. Thus, a systolic pressure of 120 mm Hg and a diastolic pressure of 80 mm Hg, is recorded as 120/80. An abnormal increase in either the systolic or the diastolic pressure is called *hypertension*, or high blood pressure.

Arteries and Veins

Blood is transported to every part of the body by the action of the heart as it pumps the blood through the network of the vascular system. The *arteries* carry blood away from the heart (Figure 6-7). Those leaving the heart are the largest. They branch into smaller arteries and finally even smaller vessels called *arterioles*. These continue to branch into smaller vessels until they branch into the *capillaries*. The *veins* return the blood to the heart (Figure 6-8). They also branch from large veins at the heart to *venules*, which finally branch into the capillaries. Thus, the cardiovascular system is a closed system. The heart pumps the blood through the arteries and arterioles to the capillaries, to the venules, and then to the veins through which the blood returns to the heart.

The force of the heartbeat forces the blood through the arteries. To cause the blood to return to the heart the inner lining of the veins forms valves that permit the blood to the flow toward the heart but prevent backflow. Also, the movement of muscles helps to cause blood to flow back to the heart.

There are two major circuits that are formed by the blood vessels. These are called *pulmonary* and *systemic*. In the pulmonary circuit, the pulmonary arteries carry blood containing carbon dioxide from the heart to the lungs. Oxygenated blood from the lungs is then returned to the heart by the pulmonary veins. This is the only time in the body in which an artery carries deoxygenated blood and a vein carries oxygenated blood.

Systemic circulation is made up of all other arteries and veins. These vessels carry oxygen and nutrients to all tissues of the body and then transport the wastes for disposal from all tissues except the lungs.

The Lymphatic System

The lymphatic system is a part of the circulatory system in that it aids in the returning of tissue fluid to the blood vessels, and its main function is to act as a transport system. It does this by collecting and transporting lymph, or fluid from intercellular spaces, by way of the lymphatic network, and then returns it to the blood. It also transports digested fats from the villi to the bloodstream and protects the body from invading microorganisms. The lymphatic system is made up of the lymphatic capillaries, two large lymph ducts, lymph organs, lymph nodes, and lymph itself.

Every cell of the body must maintain a given fluid volume. There is fluid in each cell, called *intracellular fluid*, and extracellular fluid in blood plasma. The fluid between the cells is called *interstitial fluid*.

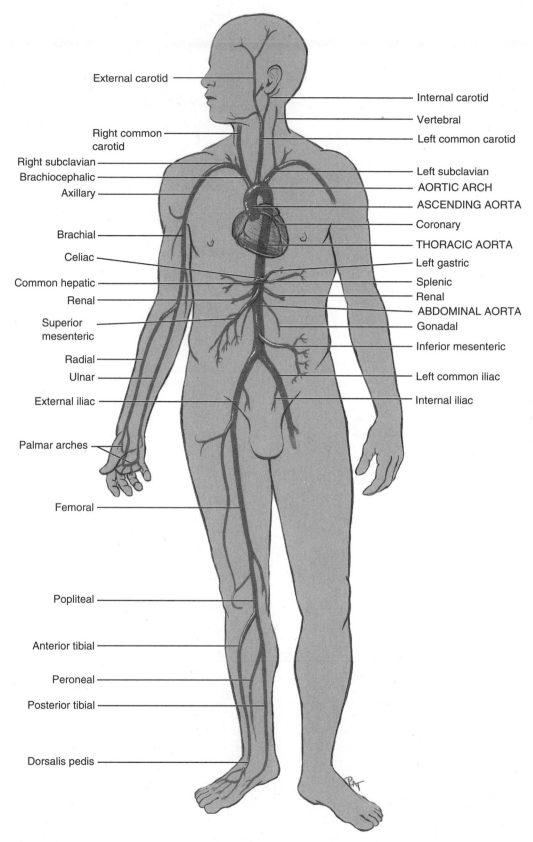

Figure 6-7
Major arteries of the body. (Reprinted with permission from Applegate, E. J. *The Anatomy and Physiology Learning System*. Philadelphia: W. B. Saunders, 1991, p 272.)

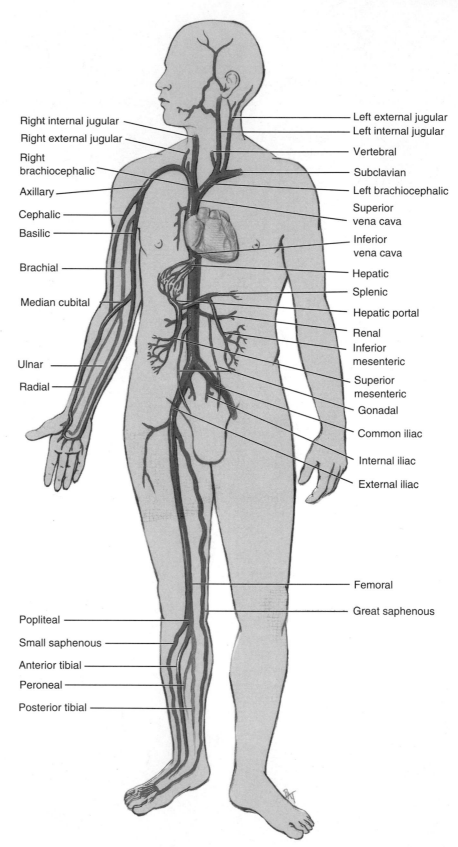

Figure 6-8
**Major veins of the body.
(Reprinted with permission
from Applegate, E. J. *The
Anatomy and Physiology
Learning System.*
Philadelphia: W. B. Saunders,
1991, p 278.)**

Right internal jugular

Right external jugular

Right brachiocephalic

Axillary

Cephalic

Basilic

Brachial

Median cubital

Ulnar

Radial

Popliteal

Small saphenous

Anterior tibial

Peroneal

Posterior tibial

Left external jugular

Left internal jugular

Vertebral

Subclavian

Left brachiocephalic

Superior vena cava

Inferior vena cava

Hepatic

Splenic

Hepatic portal

Renal

Inferior mesenteric

Superior mesenteric

Gonadal

Common iliac

Internal iliac

External iliac

Femoral

Great saphenous

Some of this fluid enters the lymph capillaries and is called *lymph*. Lymph is the clear, watery fluid found in the lymphatic vessels. It closely resembles plasma, but contains less protein.

The lymph capillaries are a series of collecting vessels that form a network throughout the body. These capillaries carry lymph from the body and then drain into the lymphatic veins. Lymphatic veins are similar in structure to blood veins, but they have much thinner walls. The lymphatic veins also have valves to prevent the backflow of fluid. These veins drain into two large ducts, the *right lymphatic duct* and the *thoracic duct*. The right lymphatic duct drains lymph from the upper extremities, the right side of the thorax, the right lung and part of the upper area of the liver, and the right side of the head and neck. It delivers the lymph to the right subclavian vein, by which it reenters the circulating blood.

The thoracic duct delivers the lymph from the rest of the body. It connects with and then empties into the left subclavian vein. In this way, lymph is returned to the circulatory system to be sent out to the tissues again.

Lymph nodes are small, rounded masses of lymphoid tissue that are scattered all over the body along the course of lymphatic vessels. They occur in larger numbers in the neck region, the axilla, the inguinal region, in the messentery of the small intestine, and the iliac, lumbar, and thoracic regions. One lymph vessel enters and another leaves each lymph node. Each node contains phagocytes which destroy microorganisms and cellular debris. Also, lymphocytes produced in the lymph nodes enter the lymph as it moves through the lymph nodes and eventually reaches the bloodstream.

Structure and Function of the Respiratory System

The main function of the respiratory system is to distribute air from the environment to the lungs, while at the same time removing the carbon dioxide that has been taken into the lungs. These two very important tasks are completed through a series of structures that make up the system. They include the *nose, pharynx, larynx, trachea, lungs, bronchus, bronchioles, alveolar duct,* and the *alveolus* (Figure 6-9). Every cell in the body requires a constant supply of oxygen in order to carry out its activities. Cells that have been deprived of oxygen die within a few minutes, but most body cells are not close to the organs of respiration, so some means of transport to supply them with oxygen is needed. The capillaries of the circulatory system supply this very important need. With the exception of some parts of the eye, no body cell is more than two cells away from a capillary. Therefore, oxygen from the lungs to the cells and carbon dioxide from the cells to the lungs, are transported by way of the blood in the capillaries.

Air is moved into and out of the respiratory system by the process of breathing. The intake of air is

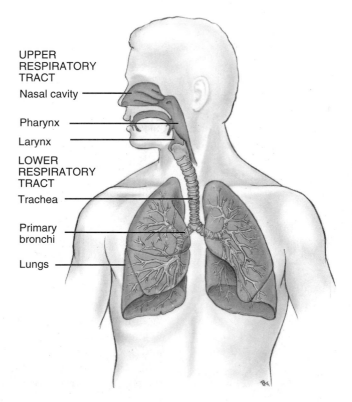

UPPER RESPIRATORY TRACT
Nasal cavity
Pharynx
Larynx
LOWER RESPIRATORY TRACT
Trachea
Primary bronchi
Lungs

Figure 6-9
The respiratory system. (Reprinted with permission from Applegate, E. J. *The Anatomy and Physiology Learning System.* Philadelphia: W. B. Saunders, 1991, p 306.)

called *inhalation*, or inspiration, and breathing out is referred to *exhalation*, or expiration.

Air enters the body through the nose. The external nose, that is, the part with which we are most familiar, is divided into two sections by a wall or septum. The openings to the outside are called *nares*.

As the incoming air enters the nose, it must first pass over ciliated mucous membrane. Tiny hairlike structures called *cilia* trap large particles of dust and debris and prevent them from gaining entrance to the nasal passages. The inner wall of each nasal cavity is folded into three ridges or *conchae*. This increases its surface area. The mucous lining entraps bacteria and particles that evaded the cilia. The air is also warmed and moistened as it flows over these folds. Thus, air entering the lungs is warm, moist, and relatively free of any bacteria and debris.

The lining of the upper fold of the nasal passage contains *olfactory receptors*. These structures are stimulated as air rushes over them, giving us the ability to sense odors. Even though our olfactory receptors have not developed to the point of being able to sense all odors, we are able to detect hundreds of individual odors and recall them. Hence, our sense of smell is important in identifying factors in the environment and in savoring food.

There are four pairs of *sinuses* that are responsible for draining the nasal cavity. These are air-filled cavities that are located in the skull. They are found in the *frontal*, *maxillary*, *ethmoid*, and *sphenoid* bones. Their function is to reduce the weight of the skull, to provide mucus for the nasal cavity, and to enhance the resonance of the voice. Sometimes the lining of a sinus cavity swells because of an allergic response or a bacterial or viral infection. This causes a condition called *sinusitis*.

The *pharynx*, or throat, is part of the respiratory system that not only functions as part of the structures necessary for breathing but also is part of the digestive system, since food passes through it to the esophagus. Air from the nasal passages also passes through the pharynx on its way to the *larynx*. There are actually seven openings into the pharynx; thus, it is truly a terminal. Not only do the two nasal passages, the mouth, the esophagus, and the larynx open into the pharynx, but also the right and left eustachian tubes, which extend from the middle ear. Air from the pharynx passes through the eustachian tube to the middle ear and exerts pressure on the *tympanic membrane*. Air also enters the outer ear and exerts pressure on the tympanic membrane from that side. In this way, air pressure on the tympanic membrane is equalized. Middle ear infections are not infrequent because bacteria from the pharynx may travel by way of the eustachian tube to the middle ear.

The *larynx* is located just below the pharynx at the upper end of the *trachea*. The opening into the larynx from the pharynx is called the *glottis*. The *epiglottis* is the structure that covers the glottis during swallowing and prevents food or liquid from entering the larynx. The larynx contains the vocal cords, which make sound production possible; therefore, it is commonly referred to as the "voicebox." The vocal cords are actually a pair of folds in the mucous lining of the larynx. Under these folds are elastic ligaments held rigidly in place by their attachment to cartilage. As air passes through the larynx, the glottis becomes narrowed, and the vocal folds, or vocal cords, vibrate, producing the voice. Many structures such as the nose, sinuses, and mouth are also involved in voice production. The vocal cords in males are usually longer and thicker, and men usually have a lower voice range than women because their vocal cords vibrate more slowly. The thinner, shorter vocal cords of the female vibrate more rapidly, thus producing a higher range of sounds.

The *trachea* is a tubelike structure, about 4 1/2 inches long and 1 inch in diameter, which extends from the larynx down to the *bronchi*. It is located in front of the esophagus. The tracheal walls are protected by C-shaped cartilage rings. These rings help to provide support and prevent collapse and obstruction of the airway. The open parts of the cartilage rings face the esophagus, making it possible for the esophagus to expand during swallowing.

The function of the trachea is to provide a passageway for inhaled and exhaled air. If it becomes obstructed for even a short time, dealth will result from asphyxiation. In fact, one of the most frequent causes of accidental death is choking on food. It can easily be distinguished from heart attack, because the victim cannot speak or breathe, usually panics, and, if not rescued, becomes pale, then cyanotic, ultimately losing consciousness.

Choking on food particles generally occurs during inspiration, when the lungs are expanded. Pressure on the diaphragm increases pressure on the air in the lungs and forces air against the lodged particles. If this occurs, the first aid procedure is to remove the object from the airway. Back blows are given first, and then, if necessary, are followed by a procedure known as the *Heimlich maneuver*. If you are required to perform either of these procedures, follow the steps outlined below.

To administer back blows:

1. Place yourself at the side or slightly behind the victim, who may be standing or sitting.
2. Place one hand on the victim's chest for support, and position his or her head at chest level or below.
3. Strike the victim with the heel of your hand over the spinal column between the shoulder blades.

4. Give four or five quick blows. If this does not dislodge the particle, begin the Heimlich maneuver at once (Figure 6-10).

To administer the Heimlich maneuver:

1. Place yourself behind the victim.
2. Wrap your arms around the victim's waist, making a fist with one hand.
3. Place the thumb side of your fist against the victim's abdomen just above the navel and below the rib cage, about 4 to 6 inches below the "V" formed by the sternum.
4. Grasp the fist with the out hand, and press it into the victim's abdomen with a quick upward thrust.
5. If necessary, repeat the procedure several times to dislodge the obstruction.

The trachea divides at the lower end to form the left and right bronchi. The *bronchi* lead from the trachea to each lung. The bronchi, like the trachea, are protected by C-shaped cartilage rings. As the bronchi enter the lungs, they branch to form smaller divisions, known as secondary bronchi. These continue to branch, forming tiny structures called *bronchioles*. The bronchioles divide into smaller and smaller structures until they become microscopic branches that eventually divide to form *alveolar ducts*. These ducts terminate into alveolar sacs, the walls of which are made up of *alveoli*.

The *lungs* are a pair of lobed organs located in the chest cavity. They extend from the diaphragm to the clavicle. The left lung is divided into two segments or lobes, and the right into three lobes. The lungs are covered with a thin tissue called the *pleura*. The inner surface of the chest cavity that houses the lungs is also lined with pleural tissue. As the chest moves during inspiration and expiration, the two pleural surfaces move smoothly, one against the other.

The lungs are actually made up of the bronchioles, the alveolar ducts, and the alveoli. Because of this structure, they give the appearance of having a spongelike consistency. The alveoli are tiny, balloon-like structures, the walls of which are only one cell thick. This makes transport of gases through the alveolar walls possible. In this way, oxygen from inhaled air enters the lung tissue, and carbon dioxide from body cells is exhaled from the lungs.

Because the alveolar walls are so delicate, you might expect that they would stick together like a deflated balloon on expiration, thus keeping them from retaining air. This does not occur because a phospholipid called *surfactant* is produced by the alveolar cells. Surfactant coats the cells and prevents them from sticking. In some diseases, the patient has an inadequate supply of surfactant, and thus the oxygen supply becomes curtailed.

The *diaphragm*, while an organ of the digestive system, is also involved in the respiratory process. This thin sheet of muscle that separates the chest and abdominal cavities is located within the chest cavity, which also contains the esophagus, trachea, bronchi, lungs, and the heart.

The Respiratory Process

Respiration is defined as the exchange of gases between organisms and the environment, that is, the taking in of oxygen, its use in tissues, and the giving off of carbon dioxide. The exchange of gases in the lungs, known as *external respiration*, and the exchange of gases in the cells, known as *internal respiration*, are phases of the respiratory process.

Movement of Air and Gas

The movement of air into and out of the lungs is governed by the same physical laws as the movement of any other gas. Gas molecules move from one area to another because of the differences in pressure. The flow is always to the area of lower pressure. Atmospheric pressure at sea level is 760 mm Hg at 0°C. If the pressure within the lung is less than 760 mm Hg, air flows into the lungs, and thus inspiration occurs. As the pressure in the lungs increases, as a result of inspiration, to more than 760 mm Hg, air flows out of

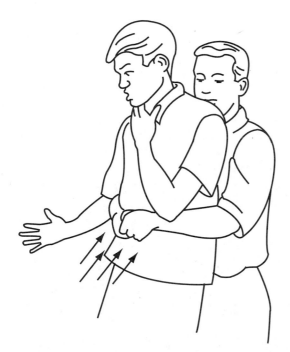

Figure 6-10
The Heimlich maneuver.

the lung, causing expiration. Therefore, in order for inspiration and expiration to occur, a difference in pressure between the lungs and the atmosphere must take place. This is accomplished by the diaphragm and chest muscles. The diaphragm contracts, moves downward, and increases the volume of the chest cavity vertically, and the chest muscles contract, thus causing the chest cavity to increase transversely. This decreases intrathoracic pressure, and air rushes in. When the diaphragm and chest muscles relax, the chest cavity decreases in size, intrathoracic pressure increases, and air rushes out.

The volume of air exchanged in breathing can be measured with a device called a *spirometer*. This information is valuable in the diagnosis and treatment of disease.

Types of Breathing

There are specific terms that we use in order to describe the different types of breathing. Recognition of these various types is important clinically. Normal, or quiet breathing, is called *eupnea*. The cessation or stoppage of breathing is called *apnea*. Abnormally increased breathing is referred to as *hyperpnea*. Finally, respiration that gradually increases in rapidity and volume until finally it has reached a climax, and then gradually subsides, eventually ceasing entirely for a few seconds, then beginning the cycle again, is called *Cheyne-Stokes* breathing.

External and Internal Respirations

External respiration deals with the exchange of the gases, oxygen and carbon dioxide, between the alveoli of the lungs and the blood in the capillaries. Air enters and leaves the lungs because of differences in air pressure and the pressure in the chest cavity. In external respiration, the transfer of gases is again the result of differences in pressure. When we discuss the exchange of these gases, we must take into account three types of pressure. These include the *partial pressure* (P), the *partial pressure of oxygen* (PO_2), and the *partial pressure of carbon dioxide* (PCO_2).

Air that is rich in oxygen is taken into the alveoli

of the lungs. The PO_2 of alveolar air is greater than the PO_2 of the blood in the capillaries surrounding the alveoli. Thus, oxygen will leave the alveoli and enter the capillaries because it will move down its pressure gradient.

In internal respiration, gases are exchanged between the blood and the body cells. When the oxygen-rich blood reaches the cells, the PO_2 of the capillary blood is greater than the PO_2 of the cells. Therefore, oxygen will leave the blood and enter the cells. There it combines with glucose in the cells to release energy. Carbon dioxide is given off in this process. The PCO_2 of the cell is greater than the PCO_2 of the capillary blood, and carbon dioxide moves from the cells to the blood. Again, the movement is governed by the pressure differential between the cell and the capillary. The PCO_2 of the capillary blood is greater than the PCO_2 of the alveoli. Therefore, carbon dioxide moves into the alveoli and is ultimately expired. It is the pressure differential that makes it possible for the flow of gases in each direction.

Some oxygen is carried in the blood plasma, but most oxygen combines chemically with the hemoglobin of the red blood cells in order to form the compound oxyhemoglobin. Almost all carbon dioxide that is carried in the blood has been dissolved in the plasma; however, some is transported by the red blood cells.

Summary

In this chapter, we talked about the various organs and structures that make up the cardiovascular system. We determined that these included the cellular structures that make up the blood, the heart, the blood vessels, and lymphatic system, and the individual structures that make up the respiratory system. We also talked about the pulse and blood pressure and the role each plays in the cardiovascular system. Finally, we discussed the actual respiratory process, the difference between internal and external respiration, and how the exchange of oxygen and carbon takes place in the body.

Review Questions

1. Briefly explain what *agglutination* means.

2. What does *coagulation* mean?

3. _____ respiration is the process of breathing out; _____ respiration is the process of exchanging gases between the lungs and the blood.

4. The movement of leukocytes through the unbroken capillary wall is called:

   a. agglutination

   b. diapedesis

   c. fibrinolysis

5. The mechanism by which blood clots are dissolved is called:

    a. agglutination

    b. diapedesis

    c. fibrinolysis

6. A blood clot that has dislodged from its place of origin is called:

    a. embolus

    b. hemorrhage

    c. thrombus

7. _____ deals with the study of blood and its components.

8. The liquid part of the blood that has been prevented from clotting by the addition of an anticoagulant is called:

    a. white blood cell

    b. red blood cell

    c. plasma

9. Another term for a blood clot is a:

    a. embolus

    b. thrombus

Common Disorders of the Cardiovascular System

Performance Objectives

Upon completion of this chapter, you will be able to:

1. Describe some of the more common and frequently seen disorders of the cardiovascular system, including those associated with congenital, inflammatory, and degenerative disease processes.
2. Explain what occurs during a myocardial infarction.
3. Explain what occurs during heart failure.
4. Describe what occurs during ischemia and a cerebrovascular accident.
5. Explain the disease process of an aneurysm.
6. Define what hypertension is.
7. Identify and briefly discuss some of the more common and frequently seen disorders of the respiratory system.

Terms and Abbreviations

Anemia   deficiency in the number of red blood cells being produced.

Aneurysm   an abnormal dilatation of a blood vessel that causes a "bulging out" of the vessel wall.

Arteriosclerosis   thickening, hardening, and loss of elasticity of an artery.

Atherosclerosis   an accumulation of fats and other substances in the arteries.

Congenital   pertaining to a condition being present at birth.

Dyspnea   difficult or labored breathing.

Edema   abnormal accumulation of fluid in the connective tissues.

Hemoptysis   coughing up of blood.

Hypertension   abnormally high blood pressure.

Hypotension   abnormally low blood pressure.

Leukemia   disease characterized by the production of an uncontrolled number of leukocytes.

Necrosis   the death of a tissue.

Pericarditis   inflammation of the pericardium.

Disorders of the cardiovascular system, including those affecting primarily the heart, are still considered among the most widespread causes of death in the United States. These diseases account for more than 55 percent of all reported deaths of the American population. The sad fact is that many of these deaths could have been avoided if detection and treatment had begun early on in the illness.

Cardiovascular diseases are classified according to their pathology and origin. There are nine categories in the classification. These include congenital anomalies, rheumatic heart disease, inflammatory conditions, arteriosclerosis, aneurysms, embolisms, neoplasms, peripheral vascular diseases, and ischemic heart disorders.

Clinical Manifestations Affecting Heart Disease

In most conditions affecting the heart, the patient's symptoms generally depend upon two manifestations. The first is the nature of the cardiopathology, and the second are the resultant physiological disturbances in circulation. In most cases, patients who suffer from some type of cardiac disorder also exhibit signs and symptoms of discomfort involving breathing, pain, edema, palpitations, hemoptysis, syncope, and in some instances, abdominal pain, discomfort, or other clinical manifestations of heart disease.

Predisposing Factors Affecting Heart Disease

As we have already noted, several cardiopathic factors, or symptoms, generally accompany heart disease. The most common of these are dyspnea, chest pain, edema, palpitations, and hemoptysis. The term *dyspnea* refers to an undue breathlessness and an awareness of discomfort associated with one's breathing. Most cardiac patients exhibit an increase in their effort to breathe. This is primarily because of a reduction of lung capacity resulting from pulmonary venous congestion. Dyspnea from heart disease is usually quite rapid and shallow, and the threshold, or tolerance for dyspnea, seems to vary with the individual.

In most patients suffering from a cardiac condition, we may see any one of four specific types of dyspnic manifestations. One type, called *exertional dyspnea*, causes a breathlessness upon moderate exertion, which is usually relieved by rest. This is most often seen in patients with congestive heart failure and those diagnosed with a chronic pulmonary disease. Another type, known as *orthopnea*, creates a shortness of breath when the patient is lying down. In this situation, relief can only be achieved by promptly having the patient sit in an upright position. Orthopnic dyspnea is generally caused by a stasis of blood causing accumulation in the lungs, often an underlying cause of left ventricular failure or mitral valve disease.

A third, less common type of dyspnea, which seems to come on suddenly, usually at night while the patient is lying down, is called *paroxysmal nocturnal dyspnea*. This is a condition that is primarily a result of the patient experiencing left ventricular insufficiency, pulmonary edema, and mitral stenosis.

The least frequently seen, and perhaps the worst type of dyspnic manifestation is called *Cheyne-Stokes respiration*. In this condition, there is periodic breathing that is characterized by a gradual increase in the depth of respirations. This is followed by a decrease in respiration, ultimately resulting in apnea. In other words, there are periods of increased respirations, called *hyperpnea*, with alternating periods of *apnea*, that is, no breathing at all. Cheyne-Stokes respiration is usually considered a serious sign and is primarily associated with a patient diagnosed with left ventricular failure and in some cases, cerebral vascular disease.

Like dyspnea, chest pain is generally considered one of the key signs of impending cardiac or cardiovascular problems. For the patient suffering from heart disease, chest pain typically originates from ischemia, which is caused by stimulation of afferent nerve endings in the myocardium of the heart. This results in an oxygen deficiency in the cardiac muscle caused by coronary heart disease.

Chest pain is predominantly characterized as excruciating or sharp precordial pain over the heart area and is generally aggravated by deep breathing. Anxiety may also be a predisposing factor to the common cause of chest pain suffered by cardiac patients.

Like dyspnea and chest pain, *edema* , which is an abnormal accumulation of serous fluid found in the connective tissues, is another symptom often seen in patients suffering from cardiac problems. It is generally caused by a buildup of salt, or sodium retention, and in heart patients edema is most often associated with congestive heart failure.

Palpitations, another symptom associated with cardiac disease, is defined as a rapid, forceful, or irregular heartbeat that is felt by the patient. Those patients suffering from palpitations usually complain of a pounding, jumping, stopping sensation in the chest. In cardiac disorders, palpitations are almost always a direct result of an enlarged heart and disturbances in the heart's rhythm.

A less frequently seen symptom of heart disease is *hemoptysis*, which is the coughing up of blood. In cardiac patients, small quantities of dark, clotting blood usually indicate the presence of mitral stenosis, whereas a mixture of blood and pus may indicate pulmonary suppuration.

Disorders of the Heart

Heart conditions that are present at birth are called *congenital anomalies*. Two of the most common of these are *tetralogy of Fallot* and *patent ductus arteriosus*. Patent ductus arteriosus is a congenital lesion found in the growing fetus. The ductus arteriosus connects the pulmonary artery and the aorta, thus bypassing the lungs, which are not needed in utero.

Shortly after birth, the ductus should close to allow full utilization of the lungs. If the vessel remains open, blood laden with carbon dioxide can enter the aorta, thereby reducing the amount of oxygen being supplied to the tissues. This disorder can usually be corrected by surgery.

In tetralogy of Fallot, four lesions are present in the fetus's heart that impair the supply of oxygen to the outlying tissues. These include a stenosis or narrowing at the pulmonary artery, consequent right ventricular hypertrophy, interventricular septal defect, and a malpositioned aorta. Like patent ductus arteriosus, this condition can be corrected surgically early in the newborn's life.

Disorders that are generally present in the three layers of the heart are usually *inflammatory*. The most common of these include *endocarditis*, *pericarditis*, and *myocarditis*.

Endocarditis is an inflammation of the outside lining of the heart, or the endocardium, which may be the result of an invasion of microorganisms or an abnormal immunological reaction. Most often, it is confined to the external lining of the valves; however, in some cases, it may also affect the lining membrane of the chambers.

Pericarditis is an inflammation of the pericardium. In cardiac patients, it is usually associated with a myocardial infarction, neoplasm, or trauma to the heart, and it almost always gives rise to symptoms such as moderate fever, precordial pain and tenderness, dyspnea, and palpitations.

Myocarditis refers to an inflammation of the myocardium and can be associated with a number of other conditions, such as infections, ingestion of poisons, heat stroke, and burns. It also occurs frequently after the patient has had a bout with rheumatic fever or diphtheria.

Another common condition affecting the heart is *arteriosclerosis*. In this disorder, the interior walls of the blood vessels, especially the arteries, are subject to a buildup of hardened materials. It is because of this buildup that we most often refer to this disorder as "hardening of the arteries."

There are two major types of arteriosclerotic diseases. The first, called *atherosclerosis*, is characterized by an accumulation of cholesterol within the arteries. In the second type, called *arteriosclerosis*, coronary circulation is blocked, causing an ischemic heart disease to develop.

The major transient disorder of arteriosclerotic disease is called *angina pectoris*. Here the victim suffers occasional chest pain that is associated with temporary loss of blood supply to the myocardium. In more serious cases, the arteriosclerotic plaque, or deposit, may cause a complete blockage of a coronary artery. This, in turn, can lead to the death of the

heart's muscle tissue, or what is referred to as a *myocardial infarction*.

Myocardial Infarction

A myocardial infarction, commonly referred to as a "heart attack," is a direct result of a coronary artery becoming occluded. The severity of the infarction will depend greatly upon the state of the collateral circulation and the location of the occlusion. Unless blood flow is reestablished to the ischemic or dead tissue, more and more cells will succumb to the effects of anoxia, or lack of oxygen. Approximately 20 minutes after the occlusion has occurred, the first dead, or *necrotic*, cells begin to appear. Until this point, recovery would have been rapid with a reestablished blood flow, but necrosis is irreversible. On the electrocardiogram, ischemia of tissues surrounding the infarction causes a reversal of the T-wave. Once the depolarization process has changed, the repolarization process is also altered.

Because of severe ischemia and lack of nutrients, the tissue immediately surrounding the center of the infarction becomes nonfunctional. It receives its blood supply from the collateral circulation. This is sufficient to keep it alive, but insufficient to maintain the membrane's integrity.

Nonfunctional or injured cardiac cells will begin to repolarize with the rest of the heart. However, a loss of membrane integrity makes it almost impossible for them to hold their charges. These charges, or ions, will then leak away from the cell. This exodus of ions from the injured tissue is called a *current of injury*.

Heart Failure

A condition in which the heart is no longer able to meet the body's demands is called *heart failure*. In either left heart failure or right heart failure, blood may pool in the body's tissues, causing a buildup or accumulation of fluid in the abdomen and the extremities. The lungs also become hypoxic, because of the lack of blood supply. Left heart failure causes pulmonary edema in the lungs and hypoxia of the systemic tissues.

Disorders of the Cardiovascular System

Although there are many disorders that may affect the entire cardiovascular system, few are seen without some involvement of the heart. The most common of these conditions include *varicose veins*, *ischemia*, *cerebrovascular accident*, *aneurysms*, and *hypertension*.

Predisposing Factors Affecting Cardiovascular Disease

As with disorders affecting the heart, diseases of the cardiovascular system usually manifest themselves by predisposing factors or specific pathophysiologic symptoms. These include coldness, generally because of a deficiency in the blood supply to a part, even though the environment is warm; *pallor* or paleness, caused by a diminished blood supply, causing a lack of color in the individual afflicted; *rubor*, or redness, caused by impaired circulation; *cyanosis*, or bluish coloring of the skin, generally perceived as an indication that less than a normal amount of oxygen is in the blood; and finally pain, which is primarily from an inadequate blood supply.

Varicose Veins

Varicose veins is a condition in which there is an enlargement and twisting of the superficial veins. They can occur in almost any part of the body, but are most commonly observed in the lower extremities and in the esophagus. The varices are caused by incompetent venous valves that may be acquired or congenital. Their development is promoted and aggravated by pregnancy, obesity, and occupations requiring prolonged standing. Esophageal varices are caused by portal hypertension that accompanies cirrhosis of the liver.

Ischemia and Cerebrovascular Accident

Two areas most frequently affected by arteriosclerosis are the cerebral and coronary vascular regions. Deposits in the intracranial vessels may result, causing a condition known as *ischemia*, or lack of oxygen to the brain tissue. A cerebrovascular accident, or "stroke," is a general term used most often to describe cerebrovascular conditions that accompany either ischemic or hemorrhagic lesions. These conditions are usually secondary to atherosclerotic heart disease, hypertension, or a combination of both.

Aneurysms and Hypertension

An *aneurysm* is defined as a local dilation of a blood vessel that bulges out from the vessel walls. It may be caused by an infectious process, such as syphilis, or as a direct result of another condition, such as arteriosclerosis, congenital weakness, or trauma. Aneurysms may occur in several shapes and are described as sacular or dissecting. These lesions may eventually rupture and break open, thus resulting in death from hemorrhage.

Hypertension, or high blood pressure, is a major class of cardiovascular disease. There are three types of hypertension: *essential*, *secondary*, and *renal*. There is no known cause of essential hypertension; however, it is still considered a common health problem of the cardiovascular system. Secondary hypertension, on the other hand, is primarily associated with toxins, central nervous system lesions, and disturbances of the endocrine system, and therefore is not seen as often as essential hypertension. Renal hypertension is caused by an excessive amount of sodium buildup in the kidneys and is a problem often seen prior to the onset of arteriosclerosis. Hence, it is considered one of the most commonly treated disorders of the cardiovascular system.

Disorders of the Respiratory System

Many of the disorders affecting the heart and cardiovascular system also affect the respiratory system. However, those most commonly seen affecting only specific organs of respiration include asthma, atelectasis, bronchiectasis, the common cold, influenza, emphysema, laryngitis, pharyngitis, pleurisy, pneumonia, and tuberculosis.

Asthma

Asthma is a condition accompanied by shortness of breath with wheezing caused by an obstruction of the flow of air in small bronchi or bronchioles. This is the result of swelling or spasm of the bronchial tubes or their mucous membranes. Since the walls of the bronchioles contain no cartilage, muscle spasms can close the airways.

Atelectasis and Bronchiectasis

Atelectasis refers to a collapse of part or all of a lung with incomplete expansion of the alveoli. *Bronchiectasis* is caused by a dilation of the bronchi or bronchioles.

The Common Cold and Influenza

The *common cold* is considered the most widespread of all communicable diseases. It is generally characterized by swollen and inflamed mucous membrane of the nose and throat. *Influenza* is a more acute, contagious, viral respiratory infection that is characterized by an inflammation of the upper respiratory tract, general aches, and a fever.

Emphysema

Emphysema is defined as a swelling or distention of air passages and alveoli. In this condition the most visible characteristic and most often seen symptom is the "barrel chest," a condition that is a result of the alveoli remaining filled with air during expiration.

Laryngitis and Pharyngitis

Laryngitis is an inflammation of the larynx that may result in hoarseness or loss of voice if the vocal cords become inflamed and swollen. *Pharyngitis*, a condition commonly referred to as a "sore throat," is the result of an inflammation of the pharynx.

Pleurisy and Pneumonia

Two conditions affecting the lungs are *pleurisy* and *pneumonia*. Pleurisy is an inflammation of the pleura or lining of the lungs and chest cavity. The resulting swelling causes the linings to rub, causing friction and pain. Pneumonia, on the other hand, is both an infection and an inflammation that affects the alveoli, and may be caused by viruses, bacteria, or chemical irritants.

Tuberculosis

A condition of the respiratory system less frequently seen since the onset of antibiotics is *tuberculosis*. In this disorder, there is an inflammation of the lungs and pleurae caused by the bacterium *Mycobacterium tuberculosis*. Although tuberculosis almost always occurs in the lungs, occasionally it may also affect other parts of the body.

Summary

In this chapter, we identified and discussed some of the more common disorders of the cardiovascular and respiratory systems, including those associated with congenital, inflammatory, and degenerative disease processes. In addition to identifying these disorders, we specifically discussed what occurs during a myocardial infarction, heart failure, and a cerebrovascular accident. We also talked about the disease process that occurs during an aneurysm, hypertension, and some of the more commonly seen conditions affecting organs of respiration.

Review Questions

1. A deficiency in the number of red blood cells being produced is called _____.

2. A thickening, hardening, and loss of elasticity of an artery is called:

   a. atherosclerosis

   b. arteriosclerosis

3. An accumulation of fats and other substances in the arteries is called:

   a. atherosclerosis

   b. arteriosclerosis

4. What is the name of a disease which is characterized by the production of an uncontrolled number of leukocytes?

5. _____ pertains to a condition that is present at birth.

6. A term used to describe difficult or labored breathing is:

   a. edema

   b. dyspnea

   c. pseudomonia

7. An abnormal accumulation of fluid in the connective tissues is called:

   a. edema

   b. dyspnea

   c. pseudomonia

8. An abnormally high blood pressure is called:

   a. hypertension

   b. hypotension

9. An abnormally low blood pressure is called:

   a. hypertension

   b. hypotension

Measuring Vital Signs

_____
_____
_____
_____

_____

Performance Objectives

Upon completion of this chapter, you will be able to:

1. Briefly explain the purpose and function of vital signs.
2. Identify each of the vitals signs and briefly discuss the role each plays in the proper functioning of the body.
3. Describe variations of the body's vital signs.
4. Describe and be able to demonstrate how to properly obtain, measure, and record a patient's vital signs.

Terms and Abbreviations

Blood pressure   the amount of force exerted by the heart against the walls of the arteries as it contracts and relaxes.
Pulse   the beat of the heart as it is felt through the walls of the arteries.
Respiration   the act of breathing in oxygen and breathing out carbon dioxide.
Sphygmomanometer   instrument used to measure the blood pressure.

Stethoscope   instrument used to listen to the beats of the heart as they are heard through the walls of the arteries.
Temperature   the degree of body heat that is a direct result of the balance maintained between heat produced and heat lost by the body.
Vital signs   important signs or measurement of the body's state of health; include the temperature, pulse, respiration, and blood pressure.

Whether you are working in the laboratory, the cardiology department, or the respiratory therapy department, as a member of the cardiovascular technology health care delivery team, there is a very strong possibility that at some time you will be responsible for obtaining, measuring, and recording the patient's vital signs. After all, one of the very best tools the doctor has for evaluating the patient's cardiovascular condition is by noting any changes or variations in his or her blood pressure, temperature, pulse, or respirations.

The vital signs are considered among the best and most measurable signs for determining one's state of health, and any variation in the norm of any individual or all of the vital signs can provide the physician with his or her first indication that there may be something wrong with the patient's cardiovascular system.

Blood Pressure

Blood pressure, according to most physicians, is considered the most significant of all the vital signs. It is the amount of force being exerted by the heart against the walls of the arteries while the heart is contracting and relaxing. It consists of two readings: the *systolic pressure*, which is created as the force of blood is being pushed against the arterial walls while the ventricles of the heart are in a state of contraction, and the *diastolic pressure*, or the pressure that occurs when the ventricles are in a state of relaxation. When recording the blood pressure, it is measured in millimeters of mercury (mm Hg). The upper number is recorded as the systolic pressure, and the lower number is recorded as the diastolic pressure.

Variations and Abnormal Blood Pressure

Like the other vital signs, blood pressure can vary according to the patient's age and sex and whether or not he or she exercises, smokes, or drinks. Other factors, such as obesity, the taking of certain medications, and the patient's emotional state, also have a bearing on blood pressure. In some cases, blood pressure can increase when the patient is standing, or when it is being measured in the right arm as opposed to the left.

Normal blood pressure generally ranges between 110 to 140 systolic and 70 to 90 diastolic. The average, or what is considered the "normal" blood pressure reading for most healthy adults is 120/80 mm Hg. Because of the loss of elasticity and the buildup of fatty deposits within the walls of the arteries, blood pressure tends to increase with age. Children, on the other hand, generally tend to have a lower blood pressure reading.

Any time there is a drastic change in the patient's blood pressure, there is cause to worry. If, for example, the blood pressure drops below 110/70 mm Hg, the doctor may be concerned with a condition known as *hypotension*, or abnormally low blood pressure. This is generally difficult to diagnose because there are few symptoms associated with it. An abnormal increase of the blood pressure over 140/90 mm Hg, or *hypertension*, on the other hand, may also give rise to worry. Hypertension is usually easier to diagnose because it is almost always accompanied by headaches, irritability, blurred vision, nosebleed, nausea and vomiting, and dizziness.

Measuring and Recording the Blood Pressure

Two instruments are used to measure the blood pressure. They are the *stethoscope* and the *sphygmomanometer* (Figure 8-1). The stethoscope consists of two earpieces, tubing, and a diaphragm, or bell, and is used to listen to the heart beating as it is heard through the walls of the artery. The sphygmomanometer utilizes an apparatus known as a *manometer*, which is the actual tool of measurement for obtaining the blood pressure. With the assistance of a cuff, an inflation bulb, and a pressure control valve, the

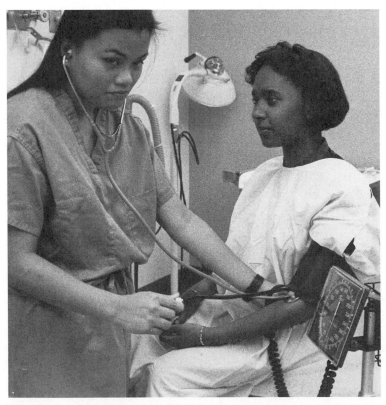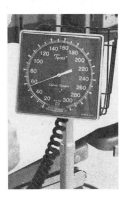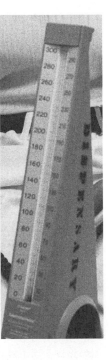

Figure 8-1
Stethoscope and sphygmomanometer.

sphygmomanometer is wrapped around the patient's arm over the brachial artery and then secured in place. The stethoscope is used to listen to the beats of the heart, at the brachial artery, while the sphygmomanometer is pumped up.

Procedure for Obtaining the Blood Pressure

To properly obtain the blood pressure, you should:

1. Gather the necessary equipment. This includes the sphygmomanometer, the stethoscope, and cotton balls or alcohol wipe pads to clean the earpieces.
2. Wash your hands and clean the earpieces of the stethoscope.
3. Position the patient in a sitting position with his or her arm supported. If the patient is wearing long sleeves, expose the arm by rolling up the sleeve approximately 5 inches above the elbow or removing the arm from the sleeve if necessary.
4. Gently place the deflated cuff evenly, yet snugly, around the patient's arm with the lower edge about 1 to 2 inches above the antecubital space, or the inside of the elbow.
5. Center the cuff over the brachial artery before securing it with clasps or Velcro.
6. Locate the brachial pulse in the antecubital space by palpating it with your fingertips. Never use your thumb, since it has a pulse of its own and may therefore be deceiving when you are "feeling" for the brachial pulse.
7. Place the earpieces of the stethoscope in your ears and place the diaphragm or bell over the brachial artery, making sure neither one is touching the cuff.
8. With the other hand, close the air valve on the bulb by gently turning the thumb-screw in a clockwise direction; pump the air into the cuff until the level of the mercury is 10 to 20 mm Hg above the palpated systolic pressure or about 180 mm Hg.
9. Turn the thumbscrew counterclockwise to release the air at a slow rate so the pressure falls at a rate of about 2 to 3 mm Hg per second.
10. Listen carefully for the first tapping sound; this represents the systolic pressure. Note this number on the scale of the sphygmomanometer.
11. Continue to deflate the cuff while listening to the sounds. Read the scale again when the second sound becomes dull or muffled; this second sound represents the diastolic pressure.
12. Keep deflating the cuff until you no longer hear any sounds.
13. After you no longer hear any sounds, open the valve completely and rapidly deflate the cuff. Remove the cuff from the patient's arm.
14. Record the results on the patient's chart, noting any unusual occurrences that you may have heard or seen, and identify on which arm the blood pressure was obtained.
15. Wash your hands.

Temperature, Pulse, and Respiration

Measuring the Temperature

Obtaining an accurate measurement of the patient's temperature, pulse, and respirations is just as important as obtaining the blood pressure. As with blood pressure, many factors also affect the patient's temperature, pulse, and respirations. These may include the time of day in which the measurements are taken, the sex and age of the patient, the emotional status and the degree of involvement in physical activities, and even the weather.

A patient's temperature is almost always obtained at the same time as the pulse and respiration. There are three methods that are acceptable for measuring the body's temperature. The most common of these is the oral method, in which a thermometer is placed under the patient's tongue, and left in place for 3 to 5 minutes before it is read.

The most accurate method for obtaining the temperature is the rectal method. It involves placing the thermometer into the patient's rectum, and leaving it in place for approximately 5 minutes. The least accurate mode of obtaining an accurate temperature is the axillary method. This is accomplished by placing the thermometer under the axilla, or armpit, and leaving it in place for approximately 10 minutes. For children, the method of choice is usually the rectal method and for children or adults who have difficulty holding an oral thermometer in place, the axillary method is considered most desirable. Whatever method is used, you must always remember to obtain the right thermometer (Figure 8-2).

Normal readings for body temperature usually vary 1 degree either way for oral, axillary, and rectal readings. The average normal reading for a healthy adult using the oral method, is 98.6° Fahrenheit (F). Using the axillary method, the average normal reading is approximately 97.6°F, and the normal reading using the rectal method is approximately 99.6°F.

Procedure for Obtaining an Oral Temperature

To properly obtain an oral temperature, you should:

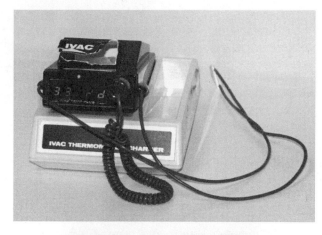

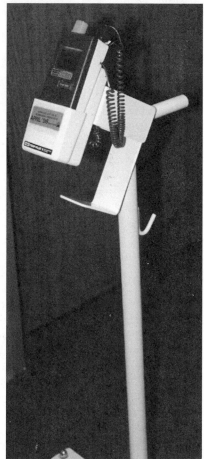

Figure 8-2
Types of thermometers.

1. Gather the necessary equipment. This will include either an oral glass thermometer, a sheath-covered thermometer, a plastic thermometer, or an electronic thermometer; some tissues; a watch with a second hand; and a piece of paper and pencil to write down the reading.
2. Wash your hands.
3. If you are using a glass thermometer, remove it from its holder and wipe it with a clean tissue. Check to be sure that the thermometer is intact.
4. Read the mercury column. If it does not read below 96°F, shake it down. Make sure you are standing away from any objects. Grasp the stem of the thermometer and gently shake it with a downward motion.
5. Insert the bulb end under the patient's tongue, toward the side of the mouth. Instruct the patient to hold the thermometer in place for 3 minutes.
6. Remove the thermometer, holding it by the stem. Wipe it from the stem end toward the bulb, and discard the tissue.
7. Hold the thermometer at eye level and locate the column of mercury. Read to the closest line and record this number on your piece of paper.
8. Wash the thermometer in cold water and soap before returning it to its proper place.
9. Wash your hands.

Procedure for Obtaining a Rectal Temperature

To properly obtain a rectal temperature, you should:

1. Gather the necessary equipment. This will include a glass rectal thermometer or the electronic thermometer with a plastic probe, a lubricant, such as K-Y jelly, and some tissues.
2. Wash your hands.
3. Put on gloves, and if you are using a glass thermometer, remove the thermometer from its holder and wipe it with a clean tissue. Make sure the thermometer is intact. Place a small amount of lubricant on a tissue.
4. Read the mercury column to make sure it registers at 96°F. If necessary, shake it down in the same manner as described in obtaining an oral temperature.
5. Apply a small amount of lubricant to the bulb end of the thermometer. Separate the buttocks with one hand and insert the thermometer about 1 1/2 inches into the rectum. Hold the thermometer in place for approximately 5 minutes.
6. Remove the thermometer, holding it by the stem, and wipe it clean from the stem end toward the bulb end and discard the tissue. Wipe the lubricant from the patient with a clean tissue.
7. Hold the thermometer at eye level and locate the column of mercury. Read to the closest line and then record your findings on a piece of paper.
8. Wash the thermometer in cold water and soap before returning it to its proper place.
9. Wash your hands.

Procedure for Obtaining an Axillary Temperature

To properly obtain an axillary temperature, you should:

1. Gather the necessary equipment. This will be the same equipment as for taking an oral temperature.
2. Wash your hands.
3. Wipe the area dry and place the thermometer in the patient's axillary. Instruct the patient to keep the thermometer close to the body. Leave the thermometer in place for approximately 10 minutes.
4. Remove the thermometer and wipe it clean. Read to the closest line and record this number on a piece of paper.
5. Clean and replace the thermometer in the same manner as you did with the oral thermometer.
6. Wash your hands.

Measuring the Pulse

The purpose of obtaining the measurement of a patient's pulse rate is to determine the strength, rate, and rhythm of the heartbeat as it is felt through the walls of the arteries. Such a pulsation, found in the arteries, is produced by the movement of blood being forced through them by the contractions of the heart.

The pulse is measured with regard to its individual *rate*, *rhythm*, and *volume*. The rate is a reflection of the number of pulsations, or beats, counted for a given period of time; usually a minute. The *pulse rhythm* refers to the intervals of time between each pulse. These intervals of time are generally described as regular, irregular, or skipping. *Volume* is a term used to describe the strength of the pulsations, that is, whether it is full, strong, bounding, weak, or thready. A normal pulse is most often described as being regular and strong.

A person's pulse, just like his or her blood pressure and temperature, can also be influenced by many different factors, such as age, sex, body size, metabolism, exercise, and even one's emotional state. For a normal, healthy adult, the average pulse ranges from 60 to 80 beats per minute, with 72 considered the norm. Children tend to have a much faster metabolism than do adults. The average range for a normal healthy child from age 1 to 7 usually runs between 80 to 120 beats per minute, while children over the age of 7 generally range from 80 to 90 beats per minute. Newborns and infants have the greatest number of pulsations, with the average ranging between 130 to 160 beats.

A pulse can only be measured at a site in which it can be felt through the walls of the arteries. Al-though there are many locations on the body where the pulse can be obtained, the location of choice is usually at the radial artery, that is, the inside of the wrist. Other locations include the brachial artery, which is located over the inner aspect at the bend of the elbow, the temporal artery, which is found at the side of the forehead at the temple, the popliteal artery, at the back of the knee, the dorsalis pedis artery, at the upper surface of the foot between the ankle and the toes, and the carotid artery, located on both the right and left sides of the anterior neck, which is most often the artery of choice for palpitation during cardiopulmonary resuscitation. In some instances, the pulse may also be taken at the apical site, which is located betwen the fifth and sixth ribs and approximately 2 to 3 inches to the left of the breastbone (Figure 8-3).

Procedure for Obtaining a Radial and Apical Pulse

To properly obtain a radial pulse, you should:

1. Gather the necessary equipment. This will include a watch with a second hand and a piece of paper and pencil, to record the pulse.
2. Wash your hands.
3. Identify the patient by name and identification bracelet and explain the procedure.
4. Position the patient in a sitting or lying position with the arm being used supported.
5. Hold the patient's wrist by placing your first three fingers on his or her wristbone over the radial artery. Gently apply light pressure so you can feel the pulsations. Be sure not to use your thumb to palpate the pulse, since it has its own pulse.
6. While holding the patient's wrist, count the pulse for one full minute. Note the rate, rhythm, and volume of the pulse.
7. After you have counted the pulse for a full minute, record the number, noting the rhythm and volume. Indicate at what site the pulse was obtained.
8. Wash your hands.

If you are required to obtain the patient's apical pulse, you will need to use a stethoscope, since this type of pulse can only be measured by listening to the heartbeat, and then determining the number of beats and the rhythm and volume at which these beats are produced. Once you have determined that the pulse will be obtained at the apical site, you should:

1. Gather the necessary equipment. This will include a stethoscope, alcohol and cotton balls or an alcohol wipe, a watch with a second hand,

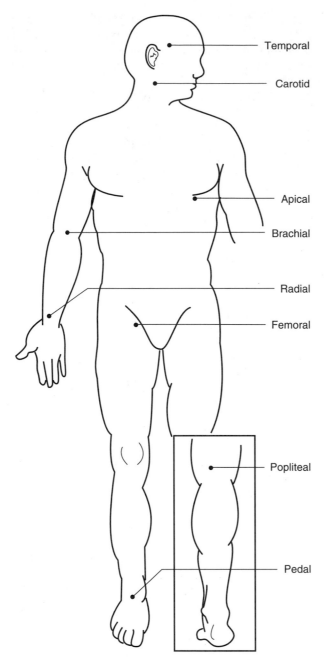

Figure 8-3
Locations of pulse sites.

Labels: Temporal, Carotid, Apical, Brachial, Radial, Femoral, Popliteal, Pedal

the heart, which is located in the fifth intercostal space 2 to 3 inches to the left of the breastbone.

7. Listen for the heartbeat and count the number of beats for one full minute, noting the number, rhythm and volume of each beat.
8. After you have listened to the beats for a full minute, record the apical pulse, indicating the site used with the letter A enclosed in a circle.
9. Clean the earpieces of the stethoscope and return it to its proper place.
10. Wash your hands.

Measuring the Respirations

When we define the term respirations, we are actually referring to the process of breathing in oxygen and breathing out carbon dioxide. Such a process takes place in the respiratory control center which is located in the medulla oblongata, found in the lower portion of the brainstem. All "healthy" respirations occur automatically; however, the very act of breathing in an out is considered to be under voluntary control. That is why a person may attempt to hold his or her breath for a period of time, but eventually must stop to allow a breath to be taken.

The act of breathing in and out actually involves two individual processes. These are referred to as *external respiration* and *internal respiration*. External respirations take place during the exchange of respiratory gases between the alveoli of the lungs and the blood. Internal respiration occurs during the exchange of respiratory gases between the body cells and the blood.

Like the pulse, when the respirations are measured, they are usually counted for one full minute, with special attention paid to the *rate*, *depth*, and *rhythm* of each respiration. The rate refers to the number of respirations per minute. It is generally described as being normal, rapid, or slow. The depth of the respirations depends upon the amount of air being inhaled and exhaled and is recorded as being shallow or deep. The rhythm is defined as the intervals of each respiration and may be described as being regular or irregular in rate and depth.

Like the other vital signs, the number of times in which a person takes in a breath of oxygen and breaths out carbon dioxide is influenced by many different factors, such as his or her age, emotional state, increase in muscular activity, such as exercise, whether or not the person is taking specific medications, and the presence of any diseases of the lungs or any other organs of the cardiovascular system. In some cases, certain changes in the climate and atmosphere may also affect the rate and depth of the respirations.

and a piece of paper and a pencil to record your findings.
2. Wash your hands.
3. Identify the patient by name and with his or her identification band and explain the procedure.
4. Position the patient in a sitting or lying position.
5. Clean the earpieces of the stethoscope with the alcohol.
6. Warm the diaphragm of the stethoscope with your hands and then place the earpieces into your ears. Place the diaphragm over the apex of

Procedure for Obtaining a Respiratory Rate

Obtaining a patient's respiratory rate is almost always done at the same time the blood pressure, temperature, and pulse are taken. This often occurs when the temperature is being obtained by the oral method. By inserting the oral thermometer into the patient's mouth, you are free to watch the patient's chest expand and lower as each breath is taken, usually without the patient trying to control the number of breaths being inhaled and exhaled. To obtain the respiratory rate, you should:

1. Gather the necessary equipment. This will include a watch with a second hand and a piece of paper and pencil to record the respirations.
2. Wash your hands.
3. Identify the patient by name and the identification band and explain the procedure.
4. Position the patient in a sitting or lying position.
5. Place three fingers on the patient's wrist as if you were going to take his or her pulse. As you are holding the patient's wrist, count each breathing cycle, that is, each time the patient inhales and exhales, as one full breath, by watching the rise and fall of the patient's chest or upper abdomen.
6. Count the number of respirations for one full minute. Then record the rate, depth, and rhythm of the respirations.
7. Wash your hands.

Summary

In this chapter, we discussed the purpose and function of the vital signs. We noted that these important signs, that is, the blood pressure, temperature, pulse, and respirations, are one of the best indicators for the physician to use in determining the patient's overall state of health. We also talked about specific variations of these vital signs, as well as what the normal ranges are for each individual sign. Finally, we explained the procedure for obtaining each of these signs, concluding that they are almost always obtained at the same time, when the patient is least able to influence their outcome.

Review Questions

1. The amount of force exerted by the heart against the walls of the arteries as it contracts and relaxes is called:

   a. pulse

   b. respiration

   c. blood pressure

2. The beat of the heart as it is felt through the walls of the arteries is called:

   a. pulse

   b. respiration

   c. blood pressure

3. Briefly explain the concept of *vital signs*.

4. An instrument that is used to listen to the beats of the heart as they are heard through the walls of the arteries is called a:

   a. sphygmomanometer

   b. stethoscope

   c. audioscope

5. What is the name of the instrument used to measure the blood pressure?

6. Give at least three examples of factors influencing a person's blood pressure:

   a. _____

   b. _____

   c. _____

7. Why is it important never to use your thumb to feel for a patient's pulse?

8. Identify at least three locations in which a pulse rate can be taken:

   a. _____

   b. _____

   c. _____

9. What method of taking a patient's temperature is most often used with small children?

   a. rectal

   b. axillary

   c. oral

10. What method of taking a patient's temperature is considered the most accurate?

    a. rectal

    b. axillary

    c. oral

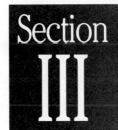

Section
III

Electrocardiography: Basic Concepts and Applications

9

Principles of Electrocardiography

Performance Objectives

Upon completion of this chapter, you will be able to:

1. Discuss the purpose and function of electrocardiography.
2. Identify the members of the ECG department and briefly discuss the education, training, duties, and responsibilities of each.
3. Briefly discuss the anatomy and physiology of the heart and their relationship to electrocardiography.

Terms and Abbreviations

Angiocardiography   an x-ray examination of the heart and great blood vessels that follows the course of an opaque fluid that has been injected into the bloodstream.

Aorta   the main trunk artery that receives blood from the lower left chamber of the heart, which is responsible for supplying blood to all the lesser arteries that branch out through all parts of the body except the lungs.

Arrhythmia   an abnormal rhythm of the heart beat.

Artery   blood vessel of systemic circulation that carries blood away from the heart to all parts of the body.

Atrium   one of the two upper chambers of the heart; also called the *auricle*.

Cardiac   pertaining to the heart.

Coronary arteries   the two arteries arising from the aorta and arching down over the top of the heart and responsible for conducting blood to the heart muscle.

ECG   abbreviation for electrocardiograph; a graphic record of the electric currents produced by the heart.

Electrocardiograph   an instrument that records electric currents produced by the heart.

Infarct (infarction)   an area of tissue damaged or dead as a result of an insufficient blood supply.

Mitral valve   also called the *bicuspid valve*; consists of two cusps of triangular segments, located between the upper and lower chambers of the left side of the heart.

Tricuspid valve   a valve consisting of three cusps of triangular segments located between the upper and lower chambers of the right side of the heart.

Vein   any one of a series of vessels of the vascular system that carries blood from the various parts of the body back to the heart.

Vena cava   the main vein returning blood from the body to the right atrium.

Ventricle   one of the two lower chambers of the heart.

Before you can understand the purpose of the electrocardiograph and the role the electrocardiographic or ECG technician plays in securing this scientific measurement, it is important that you undersand what exactly an electrocardiographic tracing represents. An electrocardiographic tracing, sometimes referred to as an ECG, utilizes an electronic device called an *electrocardiographic machine* in order to measure or record the electrical charges that occur during a complete heartbeat. These readings help the doctor to diagnose any irregularities or changes in the patient's heart action, and they are usually performed routinely as the patient ages as well as before or after surgery, and as a diagnostic tool in assisting the physician in caring for the patient.

The ECG Department

Although many physicians perform electrocardiograms in their offices, the majority are done in the hospital or in outpatient facilities or clinics. In the hospital, the ECG department may be housed as a separate unit or as part of another department. Many smaller hospitals house both their respiratory therapy and their ECG units in one combined area, often referred to as the *cardiopulmonary department*.

Both the size of the department and the number of ECGs performed generally affect the number of people associated with the ECG department. In many larger facilities, there are usually four levels of trained personnel found within the department. These levels include the ECG technician I, the ECG technician II, the cardiovascular technician, and the cardiologist. In addition to these positions, there may be other members of the staff who are more specialized in their roles. These may include a treadmill technician, a Holter recorder scanning technician, an echocardiograph technician, and a cardiac catherization technician.

The Cardiologist

The cardiologist is a medical doctor who specializes in the care and treatment of patients with conditions affecting the heart and the cardiovascular system. This person is responsible for both ordering and interpreting all medical tests that might be necessary for the accurate diagnosis and treatment of heart disorders. The cardiologist is also responsible for overseeing the smooth running and performance of all aspects of the ECG department, and in many cases, is also responsible for overseeing both the coronary care and intensive care units and the emergency room of larger hospitals.

The ECG Technician

The ECG technician works under the direction of the cardiology supervisor or the cardiologist, and is responsible for performing routine ECGs as well as any related procedures, as defined by the employing facility. This person is also responsible for operating equipment, as well as performing specific tests and procedures that may be necessary for patient treatment within the hospital, physician's office, or clinic.

Responsibilities of the ECG technician may vary according to the level of training and the environ-

ment in which the technician works; however, there are certain tasks that almost all ECG technicians are expected to perform. These include preparing patients for testing, operating the electrocardiograph machine, and recording the 12-lead ECG rhythm strips in a manner that provides reliable tests for the physician's interpretation. Additional responsibilities may include, but are not limited to, cutting and mounting the ECG strips, retrieving previous ECG recordings and attaching the new tracings to the patient's chart, filing paperwork as may be required, maintaining equipment and ordering supplies, preparing copies of a patient's ECG tracing, distributing ECG reports for patient's charts and copies to physician's offices, forwarding charges for services to billing departments, and notifying a supervisor immediately of any deviation from a patient's normal or average ECG reading.

Anatomy and Physiology

Since the anatomy and physiology of the heart and the cardiovascular system play a very important role in how the heart, arteries, and veins function, it is important that you also gain a basic understanding of how these structures work.

The Human Heart

The human heart is an organ approximately the size of a man's fist. It is a hollow muscle divided into four chambers, and its main function is to pump blood. It is located in the *mediastinum*, or the middle section of the thorax, or chest, between the lungs, with its *apex*, or pointed end, resting on the diaphragm (Figure 9-1).

Each heart chamber is separated by valves that act as "gates," opening in only one direction. This keeps the blood flowing one way and prevents it from backing up. When the heart beats or contracts, two of the valves, the *tricuspid* valve and the *mitral*, or *bicuspid, valve*, close. When the heart relaxes, the other two valves, the *aortic* and the *pulmonary valves*, close. When a valve closes, it makes a sound. This is the characteristic "lub-dub" that is heard by a stethoscope when the valves close.

The Pericardium

The heart is contained within a sac called the *pericardium*. This sac is filled with pericardial fluid, which moistens the lining of the pericardium and the epicardium, or outer surface of the heart. Normally, there is approximately 10 to 20mL of thin, clear pericardial fluid that moistens the contracting surfaces of

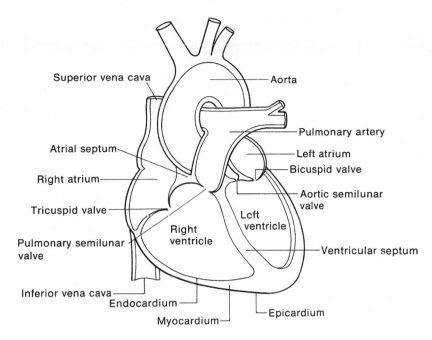

Figure 9-1
The human heart. (Reprinted with permission from Bonewit, K. Clinical Procedures for Medical Assistants, 3rd ed. Philadelphia: W. B. Saunders, 1995, p 442.)

the epicardium and the inner surface of the pericardium.

The Septum, Ventricles, and Atrium

The four chambers of the heart are separated by a structure called the *septum*, or muscle wall. The two lower chambers, called the *ventricles*, are responsible for pumping blood away from the heart, while the two upper chambers, the *atria*, are responsible for receiving the blood coming to the heart. The valves, as we have already discussed, are the structures that maintain the control of the blood flowing through the entire heart.

The left ventricle does much more work than the right ventricle, and as a result, has the thickest wall. It is responsible for pumping oxygenated blood to all parts of the body, except for the lungs, and eventually empties its blood directly into the aorta. Because the left ventricle pumps blood a very long way, it is referred to as a *high-pressure pump*.

At the same time as the left ventricle is pumping oxygenated blood to all parts of the body, blood is entering the right atrium from all parts of the body and emptying into the right ventricle via the tricuspid valve. The right ventricle pumps the nonoxygenated blood to the lungs via the pulmonary artery. The right ventricle is a *low-pressure pump*, and therefore has a thinner wall than does the left ventricle.

The interventricular septum is also a thick wall. It is responsible for separating the left and right ventricles. This wall will constrict during a heartbeat in order to provide a rigid structure during the heart contraction. If this did not occur, the high pressure that develops in the left ventricle during the contrac-

tion would cause a thin septum to bulge into the low-pressure right ventricle and eventually would interfere with its operation.

The Heart Valves

The heart valves, as we have already noted, have the major responsibility of preventing the blood from backing up as it flows through the heart. There are two types of valves found in the heart: the *atrioventricular* valves, which are the tricuspid and the mitral valves, and the *semilunar valves*, which are the pulmonary and aortic valves. All heart valves are mechanical structures that are made in such a way as to permit the blood to flow only one direction within the circulatory system.

Cardiac Muscle Cells

When we learn about the anatomy and physiology of the heart and how it relates to the electrical activity occurring during the heart's contraction and relaxation phases, it is also important that you understand the role the cells of the cardiac muscles play in the heart's activity.

The cells are most concerned with the mechanical activity of the heart; therefore, they are all similar in their appearance. The principal function of all cardiac muscle cells is to contract. Cardiac muscle cells make up three major layers, or portions, of the heart. The inner layer, which is responsible for lining the chambers of the heart, is called the *endocardium*. It is a thin, shiny, smooth membrane that lines or covers the heart valves and is therefore continuous with the lining of the large blood vessels.

The outer layer of the heart is called the *epicardium*, which is made up of thick muscular cells, while the middle layer, called the *myocardium*, is constructed of interlacing cardiac muscle fibers. Because of the consistency of the muscle fibers comprising the myocardium, this is the layer responsible for causing the heart to contract.

Blood Vessels and Circulation

Although there are many different types, sizes, and varieties of blood vessels contained within the human body, all of them may be classified into three major groups: *arteries*, which are responsible for carrying oxygenated blood away from the heart; *veins*, which carry nonoxygenated blood toward the heart, and *capillaries*, which are microscopic structures most responsible for allowing the rapid exchange of substances between the blood and the tissue cells.

Arteries

Arteries are blood vessels that carry oxygenated blood away from the heart, with the one exception being the pulmonary artery (Figure 9-2). The largest of all arteries in the human body is called the *aorta*, which measures approximately 25 mm, and is about 250 mm in diameter. As other arteries branch off the aorta, they become smaller and smaller until they reach the tissue level, at which time they become *arterioles*, which are approximately 30 micrometers, or 0.001 mm, in diameter.

All arteries consists of three layers of tissue: the *tunica adventitia*, which is the outer layer, consisting of tough, fibrous connective tissue; the *tunica media*, or middle layer, composed of smooth muscle and fibrous and elastic tissue, and which permits the vessel to dilate; and the *tunica intima*, or the inner layer, which consists of a layer of endothelial cells.

Veins

Veins, unlike arteries, are most concerned with carrying the nonoxygenated blood from the capillaries toward the heart. Although consisting of the same three layers as found in the arteries, in veins the layers are much thinner and contain fewer elastic fibers. In contrast to the walls of the arteries, which if cut will remain open, the walls of the veins, once cut, will then collapse (Figure 9-3).

Capillaries

Capillaries are most responsible for the rapid exchange of substances between the blood and the tissue cells. They are tiny, microscopic vessels composed of a single layer of endothelial cells. Capillaries function at the cellular level, that is, they transport and diffuse essential materials to and from the body's cells and the blood.

Circulation

There are two systems involved in the circulation of blood and other body fluids within the body. They are the pulmonary system and the systemic system. Pulmonary circulation includes the blood vessels to and from the lungs, with the exception of the bronchiolar arteries, which are responsible for supplying oxygenated blood to the lung tissue. During pulmonary circulation, the pulmonary artery delivers blood from the heart to the lungs, while the pulmonary veins deliver the blood from the lungs to the left atrium of the heart. The pulmonary circulation is different from systemic circulation in that it is a low-pressure system and has only vessels in which an artery, the pulmonary artery, carries nonoxygenated blood, whereas the veins carry oxygenated blood.

The systemic system differs from the pulmonary circulation in that it includes all other blood vessels, beginning with the aorta, which eventually branches into smaller arteries and finally arterioles. The system also includes microscopic capillary exchange vessels as well as venules, which are microscopic veins responsible for collecting returning nonoxygenated blood from the capillaries, which eventually empty into the veins when transporting nonoxygenated blood to the vena cava and finally to the right atrium.

The Lymphatic System

Not only is blood responsible for supplying the cells of the body with food and oxygen, but it also plays a role in removing waste products. This exchange takes place at the capillary level. The tissue fluid that bathes the cells and acts as a connecting link between the blood and the cells is called *lymph*. Lymph is formed when certain parts of the blood plasma pass through the capillary walls into the tissue spaces and is continually being drained from the tissue spaces through a system of tubules called the *lymphatic system*.

The lymphatic network begins as tiny lymph capillaries, which are similar to the blood capillaries. These vessels eventually become larger lymphatic vessels that parallel the veins. The lymphatic vessels eventually converge and empty into the lymphatic ducts.

Two major ducts are present in the lymphatic system. The first, called the *lymphatic duct*, is responsible for draining lymph from the head, neck, and right

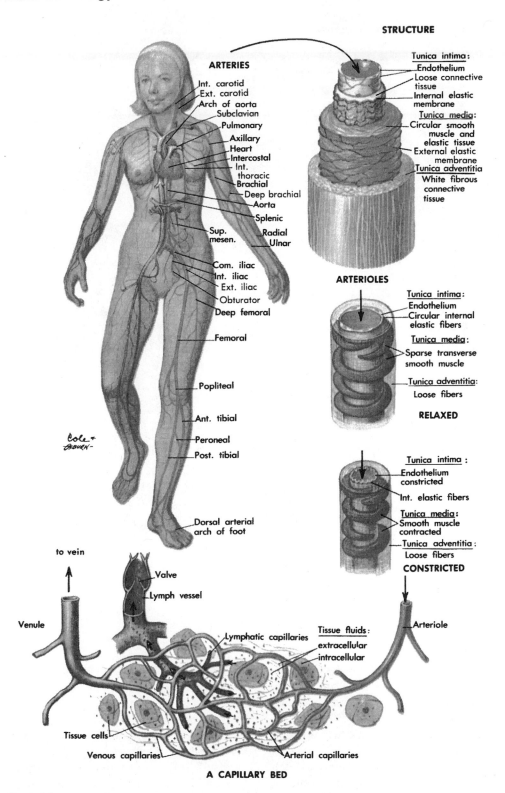

ARTERIES

Int. carotid
Ext. carotid
Arch of aorta
Subclavian
Pulmonary
Axillary
Heart
Intercostal
Int. thoracic
Brachial
Deep brachial
Aorta
Splenic
Sup. mesen.
Radial
Ulnar
Com. iliac
Int. iliac
Ext. iliac
Obturator
Deep femoral
Femoral
Popliteal
Ant. tibial
Peroneal
Post. tibial
Dorsal arterial arch of foot

STRUCTURE

Tunica intima:
Endothelium
Loose connective tissue
Internal elastic membrane
Tunica media:
Circular smooth muscle and elastic tissue
External elastic membrane
Tunica adventitia
White fibrous connective tissue

ARTERIOLES

Tunica intima:
Endothelium
Circular internal elastic fibers
Tunica media:
Sparse transverse smooth muscle
Tunica adventitia:
Loose fibers
RELAXED

Tunica intima:
Endothelium constricted
Int. elastic fibers
Tunica media:
Smooth muscle contracted
Tunica adventitia:
Loose fibers
CONSTRICTED

to vein
Valve
Lymph vessel
Venule
Arteriole
Lymphatic capillaries
Tissue fluids:
extracellular
intracellular
Tissue cells
Venous capillaries
Arterial capillaries

A CAPILLARY BED

Figure 9-2
Major arteries of the body. (Reprinted with permission from Bonewit, K. *Clinical Procedures for Medical Assistants,* 3rd ed. Philadelphia: W. B. Saunders, 1995, plate 8.)

STRUCTURE

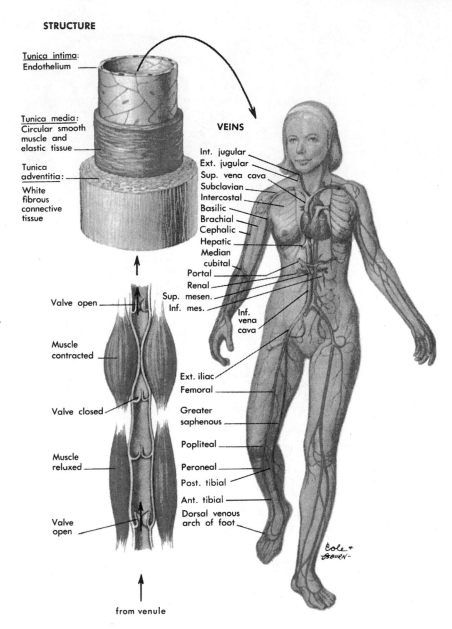

Tunica intima:
Endothelium

Tunica media:
Circular smooth
muscle and
elastic tissue

Tunica
adventitia:

White
fibrous
connective
tissue

VEINS

Int. jugular
Ext. jugular
Sup. vena cava
Subclavian
Intercostal
Basilic
Brachial
Cephalic
Hepatic
Median
cubital
Portal
Renal
Sup. mesen.
Inf. mes.

Inf.
vena
cava

Figure 9-3
**Major veins of the body.
(Reprinted with permission
from Bonewit, K.** *Clinical
Procedures for Medical Assistants,* **3rd ed. Philadelphia:
W. B. Saunders, 1995,
plate 7.)**

Valve open

Muscle
contracted

Valve closed

Muscle
reluxed

Valve
open

Ext. iliac
Femoral

Greater
saphenous

Popliteal

Peroneal

Post. tibial

Ant. tibial

Dorsal venous
arch of foot

from venule

chest. The second major duct is called the *thoracic duct*. It is responsible for draining lymph from the remainder of the body. Once both ducts have completed their respective tasks, each empties lymph into both the right and left jugular veins.

The lymphatic system is the only means by which protein, or albumin, may leave the vascular compartment to be returned back to the blood. This is because protein diffusion, or breakup, does not occur within the capillaries. If this protein were not removed by the lymph, it would then accumulate in the tissue space and eventually produce edema, or swelling. In addition to protein drainage, the lymphatic system also filters the lymph and removes any foreign particles such as bacteria.

Coronary Circulation

Coronary circulation is the flow of blood throughout the coronary arteries. These arteries are responsible for carrying oxygenated blood to the heart muscle itself. This blood supply is then carried off of the aorta, which is the main artery found in the heart and located just above the aortic valve.

After the oxygenated blood is carried to the myocardial tissue by both the left and right coronary arteries, the oxygen is exchanged for carbon dioxide and the returning nonoxygenated blood is returned by the coronary veins, which are responsible for emptying into the coronary sinus. This in turn empties into the right atrium.

Because the heart requires a constant supply of oxygenated blood to maintain energy for a constantly beating heart, the function of the coronary arteries is to provide the heart with the oxygenated blood. If the arterial supply is cut off, the heart will suffer a lack of oxygen, thus resulting in what is referred to as a *myocardial infarction*, or heart attack, caused by the death of the heart tissue. Therefore, the maintenance of coronary arterial blood supply is vital to sustaining life.

Innervation, Blood Flow, and Blood Supply

The heart receives nerve fibers from the sympathetic nerves, which terminate upon the *sinoatrial node (SA node)* and the *atrioventricular node (AV node)*. In addition, because these nerves also terminate at the myocardium, the heart also receives a certain amount of blood supply from the parasympathetic nerves. Like the sympathetic nerves, the parasympathetic nerves also terminate at the SA and AV nodes.

All cardiac muscle cells have an inherent, or characteristic, rate of contraction called *depolarization*. What this means is that the heart maintains a beat unless other stimuli are received. The sympathetic and parasympathetic nerves can therefore influence the heartbeat rate, but in opposite directions.

Parasympathetic nerves also have the capacity to cause the heart rate to decrease, while the sympathetic nerves have the opposite influence, that is, they may cause the heart rate to increase. The two share the dual responsibility of balancing the heart rate and thereby maintain a normal heart rate, usually between 60 to 100 beats per minute for an average healthy adult.

During exercise, or any other strenuous activity, the heart rate increases because of the sympathetic nerve activity. In addition to affecting the heart's rate, these nerves may also cause the heart to contract with greater force. The parasympathetic nerves have no influence on the strength of the heart's contractions.

The Cardiac Cycle

As we previously stated, the normal, healthy heart beats approximately 60 to 100 times per minute. This number is referred to as the *heart rate*, and is reflected in what we call the *cardiac cycle*. Although there are a number of events that take place during a cardiac cycle, the most important point to remember is that the cardiac cycle is the time when the cardiac muscle contracts, forcing the blood to move out through the arteries, and eventually causing the mus-

cles of the ventricles to relax. The cardiac cycle is both a muscular contraction and a muscular relaxation. At the end of the contraction, the muscles begin to relax. This causes the incoming arterial blood to expand the muscle fibers and the relaxed muscle fibers to lengthen. Within normal limits, the longer the muscle fibers lengthen, the greater will be the contraction.

The state of the heart when the myocardium completes its contraction is referred to as *systole*. As the myocardium begins to relax, it becomes dilated by the inrushing arterial blood. This is called *diastole*. Both the atrial and the ventricular myocardium exhibit systole and diastole, and the cardiac cycle cannot be complete until the atrium finishes its contraction before the ventricles begin their phase.

Blood Pressure and the Cardiac Cycle

Blood pressure is the time spent during the heart contraction and relaxation. Systole, as we have already stated, is the time when the myocardium completes its contraction, but also it is defined as the maximum pressure formed during a ventricular contraction. Diastole, on the other hand, is not only created by an inrushing of arterial blood as the myocardium begins to relax, but it is also the minimum amount of pressure exerted during the ventricles' relaxation phase.

Blood pressure is measured in millimeters of mercury (mm Hg). Thus, in a blood pressure of 120/80, the 120 represents the systolic pressure, or the time in which the heart is contracting, and the 80 represents the diastolic pressure, or the time in which the heart is relaxing.

The Conduction System and the Cardiac Cycle

During the time in which the heart is pumping blood from its origination point to all parts of the body, electrical impulses are also being created by certain anatomical structures located within the heart itself. It is these electrical impulses that are measured during the electrocardiogram ordered by the physician.

The structures creating the electrical impulses or stimuli make up the *conduction system*. They include the *sinoatrial*, or *SA, node*; the *atrioventricular*, or *AV, node*; the *bundle of His*; and the *Purkinje fibers* (Figure 9-4).

The SA node is located in the right atrium at the opening of the superior vena cava. It is made up of a group of cells responsible for generating electrical impulses spontaneously and repeatedly. It is for this reason that it is most commonly referred to as the

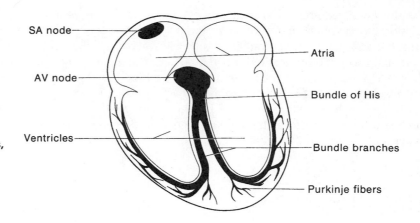

Figure 9-4
Conduction system of the heart. (Reprinted with permission from Bonewit, K. *Clinical Procedures for Medical Assistants,* 3rd ed. Philadelphia: W. B. Saunders, 1995, p 443.)

"pacemaker" of the heart. It is stimulated by both sympathetic and parasympathetic nerves, which in turn regulate the heart rate.

The cells of the SA node have the ability to generate a small electrical charge, which in a normal, healthy person, fire off in short, rhythmic bursts, much like the flashing of an automobile turn signal. Each short burst of electrical current then depolarizes the muscle cells, causing the atrial muscle to contract. As the electrical current begins to cause the atrial muscle to contract, it also spreads along each muscle fiber toward the AV node.

The AV node is located in the right atrial muscle tissue at the junction of the atrium and the intraventricular septum. It is most responsible for receiving parasympathetic and sympathetic nerve fibers. As the electrical current is generated and spread from the SA node, it causes the AV node to "fire off." Once the AV node picks up the electrical charge, it then relays the current to the *bundle of His.*

Consisting of both a right and left branch, the bundle of His is located in the intraventricular septum near the base of the heart. Alongside each of the branches, the AV bundles give off small fibers that project into the ventricular muscle fibers. Once the electrical charge has been sent from the AV node to the bundle of His, it is then relayed into each AV bun-

dle. Finally, the electrical current spreads from the AV bundle into the small fibers, called *Purkinje fibers,* eventually causing the cardiac muscles to contract. It is important to note that the electrical stimulus that has been conducted from the SA node all the way to the muscle fiber occurs in hundredths of a second.

Electrical Activity

Electrical signals that are generated by the conduction system are recorded on the electrocardiograph machine as a series of waves, intervals, and segments, each of which pertains to a specific occurrence during the beating of the heart. These include the *P wave,* which represents the depolarization of the atrial myocardium; the *QRS wave,* sometimes called the *QRS complex,* in which depolarization of the ventricular myocardium is taking place, the *PR interval,* which represents the beginning of the excitation of the atrium to the beginning of the ventricular excitation, and the *ST segment,* which has no deflection from the baseline but in an abnormal state may be elevated or depressed (Figure 9-5).

Electrical events occurring during the cardiac cycle can be considered as the cycle beginning with the P wave in the electrocardiogram. At this point, the SA node has fired and the electrical current has

Figure 9-5
Heart action during ECG cycle.

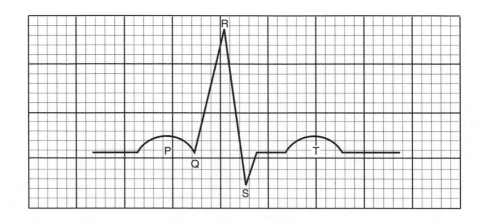

begun to spread to the atrial myocardium. The atrium then depolarizes and contracts, which causes the P wave in the electrocardiogram. During atrial systole, the atria contract, forcing blood from both atria into their respective ventricles. Next, the electrical current spreads to the AV node, bundle of His, and Purkinje fibers, during the interval from the end of the P wave, until the Q wave appears. This entire process is known as *atrial systole*.

During atrial systole, the QRS waves represent the depolarization of the ventricular myocardium. This is when the first heart sound is heard, or the "lub." This sound represents the closing of the mitral and tricuspid valves. Also, during this period, the ventricular pressure begins to increase, and when it reaches the systolic pressure, the aortic valve opens. After the S wave and at the exact moment of the aortic valve opening, the heart cycle is in what we refer to as its *rapid ejection phase*. What occurs during this time is a rapid emptying of the ventricle, which in turn causes the atrial pressure to begin to rise to its highest level, and the ventricular myocardium, at the same time, to begin to make itself ready to repolarize, cause the T wave to form on the ECG.

At the end of the T wave, the ventricle is beginning to relax and start ventricular diastole. At the exact time in which this is occurring, the atrial pressure in the aorta starts to exceed the pressure in the ventricle. The ventricle pressure then falls until such time as the atrial pressure exceeds the ventricular pressure. At that exact moment, the mitral and tricuspid valves open and the heart is in what we refer to as its *rapid filling phase*, which is the time during which the ventricles fill up with the blood.

The PQRST Complex

The electrical activity in the heart that leads to the contraction of the heart muscle is displayed as a *PQRST pattern*, or *complex* on the electrocardiographic paper. Each of these patterns or complexes, represents the electrical activity occurring during the contraction phase of the heart muscle. Therefore, each PQRST phase represents one complete heartbeat. A cardiologist or trained health care professional can study the various parts of the complex and can determine any possible diseased or abnormal conditions present in the heart. Because of the importance of this pattern, it is extremely important that you as the technician make sure that the complex is centered on the paper and large enough so that all parts of it can be studied.

To make it easier for you to understand, let us take a look at the individual parts of the complex. To start with, the P wave, or the point at which depolarization begins to take place, indicates the spread of the impulse generated by the SA node over the atrium. It is therefore referred to as *depolarization of the atrium*. The PR interval is the period of time from the onset of the P wave to the beginning of the QRS complex. This includes the time required for atrial depolarization and repolarization as well as the time necessary for the initial impulse from the SA node to arrive at the AV node.

The PR segment represents the period of time from the end of the P wave to the onset of the QRS complex. Normally this is an isoelectric period on the ECG. The QRS complex represents the electrical voltages during the depolarization of the ventricles as the impulse begins to spread through the bundle of His, bundle branches, and the Purkinje fibers. The ST segment represents the interval between the end of the ventricular depolarization and the beginning of ventricular repolarization. Physiologically, this is the interval between the ventricles contracting and their recovery. During the ST interval, the ventricles also begin to recover from their contraction.

Finally, the QT interval represents the time interval from the beginning of ventricular depolarization to the completion of ventricular repolarization. Physiologically, the QT interval represents the beginning of the ventricular contraction to the complete recovery of the ventricles. The U wave, considered the "afterpotential" of the T wave, represents the repolarization of the ventricular Purkinje fibers. However, the precise significance of the U wave is not completely understood.

How the Whole Cardiac Cycle Works

Now that we have discussed both the anatomy and the function of the cardiac cycle, let's try to summarize exactly what is happening during this most vital period. To begin with, the SA node, or the "pacemaker" of the heart, fires, causing both the atrium to contract and the blood to be forced into the ventricles. The ventricular myocardium is then stimulated and contracts, causing the "lub," or first sound of the heartbeat, by the closing of the mitral and tricuspid valves, as a result of the increasing ventricular pressure.

Rapid ejection of blood from the ventricles into the arteries then takes place, causing the atrial pressure to rise to its maximum level, which in turn causes the ventricles to begin to relax. Atrial pressure is still high when the ventricular pressure begins to decrease. Immediately following this process, the "dub," or second sound emitted by the heartbeat, occurs as the pulmonary and aortic semilunar valves snap shut, thereby preventing blood from flowing back into the ventricles.

Summary

In this chapter, we took our first look at the role the cardiology department plays in caring for a patient suffering from a disorder of the circulatory or cardiovascular system. We also talked about the various members of this department, including the cardiologist and the ECG technician. Finally, we spent some time discussing the basic anatomy and physiology of the heart and cardiovascular system, including not only the actual structures but also the conduction system and the role it plays in the cardiac cycle.

Review Questions

1. An x-ray examination of the heart and great blood vessels that follows the course of an opaque fluid injected into the bloodstream is called:

   a. arteriolography

   b. angiocardiography

   c. myocardiography

2. A blood vessel that carries blood from all parts of the body back to the heart is called:

   a. artery

   b. vein

   c. capillary

3. A blood vessel that carries blood away from the heart to all parts of the body is called:

   a. artery

   b. vein

   c. capillary

4. What is the term used to describe an abnormal rhythm of the heartbeat?

5. What is the term used to describe an area of tissue damaged or dead as a result of an insufficient blood supply?

6. What is the name of the procedure that is used to record the electrical currents of the heart?

7. A _____ is a medical doctor who specializes in the care and treatment of patients with conditions affecting the heart and the cardiovascular system.

8. What is the name of the structure in which the heart is contained?

9. How many chambers does the heart have?

   a. 2

   b. 4

   c. 6

10

Preparation and Monitoring of Electrocardiograms

Performance Objectives

Upon completion of this chapter, you will be able to:

1. Discuss the role of the ECG technician as it relates to patient care and recording of the electrocardiogram.
2. Identify and describe the various types of equipment and supplies used in the monitoring and recording of electrocardiograms.
3. Explain how the ECG technician can most effectively deal with meeting the physicial and psychosocial needs of the cardiac patient.
4. Explain the purpose and function of the standard 12-lead electrocardiogram.
5. Explain the purpose and function of a three-channel computerized electrocardiogram.

Terms and Abbreviations

Communication   a two-way process in which information, facts, or feelings are shared with others; it may be either the verbal, written, or nonverbal.

Confidentiality   the noncommunication of information from one person to another.

Ethics   standards and principles inherent in the science and art of medicine.

Negligence   the failure to perform a task in a manner or in a way in which another individual of the same training or background would perform the task.

Malpractice   the performance of a task for which an individual has not been properly trained; unskillful or incorrect medical or surgical treatment.

As a member of the allied health community, you are as responsible for your own actions as the others who make up the health care delivery system. Therefore, as with all health care providers, your role as an ECG technician involves working within an environment in which communication, professionalism, safety, and ethics are all equally important.

Understanding the Role of the ECG Technician

Communication

Communication in its most simplistic form, is defined as a two-way process in which information, facts, or feelings are shared with others. All communi-

83

cation must involve both a sender and a receiver, and it can be interpreted either in a verbal or nonverbal manner. Verbal or oral communication involves the utilization of both knowledge of what you are speaking about, as well as acceptable verbal skills necessary in communicating your message. This type of communication is used most frequently by the ECG technician when answering the telephone and reporting information.

Written communication involves using documentation to provide information. The two most frequently used written communications in the health care environment that you will be most concerned with include the patient's nursing care plan and the patient's medical chart.

A third type of communication that involves the transmitting of information through the use of one's body gestures rather than through speech or writing, is called *nonverbal communication.* Commonly referred to as "body language," this type of communication can often tell more about a patient and how he or she is feeling than can verbal communication.

ECG technicians communicate with many people, including patients, coworkers, supervisors, and physicians. They are responsible for both transmitting and receiving information regarding the care and observation of patients, as well as providing intercommunication among members of the hospital staff.

Communication involves the process of *observation.* This is particularly important for the ECG technician, since much of what you will be involved in deals with the direct "hands-on" performance of tasks that measures the patient's most vital signs. Observation means much more than just looking at a patient. It involves using all of your senses and noting anything that may appear unusual. It also utilizes the skills involved in communicating or reporting these findings to the person in charge of the patient, or, in some cases, to your supervisor or directly to the physician.

In observing the patient, your senses of vision and hearing are your two greatest assets. The more carefully and efficiently you make your observations, the more expertise you will develop in quickly identifying any situation that might be out of the ordinary.

Skill in observation and communication does not come easily; they require both experience and practice. As you become more involved in these processes, you will begin to learn how to make "mental notes" automatically of what you see, feel, and access regarding the patient's condition. Eventually, you may even be able to sense a problem, or perhaps even change a negative situation into a positive one. Remember, to be of any value, observations must be communicated both effectively and efficiently.

Professionalism and Attitude

Being an ECG technician not only requires skill and training, but also that you possess both enthusiasm and a concerned and positive attitude for the profession. It also requires that you be aware of the needs of others and that you carry yourself in a manner befitting a member of the health care delivery team.

Professionalism involves those characteristics and personal traits that make up an individual who is committed to performing his or her job in an accurate and efficient manner. It includes having both a positive attitude and carrying oneself in a way in which others look to you for guidance and understanding of a "job well done."

Safety and Care of the Patient

Just as important as having a good attitude and carrying out your tasks in a professional manner, is the way in which you provide for the safe care and treatment of your patient. Always remember, that safety, above all, is the single most important task that all members of the health care team must observe. The patient's safety and comfort are everyone's concern. Always try to keep in mind that the needs and feelings of a patient involve maintaining a safe environment. This includes providing for the patient's personal safety, maintenance of all equipment in good working order, and providing a safe environment for yourself and your coworkers.

Ethics and the ECG Technician

The study of ethics and legal aspects involved in working as a member of the cardiology department deals with having an understanding of those standards and principles inherent in the science and art of medicine. The code of ethics involved in health care deals with rules that act as guidelines for those individuals responsible for caring for the sick. These rules are both moral and legal and are grounded in the concept of the preservation of life.

Confidentiality

One of the most basic rules of ethics deals with what you as a member of the health care team sees and hears while working in the health care facility. Much of the information you are concerned with is considered personal, and therefore, it must be kept in strictest confidence. No matter how upset or distressed you might become, you must never allow

yourself to discuss matters that concern patients, coworkers, or physicians. The medical code of ethics forbids any member of the health care team from discussing or repeating information concerned with the everyday workings of the hospital's medical office environment, particularly if it can be used for one's own personal gain. If you believe that specific information is important to the welfare or concern of the patient, it should be reported through the appropriate channels as quickly as possible.

Dealing with Legal Aspects in Health Care

Legal aspects in the health care industry involve three very important concepts. These include *negligence*, *malpractice*, and the reporting of inappropriate acts.

Negligence, when used in the medical sense, describes an individual failing to perform a task in a manner or in a way in which another individual of the same training or background would perform the task. Failing to check out the ECG machine for proper working order prior to hooking the patient up to it, is one example of negligence on the part of the ECG technician.

Malpractice pertains to an individual performing a task for which he or she has not been properly trained. One example would be an ECG technician recording the electrocardiogram on a patient prior to receiving proper instruction on the techniques involved in performing such a task.

Because of the nature of the work performed by members of the health care team, individuals who are employed in hospitals and health care facilities must possess the highest degree of honesty, dependability, and integrity. This means that people working in medicine are expected to conduct themselves in an honest and professional manner. Therefore, any time you are witness to such acts as the misuse of drugs, alcohol, or patient harm, you have both a moral and a legal responsibility to report these acts.

Electrocardiographic Equipment and Supplies

Before we can begin to discuss the actual hands-on skills involved in recording the electrocardiogram, it is extremely important that you first understand the instrumentation and supplies used in obtaining your recording.

To begin with, we generally refer to the instrument used to record an electrocardiogram as an ECG machine. Although several different makes and models of ECG machines are currently in use, there are two basic classifications of machines that the majority of physicians and hospitals use to perform electro-

cardiograms. These include the standard 12-lead ECG machine and the 3-channel computerized ECG machine (Figure 10-1).

The standard 12-lead machine consists of five basic parts. These parts include the *electrodes*, which are made of small pieces of conductive metal used to pick up the electrical activity of the heart; the *leads*, which are the wires connected to the machine, and used for carrying impulses from the electrodes that have been placed on the patient's skin; the *amplifier*, whose purpose involves the magnification of the heart's electrical activity so that it can be recorded; the *galvanometer*, which converts the amplified electrical activity into motion; and the *stylus*, which is responsible for recording the motion onto the graph paper located in the machine.

Safety and the ECG Machine

Whenever we discuss the use of an inanimate object that uses electrical current as part of its performance, we must also address the very important issue of safety. This precaution is doubly important with the ECG machine, because improper use of the machine can have devastating effects not only on the patient's treatment, but also on his or her complete state of health.

The most hazardous part of the ECG machine, is the wires used to hook the patient up to the machine. Although you will have ample opportunity to practice placing the electrodes on patients during your training, the following information will help you to feel more at ease as you begin to learn how to "wire" the patient up correctly.

The most critical aspect of the ECG procedure is the correct attachment of the electrodes and the leads, or the wiring of each lead from the patient to the machine. If either the electrodes or the leads are not placed correctly on the patient, the ECG tracing will be both inaccurate and dangerous.

Because safety is so very important in the ECG procedure, following the safety guidelines outlined below, will assist you in properly placing the leads and the electrodes:

1. Prior to placing the leads and electrodes onto the patient, always remember to wipe the patient's skin with a cleansing agent, especially if the skin is oily, scaly, or sweaty.

2. Always apply the electrode paste or conductive solution to the patient's arms and legs.

3. Remember that the arm electrodes are placed on the fleshy part of the upper outer arm. Use a *white* lead on the right arm and a *black* lead on the left arm.

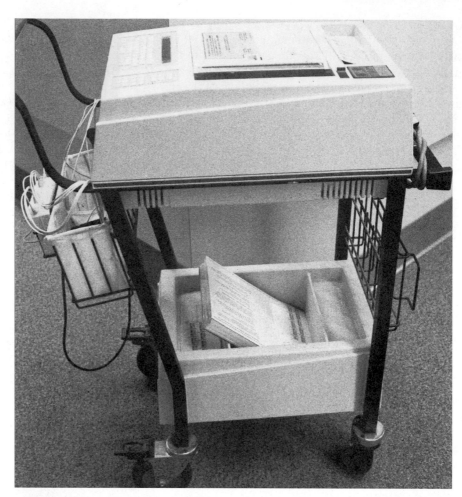

Figure 10-1
Computerized 3-channel ECG machine.

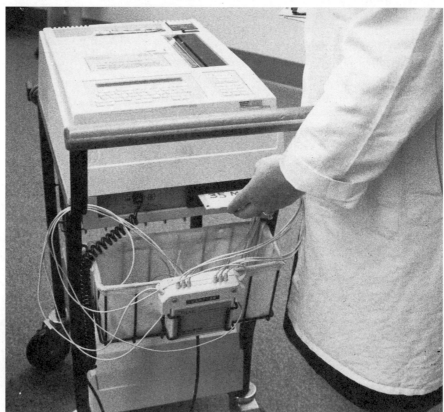

4. Always remember to place the leg electrodes on the inner lower calves. Use a *green* lead on the right leg and a *red* lead on the left leg. Remember:

right arm (RA)   *White*
left arm (LA)   *Black*
right leg (RL)   *Green*
left leg (LL)   *Red*

5. Remember that there are six leads that must be placed upon the patient's chest, all of which have specific locations; if any one of the leads is placed incorrectly, the ECG will be inaccurate. The chest leads include the following:

V_1 placed at the fourth intercostal (between the ribs) space, right sternal (breast bone) border

V_2 placed at the fourth intercostal space, left sternal border

V_3 placed at equal distance between the V_2 and V_4 leads

V_4 placed at the fifth intercostal space, left mid-clavicular (collar bone) lines

V_5 placed lateral (to the side) of the V_4 lead, at the anterior (in front of) the axillary (arm pit) line between V_4 and V_6

V_6 placed lateral to V_5 at the midaxillary line

Switches and Markers

As we have already discussed, there are several different makes and models of ECG machines currently in use. However, all machines contain many of the same basic operational parts, including the switches and markers that make obtaining the ECG possible. A good rule of thumb to remember is that whenever you are required to perform an electrocardiogram, prior to using it, always check the manufacturer's instructions that accompany it.

The switches and markers that make up the operation of the standard 12-lead machine include the *main switch control*, which is the control for turning the machine on and off, and which should never be left in the ON position; the *pilot light*, usually seen as a red light, indicating that the machine has been turned on; the *standard control* or *ST'D*, which allows the technician to standardize the machine; the *stylus head control*, which is used to adjust the stylus temperature; the *stylus position control*, which is used to move the recording up and down on the paper; the *record switch*, which utilizes four separate functions, all of which are needed in order to control the amplifier and paper drive or the speed; the *standardize button*, or *ST'D*, which must be pushed in order to put the standard mark onto the graph paper; the *marker button*, which, when pushed, places a mark or code onto the paper in order to identify the lead being recorded; the *lead selector switch*, which allows the

proper selection of the lead to be run; and the *sensitivity switch*, which controls the amplifications.

The Automated Electrocardiogram

As with all the other types of science and technology currently in use throughout the world, automation and the computer have also entered the world of electrocardiography through the 3-channel computerized ECG machine. Although there are several different types of computerized machines presently being used, the premise for all of them is the same: to provide the physician with the most accurate, state-of-the-art analysis of the patient's heart, utilizing the greatest amount of safety, in the quickest duration of time.

Like its manual standard 12-lead counterpart, the computerized machine also employs a series of switches that augment its operation. These include the *power switch*, which turns the machine on and off; five lead *select switches*, which allow the technician to select a particular lead group to be manually recorded; a *stop switch*, which when pressed stops the paper drive; the *autorun switch*, which allows the paper to be placed in the correct starting position; the *manual run switch*, which activates the paper drive, thus allowing the unit to record the lead group selected by the lead select switches; a *1-mV switch*, which is used to test the gain and damping of the unit; the *speed 25/50 switch*, found both on the standard 12-lead machine and the computerized machine, which provides the technician with the ability to move the paper at either 25 or 50 mm/s; the *filter in/out double switch*, which provides for selection of frequency responses of the unit; a *chest X 1/2 switch*, which when pressed provides for chest sensitivity or amplitude reduction by one-half; the *limb X 1/2, X 1, X 2 switch*, used by the technician for selecting the desired lead sensitivity of leads 1, 2, 3, aVF, aVL, and aVR; and the *position switch*, which is responsible for adjusting the position of the recording styluses in their respective channels.

Additional switches that are found on both the standard manual ECG machine and the computerized machine include the *stylus heat switch,* which is used to produce a solid clean line on the recording paper, the *power connection cable*, which is connected from the power jack located on the back of the machine to the grounded wall outlet; and the *patient cable*, which is the mainline connection between the patient and the machine.

Electrocardiographic Supplies

Since the purpose of an electrocardiogram is to provide the physician with a graphic picture of the heart's electrical activity, certain "modes of transport" must be utilized to provide such information. These include the use of sensors, electrolyte, and ECG graph paper.

Sensors are used to attach the patient to the lead, which in turn connects the patient to the ECG machine. In essence, the main purpose of a sensor is to act as a conductor so that the machine can record the electrical impulses made by the heart and eventually record them onto the paper of the ECG machine.

The most frequently used sensors are called *Welsh self-retaining* sensors, and in most cases, they are generally included as part of the standard accessories supplied with the electrocardiograph machine (Figure 10-2). Since there are different types of sensors currently available on the market, a good rule of thumb is never mix sensors with those of another manufacturer. Because the metal of which they are made may be dissimilar, placing different sensors on the patient could cause considerable baseline drifting or blocking.

An *electrolyte* is a substance used to assist the machine in creating conductivity from the sensor, which has been attached to the patient, to the machine, so that electrical currents or impulses produced by the heart can be traced. Electrolytes can either be a liquid substance, which is placed onto the lead before it is attached to the patient, or an electrolyte pad, which is gently attached to the inside of the sensor and then removed after the tracing has been completed.

No matter what type of electrolyte has been selected, it is important to make sure that you wipe the

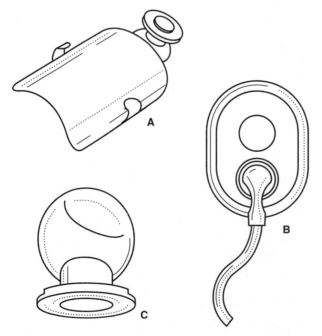

Figure 10-2
Limb sensors.

sensors clean after each application. Preferably, the sensors should be washed after use and then scoured with a kitchen cleanser. Excessive corrosion or an accumulation of electrolyte may cause the baseline to drift, thus impairing the quality of the ECG recording.

When required to perform an electrocardiogram using a liquid electrolyte, follow the guidelines outlined below. By doing so, you will correctly apply the sensors and electrolyte, thus providing you with a more accurate ECG recording:

- Prior to applying the electrolyte to the sensors, only expose the patient's arms, legs, and chest.
- Connect the patient leads to the self-retaining sensors; that means using 10 sensors for a standard 12-lead ECG.
- Squeeze a small amount of electrolyte onto the sensor site and use the sensor to spread it evenly over the sensor contact area. Always make sure you apply the same amount of electrolyte to each sensor site. If you are using the "bulb" type of sensor, gently depress the bulb when applying the sensor so as to leave only a small "dimple" when the bulb is released.
- For the arm sensors, position the sensor on a smooth, fleshy area of the upper arm. Position it so that the sensor will not press against the body or table when the patient is relaxed.
- Attach the leg sensors on a fleshy part of the lower leg, but never over the tibia.
- Be sure that the leads conform to the body's contours, with no strain being placed on the sensors. Avoid looping any excess length of lead wires.
- Plug the patient cable into the patient jack unit until it is secure.

Another supply that you must get used to working with, is ECG paper. Although automated or computerized ECG machines may use a different size and type of paper from that which is used by the standard 12-lead machine, you should remember that all ECG paper is treated in such a way as to react to the stylus heat so that a tracing can be produced upon the paper.

ECG paper is designed to be divided into two sets of squares (Figure 10-3). The sole function of the paper is to provide for total accuracy and measurement of the electrical waves, intervals, and segments as they relate to the recording of the patient's heartbeat. Each square of the paper is made up of 25 smaller squares, with each one measuring 1 mm high and 1 mm wide. When measured horizontally, each square represents the time in which each beat of the heart is recorded, that is, 0.04 seconds per square. When the square is measured vertically, each represents the amount of voltage being fired off by the heart, or 0.1 mV per square.

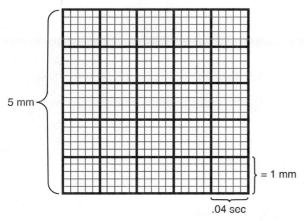

5 mm

= 1 mm

.04 sec

Figure 10-3
ECG paper.

All electrocardiographic paper consists of a black base overlying a white plastic coating. It is made that way so that when the heated stylus moves over it, a reaction occurs, causing the paper to melt, or break down the plastic coating. This leaves only the recording of the tracing. In addition to the paper being coated with plastic, it is both heat and pressure sensitive. This allows the stylus of the ECG machine to produce a clear and sharp image of the tracing.

The Holter Monitoring System

Another piece of equipment that you must become familiar with if you plan to work as an ECG technician is the Mini-Holter Transtelephonic Monitoring System (Figure 10-4). Originally developed by the Holter Data Services Company, this system was designed to provide the physician with a means to monitor a patient's ECG over a 24-hour period. The main advantage to using this device over the standard 12-lead machine is that it is able to provide a continous analysis, giving the physician important diagnostic data in the patient's own environment that were previously not available. Thus, the system allows the ambulatory monitoring of the patient for as many days as the physician determines is necessary.

Preparation and Operation of the Holter System

As an ECG technician, it is most important that you understand that the quality of the electrocardiographic transmission is directly dependent upon how well the electrodes are applied to the patient. Because this system works well on its own, and because the technician is not able to be at the patient's side for every hookup, it is important that the patient fully understand the complete procedure for hooking up the system before affixing the electrodes to their positioning sites on the patient.

As with any electrocardiogram, both the location and the manner in which the electrodes are placed onto the patient are of equal importance when hooking up the Holter system. Figure 10-5 shows the correct positioning sites of the five electrodes. Once you have determined where the electrodes are to be placed, you should follow the steps outlined below:

· Thoroughly clean the patient's skin where the electrodes are to be placed. If necessary, shave

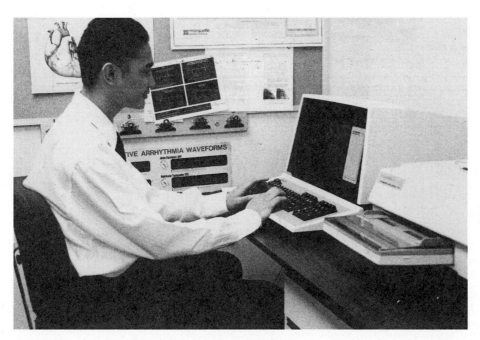

Figure 10-4
The mini-Holter system.

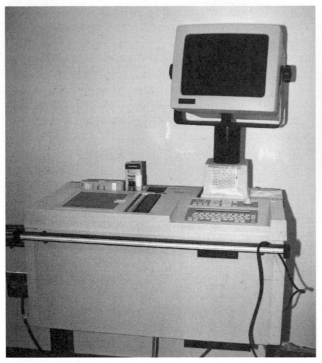
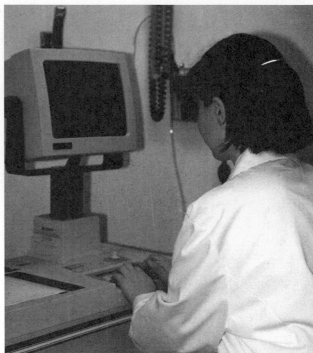

Figure 10-5
Holtor monitoring system.

any hair from the electrode site. This will help to provide a better conduction.

· Scrub the electrode site with a prep pad.
· Remove the backing on the electrode pad and place it on the patient's chest. Gently press the center of the electrode and work out toward the edge.
· Note that the color-coded electrode lead wires correspond to the colors on the Holter jacks. Place each lead wire (male end) into the female pin by color matching it to the Holter recorder. Snap the other end of the lead set to each corresponding color electrode on the patient's chest.
· Install a new 9-V battery in the Holter recorder. Listen for the five beeps that will indicate that the power is on. If the electrode buzzer beeps 20 times and there is no electrode LED flash, an electrode disconnect has occurred. Check it and connect a lead wire, making certain that no electrode has been removed from the patient.

Once you have properly connected the monitor and explained the procedure to the patient, you are ready to begin operation of the system.

The Holter system transmits the patient's electrocardiographic data via the telephone from the Holter recorder to the Holter data bank. An ST level may be changed per the physician's preference, and is normally preset at 80 mm/s, or 1.5 mm. To set the ST level, simply remove the four screws located at the back of the recorder and unhook the top lid from it. Switches can then be moved to make the change of setting. Once the indicator has been changed, the lid is replaced and all four screws should be tightened.

To transmit data from the Holter system, you should:

1. Dial the transmitter telephone number, located in the patient's chart. After a few rings, a "squeal" tone should be heard. If this tone is not heard, phone back in about 15 minutes.
2. Place the phone mouthpiece on the Holter monitor and directly over the company's printed name (Holter Data Services Company). Hold the recorder firmly to the mouthpiece.
3. Slide the transmitter switch to the ON position. After several minutes, a continous loud tone will be heard, indicating that the Holter transmission is complete.
4. Slide the transmitter to the OFF position, and wait for the five "beep" tones.
5. Remove the telephone from the face of the recorder and hang up the telephone.

Meeting the Needs of the Cardiac Patient

When working as an ECG technician, it is not enough just to know how to use the proper equipment to record an electrocardiogram, or what the various segments or intervals are of the tracing you have just completed. You must also understand the importance of your role as a caregiver. This means working with others to help meet both the physical and the psychosocial needs of the patients with whose care you have been entrusted.

All of us require necessities in life in order to help us get along and interact with others. These needs are both physical, such as the need for heat when the weather is cold, and emotional, as in needing love and understanding. For cardiac patients, who may be experiencing feelings of despair, believing that perhaps they may be reaching the end of their life, meeting the patient's everyday physical needs and helping to provide them with emotional and psychological support, can make the difference between total recovery from a cardiac condition, and death.

Human beings grow, that is, they change physically and develop psychologically from affect. All of us go through life on a continuum that begins at birth to death. However, not all of us progress at the same rate in their growth and development, and it is for this reason that the provision of both physical and emotional well-being is so vitally important to the hospitalized cardiac patient.

Understanding Human Needs

Psychological or developmental skills and physical growth vary throughout one's life, however, it is our basic human needs, that is, the need to communicate, to have one's emotional and spiritual well-being assured, and to have specific physical needs, such as food, shelter, and clothing, fulfilled that are paramount to our existence.

Each of us wants to be understood by others. We all want to be able to communicate what we feel. We meet this need both verbally and through the use of nonverbal signals, such as crying or changing our facial expressions. In addition to communicating our feelings, human beings have a great need to experience emotional well-being. In doing so, we both enhance and protect our self-esteem. In health care, how patients respond to threats to their self-esteem depends greatly upon how they interpret their own feelings of helplessness before, during, and after their illness.

Many health care providers agree that in no other study of medicine is the need to meet the patient's emotional well-being as important as it is in dealing with the cardiac patient. Many of these patients are frightened that they are approaching the end of their life. For the person suffering from a cardiac dysfunction, the constant threat of death and the pain and discomfort felt may force the patient to cry for what

appears to be no reason at all. Being able to understand and recognize the patient's fears and anxieties will help you to more effectively and efficiently communicate your desire to assist the patient during bouts with sadness and fright.

In addition to caring for the cardiac patient's emotional needs, as a member of the cardiology health care team, you have an equally important responsibility to meet the patient's physical needs. In addition to those basic needs we all require to survive—food, shelter, sleep, etc.—the cardiac patient may require special physical care. Your responsibility as an ECG technician involves being aware of these needs, particularly as they relate to special procedures the patient may be undergoing as part of his or her treatment. Whether it is providing privacy during the recording of the electrocardiogram, or providing support to a patient's family waiting outside the treatment room, the ECG technician's role is not only to perform the basic tasks involved in completing a procedure, but, just as important, to play a key role in assisting the rest of the cardiac team members in helping to meet the very special physical needs of the cardiac patient.

The Patient's Rights

According to the American Hospital Association, all patients, whether they are suffering from a cardiac dysfunction, admitted to have a baby, or receiving treatment in the out-patient center, are entitled to have their basic rights observed. This means that they have the right to know and understand that all orders the physician writes will be followed accurately and that procedures will be carried out in the way in which they should be. It also means that the patient has a right to be properly identified, according to his or her name, and to be provided with a sense of security every time you check the patient's nameband prior to carrying out a procedure.

In 1973, a document known as the "Patient's Bill of Rights" was established and adopted by all hospitals sanctioned to operate under the Joint Commission on Accreditation of Hospitals. This document stated that in order for a hospital to be allowed to operate, it must recognize, and make available, certain specified rights to each patient. It also stated that a patient could expect as part of his or her care, the following:

· The right to have considerate and respectful care.
· The right to obtain complete and current information from his or her physician, regarding the diagnosis, treatment, and prognosis, in terms the patient could be expected to understand.

- The right to receive information from the physician which is necessary to give informed consent prior to the start of any procedure and/or treatment.
- The right to refuse treatment to the extent permitted by law and to be informed of the medical consequences of such action.
- The right to every consideration of privacy concerning the medical care treatment.
- The right to expect that all communications and records pertaining to the patient's care, be treated as confidential.
- The right to expect that within its capacity, a hospital must make reasonable response to the request of a patient for services.
- The right to obtain information as to any relationship of confining hospital to other health care and educational institutions insofar as the patient's care is concerned.
- The right to be advised if the hospital proposes to engage in or perform human experimentation affecting the patient's care or treatment, and the right to refuse to participate in such projects.

- The right to examine and receive an explanation of the charges and bill, regardless of the source of payment.
- The right to know what hospital rules and regulations apply to patient conduct.

Summary

In this chapter, we dealt with the preliminary information and concepts involved with preparing to record the electrocardiogram. In doing so, we discussed the role of the ECG technician as it related to patient care and recording of the ECG tracing. We also identified and described the various types of equipment and supplies used in recording and monitoring electrocardiograms. Finally, we discussed how the ECG technician could most effectively deal with both the physical and the psychosocial needs of the cardiac patient, including seeing to it that the patient is provided with those rights inherent with being cared for in a medical or health care environment.

Review Questions

1. A two-way process in which information, facts, or feelings are shared with others is called _____ .

2. Standards and principles that are inherent in the science and art of medicine is called _____ .

3. Briefly explain the concept of *negligence* as it relates to the health care profession.

4. Briefly explain the concept of *malpractice* as it relates to the health care profession.

5. _____ involves those characteristics and personal traits that make up an individual who is committed to performing his or her job in an accurate and efficient manner.

6. Briefly explain the concept of *confidentiality* as it relates to the health care profession.

7. Give at least three rights a patient is expected to receive while being cared for in a health care facility:

    a. _____
    b. _____
    c. _____

8. Briefly explain the responsibility of the *Joint Commission on Accreditation of Hospitals* as it relates to the patient and the health care facility.

11

Recording and Measuring the Electrocardiogram

Performance Objectives

Upon completion of this chapter, you will be able to:

1. Explain the purpose and function of the standard 12-lead electrocardiogram and the three-channel computerized electrocardiogram.
2. Describe and be able to demonstrate the proper procedure for recording and mounting the standard 12-lead electrocardiogram and the three-channel computerized electrocardiogram.
3. Describe the safety precautions that are necessary whenever the ECG technician is required to record and mount either a standard 12-lead or three-channel computerized electrocardiogram.

Terms and Abbreviations

Artifact   any unwanted activity produced on the electrocardiogram that is not part of the actual measurement of the heart's electrical activity; an artifact may be produced by patient movement or by the electrocardiogram machine.

Electrocardiogram   a procedure that is used to define any electrical record of the heart's action.

As we have already discussed, an electrocardiogram, or ECG, is a tracing of the electrical impulses occurring in the heart. During the electrocardiographic process, an electrode is placed upon the patient's skin. This metal alloy conductor is responsible for both receiving and conducting the electrical impulses being "fired off" by the heart's conduction system. By using these special electrodes, the electrical activity is then recorded from different angles, which are called *leads*. The individual leads, or angles, give the physician a more complete picture of the heart. By noting an electrical disturbance in any of the leads, the physician can then determine which parts of the heart may be diseased or malfunctioning.

A complete ECG normally consists of 12 leads, with the electrodes being placed at specific locations on the body to pick up electrical voltage. The ECG is a relatively simple procedure and is used most frequently to help the physician to detect any cardiac abnormalities. The ECG is also used to record the electrical impulses of the heart as the blood is being pumped throughout the body. Tracings of electrical impulses appear as "waves" on a graph paper, creating a wave pattern reflecting the continuous phases of contractions and relaxations of the heart's four chambers.

Diseases of the heart and the cardiovascular system affect more than 40 million Americans each year, and if diagnosed early, many of these problems can be successfully treated before they have had the chance to become acute and life-threatening. The ECG is a very important procedure because it is one of the most effective ways of detecting heart disease and abnormalities. It is used primarily as a diagnostic tool. It can also be used as an invasive tool in assisting the physician to rule out any other problems associated with the heart.

Purpose and Function of the ECG

A physician is compelled to order an ECG whenever he or she believes the patient's symptoms might indicate an impending heart problem. When such symptoms occur, the ECG can help the doctor to diagnose the cause of the problem and ultimately will assist in the determination of the right course of treatment.

In addition to the ECG being used as a diagnostic tool in determining the course of treatment in a cardiac or cardiovascular disease, the procedure can also be used as a means of treatment after the patient has suffered a heart attack, has been taking cardiac medications, and as part of a routine medical checkup. Patients who have already sustained a myocardial infarction, for example, must have an ECG taken after the onset of the attack in order to determine its exact cause. In this case, the ECG helps the physician to monitor the patient's condition and assists in detecting any improvement or deterioration in the patient's condition.

Many cardiac patients are required to take certain medications on a routine basis in order to help their heart to continue to beat strongly and efficiently. When a prescribed medication is ordered by the physician, he or she normally orders routine ECGs so an evaluation can be made as to the effects of the medication and to check for any side effects.

There may be times when the physician orders an ECG as part of a routine medical checkup. In these instances, the procedure is ordered so that the patient's medical history and health status are kept current, and to reassure the patient that his or her heart is in good condition. By ordering the routine ECG, the physician can also detect any early signs or symptoms of impending heart disease.

Recording the Electrocardiogram

Whether you are required to record a standard 12-lead ECG or a computerized version, it will be necessary for you to follow basic preliminary steps before you can begin the actual recording of the ECG. These steps include those tasks necessary to ensure the proper operation of the procedure and involve checking out the proper operation of your equip-

ment, making sure that the machine has been properly hooked up to the patient, spending time talking with the patient and explaining the procedure, and providing for both the patient's physical and emotional well-being before, during, and after the recording of the ECG.

Procedural Steps for Recording the ECG

Once you have completed the preliminary steps necessary for recording the ECG, you are ready to begin the actual procedure. If you are making the recording using a standard 12-lead machine, follow the steps outlined below in order to ensure the proper completion of this task.

1. Prepare the patient's skin by removing any oil, sweat, or scales, using a nonabrasive cleansing agent. If the patient is wearing any type of necklace around his or her neck, ask that it be removed, since it may cause unwanted artifacts to be recorded (Figure 11-1).
2. Prepare the patient by applying a conductive solution or paste on the patient's arms and legs where the skin will come into contact with the electrode.
3. Apply the electrodes securely to the patient's upper arms and thighs in the same manner as outlined in wiring the patient. Apply the chest electrodes securely.
4. Connect the lead wires to each electrode. Make sure you use the correct wires.
5. Plug in the cable that connects the patient to the ECG machine.
6. Check to be certain that the stylus is in proper operation to record.
7. Start the recording.
8. Turn the machine off and move the chest electrode to another position.
9. Turn on the machine and record the tracing. Repeat step 8 above. You will move the chest electrode to a total of six positions (Figure 11-2).

If you are making your recording using the 3-channel computerized ECG machine, it is advisable that you first operate the unit and become familiar with the controls. As the patient cable will not be connected during this prestage of the recording, no ECG recordng is evident during the preliminary steps. Instead, what will be noticeable will be the isoelectric, or baseline, and standardization pulse, both of which will appear on the ECG paper. The presence and proper appearance of these markings generally indicate that the unit is functioning properly.

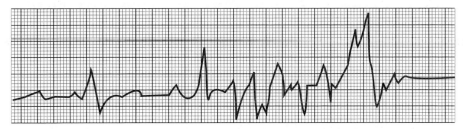

A. Loose or Broken Wires

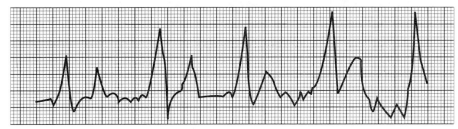

B. Baseline Shift

Figure 11-1
Types of artifacts.

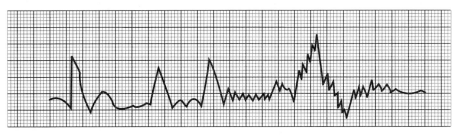

C. Patient Movement (Somatic Tremor)

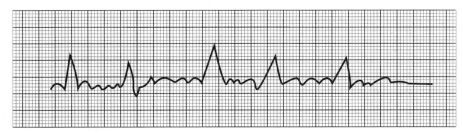

D. Electrical Interference

Procedure for Recording the 12-Lead ECG

Once the preliminary steps have been completed, you are ready to begin the actual procedure involved in recording the ECG. The general steps outlined below will help you in completing this task:

1. Assemble all the necessary equipment. This will include the ECG machine, the leads, electrodes (sensors), and the electrolyte. Notify the members of the nursing staff of the procedure, so that you will not be interrupted once you have begun.
2. Wash your hands.
3. Identify the patient and explain the procedure.

Prepare the patient for the procedure by asking that he or she remove all clothing from the waist up, including any jewelry that may be around the neck.

4. Ask the patient to lie in a supine position (on the back). If the patient wishes, a pillow can be placed under the head for comfort during the procedure.
5. Drape the patient by exposing only the area in which you will be working. While you are moving the chest leads about, make sure that you provide for the patient's privacy by covering the rest of the chest and the lower half of the body.

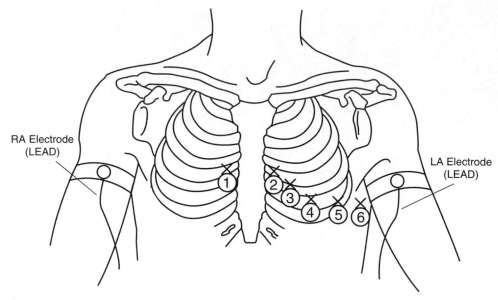

RA Electrode
(LEAD)

LA Electrode
(LEAD)

Figure 11-2
Chest lead placement.

6. Ask the patient to remain very still and to relax, since any movement may cause unwanted electrical activity or artifacts and may interfere with the recording.

7. Place the ECG machine close enough to the patient so that the power cord is away from the examination table or hospital bed and does not run under it.

8. After applying a small amount of electrolyte to the skin where the sensor will connect, place each of the limb sensors, or electrodes, in position. The two upper sensors should be placed on the upper arms, and the two lower electrodes on the lower legs, with the lead connectors pointed toward the center of the patient's body.

9. If you are using a metal disc chest electrode, position the chest strap under the patient's left side, with the concave surface of the weighted end of the strap lying against the chest wall.

10. Connect the lead wires to the sensors. Generally, these wires are color-coded, with the abbreviations *LA* (left arm), *LL* (left leg), *RL* (right leg), and *C* (chest) or *V* (ventricles), which will help you to distinguish one from the other when connecting them to the sensors.

11. Apply the electrolyte to the chest sensors and place it on the first chest lead position (V_1). Make sure that the metal disc is held in place by the weighted chest strap.

12. Connect the cable to the sensors. If there is any excess wire, coil it in a loop and fasten it with tape or a band, so that it is out of the way.

13. Position the *lead selector switch* to *ST'D*, and center the stylus. Move the *record switch* to 25 mm and check your standardization of the machine by momentarily depressing the *ST'D* button.

14. Turn the machine to *AMP OFF* and check whether the amplitude of the ST'D mark is 1 mm on the ECG paper.

15. Center the stylus and run about 10 inches or four to six cycles, of *leads I, II,* and *III,* by moving the *record switch* to *RUN* (25 mm/s) and turning the *selector switch* to each of the individual positions. If requested by the physician, insert a standardization mark between the T wave of one ECG cycle and the P wave of the next.

16. While watching for any unwanted movement or artifacts, record about 5 to 8 inches of *aVR, aVL,* and *aVF,* by turning the lead selector to the appropriate position.

17. Record about 5 to 8 inches of chest lead (V_1 to V_6), by moving the lead selector switch to its appropriate position. While recording the chest leads, make sure that the machine is turned to the *AMP OFF* position prior to moving and recording any of the chest leads.

18. Complete the recording by positioning the lead selector switch back to *ST'D* and running off approximately 12 inches. Make sure to properly identify the tracing with the patient's name, the date and time of the recording, and your initials.

19. Turn the machine to *OFF,* unplug the power cord, and disconnect the lead wires. Remove the

sensors and rubber strap from the patient, making sure to clean off any leftover electrolyte from the patient's skin.
20. Help the patient off the examination table or bed, and assist as needed.
21. Clean and return the equipment according to your hospital or facility's policy.
22. Wash your hands.
23. Record the procedure in the patient's chart, making sure to put down both the date and time of the recording.

Recording the Automated ECG

The main difference between recording the automated or computerized ECG and the standard 12-lead ECG is that the computerized machine makes the recording a great deal easier, in less time, and seemingly with more accuracy. This is primarily because the majority of the steps outlined in the standard 12-lead recording are completed automatically on the computerized unit. This leaves little room for mistakes and inaccuracy on the part of the technician. If you are required to make the recording using the computerized machine, following the guidelines outlined below will be helpful.

1. Assemble your necessary equipment.
2. Wash your hands.
3. Identify the patient and explain the procedure.
4. Begin the auto sequence operation: connect the patient cable to both the patient and to the unit; place the *POWER* switch in the *ON* position; if desired, make sensitivity, speed, or filter changes; press the *AUTO RUN* switch; the paper will be queued to the correct point and the unit will automatically record each lead group and stop when the sequence has been completed; pressing the *STOP* switch during this mode will terminate the auto sequence, thereby allowing a different selection to be made.

If it is determined that you must perform a manual sequence operation using the computerized unit, follow the steps outlined below:

1. Connect the patient cable to both the patient and to the unit.
2. Place the *POWER* switch in the *ON* position.
3. If necessary, make the appropriate sensitivity, speed, or filter changes.
4. Press the *LEAD SELECT* switch of the desired lead group.
5. Press the *MAN RUN* switch.
6. The selected lead group will be recorded until a

new lead group is selected or when the *AUTO RUN* or *STOP* switch is pressed, or when the unit is turned off.

Mounting the Electrocardiogram

The final steps in completing the recording of the ECG have to do with the proper mounting and identification of the ECG graph. The technique involved is just as important as the skills necessary in recording the tracing. The purpose of correctly mounting the ECG is to provide the physician with a sharp, concise pictorial "history" of what the patient's heart is doing; the tracing can then be inserted into the patient's medical chart for possible future use.

To properly mount the ECG, follow the steps outlined below:

1. Assemble the necessary equipment. This will include an ECG ruler, the ECG recording to be mounted, and a pair of scissors.
2. Wash your hands.
3. Label the ECG recording with the correct information. This includes the patient's name, the date and time of the recording, the patient's age, and the physician's name.
4. Unroll the ECG recording carefully, so as to avoid any possible scratches on the paper. Never, under any circumstances, fold ECG paper, since doing so can leave bend marks, making interpretation of the recording almost impossible.
5. Locate lead I. Find the correct ST'D mark, making sure it is centered between the complexes. Once lead I has been located, position the ruler so that the ST'D is centered in the middle of the length required for lead I. Use a pen or pencil to make a small mark on the upper margin at each end of the required length.
6. Gently and carefully place the ruler vertically along the end of the required length and hold it securely so that you can tear the paper evenly.
7. Slip the ruler into the lead I slot, making sure it is open and loose enough to mount the recording into it. Remove the protective cover or expose the tape or sticky surface on self-stick mounts.
8. Fold approximately one-quarter inch of the paper over the end of the ruler, making sure to hold the strip in place while sliding it into the lead I area on the slot mount. If you are using self-stick mounts, position the recording and press gently to the sticky surface.
9. Check to make sure the recording is firmly attached to the mount. On slot mounts, hold the

strip in place gently while moving the ruler.
Check to ensure that the strip is mounted neatly,
the ST'D is centerd and correct, and the complexes are clear.
10. Repeat steps 5 through 9 for the remaining leads.
Use the marked areas on the ECG ruler to
determine the length of each lead.
11. Recheck the entire mount to assure it is neat,
mounted correctly, and has the proper standards
in each lead.
12. Replace all the equipment according to your
facility's policy.
13. Wash your hands.

Summary

In this chapter, we explained the purpose and function of both the standard 12-lead ECG and the automated or computerized 3-channel ECG. We outlined
and described the various steps involved in recording
the ECG tracing on both, as well as defined some of
the safety precautions necessary whenever the technician is required to record the ECG. Finally, we discussed the purpose and function of mounting the
ECG, including the various steps involved for correctly mounting either the standard 12-lead ECG or
the computerized 3-channel ECG tracing.

Review Questions

1. Briefly define what is meant by an *artifact*.

2. A procedure that is used to define any electrical record of the heart's action is called an:

   a. electrocardiogram

   b. mylocardiogram

   c. echocardiogram

3. Diseases of the heart and the cardiovascular system affect more than _____ million Americans each year.

   a. 20

   b. 40

   c. 100

4. When is a physician most likely to order an ECG on a patient?

5. Briefly explain the procedure for performing a 12-lead ECG.

6. What is the purpose for mounting an ECG?

7. Why is it important to make sure the patient removes all jewelry prior to taking an ECG?

12

Basic Arrhythmia Recognition and Interpretation

Performance Objectives

Upon completion of this chapter, you will be able to:

1. Discuss the various components of the cardiac cycle.
2. Briefly explain how to recognize an abnormal electrocardiogram.
3. Discuss arrhythmias and identify how to interpret those of the sinoatrial (SA) node, sinus tachycardia, sinus arrest, wandering pacemaker, and sinus bradycardia.
4. Identify atrial tachycardias, atrial flutter, and atrial fibrillation, and be able to explain how to identify them on an ECG.
5. Briefly explain what occurs during premature atrial contractions.
6. Briefly explain ventricular arrhythmias and discuss how to identify and interpret the following: ventricular fibrillation, ventricular flutter, and ventricular asystole.
7. Explain the difference between right and left bundle branch blocks, and briefly define how each can be identified on an electrocardiogram.
8. Discuss first- and second-degree AV block and explain how they can be identified on the ECG.
9. Briefly explain what a premature ventricular contraction is and how it is recognized on an ECG.

Terms and Abbreviations

Arrhythmia   any abnormal heartbeat.
Bradycardia   abnormally slow heartbeat, generally below 60 beats per minute
Conduction   the time it takes for the impulse originating at the SA node to stimulate ventricular contraction.
Configuration   informs the ECG technician of the extent and location of any myocardial damage.

Normal sinus rhythm   a normal, regular heartbeat; that is, one ranging from 60 to 100 beats per minute.
Rate   the number of pulse rates and heartbeats per minute.
Rhythm   the regularity of the heartbeats.
Tachycardia   abnormally fast heartbeat, generally above 100 beats per minute.

Although your role as an ECG technician does not generally involve any type of interpretation of the ECG that you have secured, it is important that you gain a basic understanding of some of the more fre-

quently seen and recognizable arrhythmias that may appear on the ECG recording. This is an important and necessary part of your job. A technician who is aware of any irregularities or abnormalities recorded on the ECG is better able to alert his or her supervisor or the physician of any potential problems before they become full-blown disasters.

Basic Interpretation of ECGs

In learning the skills involved in basic interpretation of ECGs, there are four elements that we look for in each of the segments of the ECG recording: rate, rhythm, conduction, and configuration.

Rate pertains to the number of pulse rates and heartbeats per minute. It can be calculated either by using the apex of the wave, or the initial upstroke of the wave. To calculate the heart's rate, count the number of small squares (1 mm × 1 mm) between the R wave (to get the ventrical rate), or between the P waves (to get the atrial rate). That number is then divided into 1,500, which is a preset number used to determine rates, with the sum given as the accurate heart rate.

Another way to calculate the heart rate is to count the large squares (5 mm × 5 mm) between the R wave of one cycle to the R wave of the next cycle and then divide that number by the preset number of 300.

You can use a third way to calculate the heart rate by counting the number of cardiac cycles in 6 seconds and then multiplying that number by 10. While this method is considered the least accurate of all three, it is the easiest to use during episodes of tachycardia.

Cardiac Rhythm, Conduction, and Configuration

When we talk about the *rhythm* of the heart, we are referring to the regularity at which the heart beats. Usually a glance is enough to determine whether the rhythm is regular or irregular; however, to be more accurate, it would be better to measure the rhythm using a *caliper*, or ruler, in order to see if the distance between each R wave is equal to that of the next.

Conduction refers to the time it takes for the impulse originating at the sinoatrial (SA) node to stimulate ventricular contraction. It is found by measuring the PR interval and the QRS duration.

The *configuration* and the location of the waves on the ECG recording will tell you about the extent and location of any myocardial damage. In order to determine the configuration, you must ask yourself the following questions: (1) Are the waves similar in shape and size? (2) Do the waves point in the same direction? (3) Are the waves upright, inverted, or diphasic? (Figure 12-1).

Interpreting the Cardiac Cycle

A single cardiac cycle of the electrical activity as recorded on an ECG tracing is able to provide information that may appear in a typical normal lead. Any variation could be an indication that an abnormality may be present.

Each individual cardiac cycle is able to provide

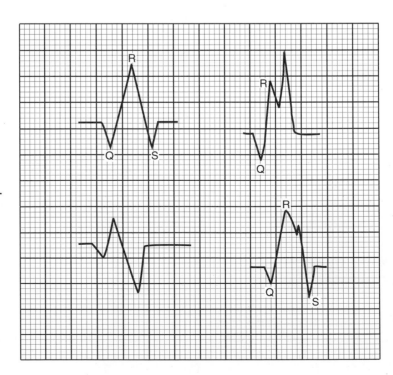

Figure 12-1
Different types of QRS configurations.

the physician with a picture or graph of certain specific actions taking place within the heart. Each one of these actions is represented by a unique or specific feature found on the ECG recording. These include the *P wave*, the *PR interval*, the *QRS complex*, the *ST segment*, the *T wave*, the *U wave*, and the *QT duration*.

The P Wave and the PR Interval

The P wave represents the contraction of the atria; normally, it should not exceed more than 0.11 seconds. It will appear upright in leads I, II, and aVf, and varies in leads III, aV_1, and V_1 through V_6.

The PR interval represents the amount of time it takes for the electrical impulse to travel from the SA node to the bundle of His. Normally it should take anywhere from 0.12 to 0.20 seconds and is best measured from the beginning of the P wave to the beginning of the QRS complex, and then multiplied by 0.04 (Figure 12-2).

The QRS Duration

The QRS duration represents the spread of the impulse through the ventricular muscle, or what is commonly referred to as *depolarization*. Normally it should take from 0.05 to 0.11 seconds and is measured from the beginning of the Q to the S, and then multiplied by 0.04. Any measurement over 0.12 seconds may be an indication of an abnormal ventricular conduction or bundle branch block, or a ventricular arrhythmia.

The ST Segment, the T Wave, and the U Wave

The ST segment represents the resting period between depolarization and repolarization. Normally it is seen as a flat isoelectric line and is measured from the beginning of the S to the beginning of the T wave. To determine if the ST segment is elevated or depressed, place the straight edge of a paper along the

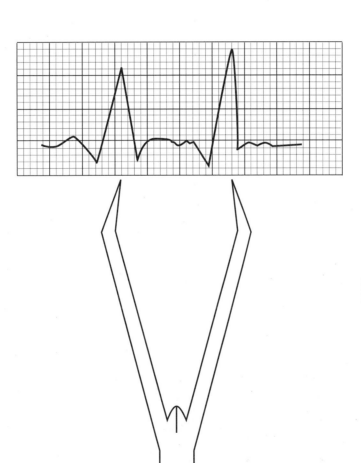

Figure 12-2
Determining the PR interval.

baseline. Above the line represents an elevation, and below the line represents a depression.

The T wave represents the recovery period of the ventricles. Normally all T waves should be the same size and shape throughout the recording. They should all point in the same direction as the QRS complexes, and should be measured from the beginning to the end of each T wave.

The U wave is a small wave, sometimes seen following the T wave, and often occurs when a patient has a potassium deficiency.

The QT Interval

The QT interval is responsible for giving the physician a better picture of the total ventricular activity occurring in the heart. It is measured from the Q to the end of the T wave, and often varies with the heart rate, sex, and age of the patient. It may also lengthen with the presence of congestive heart failure and myocardial infarction (Figures 12-3).

Recognition of Abnormal Arrhythmias

Although there are many different types of arrhythmias that can be seen on the ECG, there are some that are found more frequently than others. Since your role as an ECG technician deals more with the mechanics of recording the ECG than with recognition and interpretation of abnormal occurrences of the heart, we will concentrate on the most common arrhythmias seen on the ECG recording.

Whenever you are required to record the heart's activity through the ECG, it is important to understand that your awareness of seeing any deviation in the recording or noting anything out of the ordinary and then reporting that information to your supervisor or the physician, is as important as knowing the proper procedure for recording the ECG. Such aware-

ness is the first step in the assessment of the patient's condition and carrying out his or her needed treatment.

What Is an Arrhythmia?

When a heart beats regularly, it generally beats at a rate of 60 to 100 beats per minute. This is called *normal sinus rhythm*. When this rhythm begins to deviate, causing an abnormal increase or decrease of the beats, a chain reaction usually results, triggering what is known as an *arrhythmia*.

An arrhythmia is a medical term generally used to describe any form of abnormality of the heart, including disturbances in the heart's rate, rhythm, and conduction system. Some of the more common irregularities causing cardiac arrhythmias include sinus bradycardia; atrial flutter; right and left bundle branch blocks; sinus tachycardia; premature atrial and ventricular contractions; atrial fibrillation; first-, second-, and third-degree heart blocks; ventricular tachycardia; ventricular fibrillation; and the most fatal of all arrhythmias, ventricular asystole.

Most cardiac arrhythmias are classified according to their effect on the anatomical structure of the heart. They include arrhythmias of the SA node, atrial tachycardias, premature atrial contractions, and ventricular arrhythmias.

Arrhythmias Originating at the SA Node

Arrhythmias which originate from the SA node are considered the least dangerous of all arrhythmias. The most common of these include sinus bradycardia, sinus tachycardia, sinus arrest, and a wandering pacemaker.

A *sinus bradycardia* (Figure 12-4) is characterized as a sinus rate, still originating its impulses from the SA node, but falling below 60 beats per minute. This

Figure 12-3
The ECG complex and a typical ECG rhythm strip.

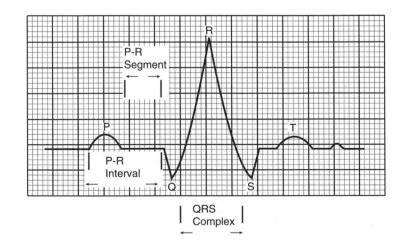

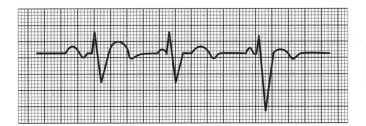

Figure 12-4
Rhythm strip showing sinus bradycardia.

type of arrhythmia is generally found in what is otherwise a healthy person, especially if he or she is an athlete who has an enlarged heart from excessive exercise. Sinus bradycardia may also be seen as an underlying heart condition, as in the case of a patient who has sustained a myocardial infarction or heart attack.

Another common arrhythmia, as we have already noted, is *sinus tachycardia* (Figure 12-5). In this condition, the heart usually beats at an abnormally fast rate, generally ranging between 100 and 160 beats per minute. Sinus tachycardia may also be experienced by otherwise normal, healthy people, and in these cases it is most often associated with anxiety or strenuous exercise.

The arrhythmia originating from the SA node that is considered the most dangerous is *sinus arrest* (Figure 12-6). Occasionally the SA node may momentarily fail, resulting in a loss of the impulse. This may be the result of an increased vagal stimulation, such as overeating, excessive consumption of coffee or cigarettes, or even taking an unusually deep "gulp" of air. If this momentary stopping of the impulse does occur, sinus arrest may result, causing a literal "standstill" of the heart.

The most confusing of arrhythmias originating from the SA node, is the *wandering pacemaker*. This confusion is present because the site of the impulse shifts. Sometimes the beats originate in the SA node; other times they may occur in the AV node or at an irritable atrial focus (Figure 12-7). A wandering pacemaker can be caused by irritated atrial tissues stemming from a rheumatic heart condition or from an infection. It can also be a result of an excessive buildup of heart medication such as digitalis. Ironically, despite its unusual configuration, a wandering pacemaker arrhythmia is rarely considered dangerous or life-threatening.

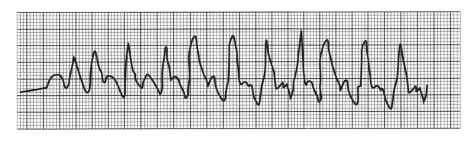

Figure 12-5
Rhythm strip showing sinus tachycardia.

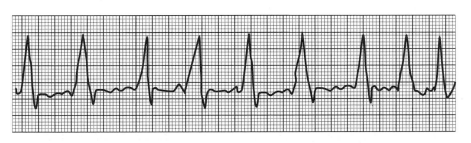

Figure 12-6
Rhythm strip showing sinus arrhythmia.

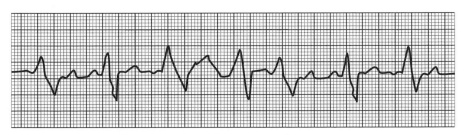

Figure 12-7
Rhythm strip showing a wandering pacemaker.

Atrial Tachycardia Arrhythmias

Arrhythmias in excess of 160 beats per minute and originating from the atrium are classified as atrial tachycardias. These include paroxysmal atrial tachycardia, atrial flutter, and atrial fibrillation.

Paroxysmal atrial tachycardia, or *PAT* (Figure 12-8) is a type of arrhythmia that can occur in otherwise healthy people. However, when such a condition is present, it is generally considered a forerunner to a very serious ventricular arrhythmia. A PAT is a very rapid regular heartbeat that begins suddenly and usually has been preceded by frequent premature atrial contractions. In some cases, the tachycardia is brief, while at other times, it can last hours.

Another atrial tachycardic condition, often misdiagnosed as a PAT because of its impulse originating from an atrial ectopic focus, is *atrial flutter* (Figure 12-9). In patients suffering from atrial flutter, the actual atrial rate ranges from 220 to 350 beats per minute, while the ventricles beat at a much slower rate, usually about 75 beats per minute. What is most interesting about this condition is that in most cases of atrial flutter, the rhythm of the ventricles is almost always regular.

Atrial fibrillation is a third type of atrial tachycardia. It is easily recognized because of its grossly irregular ventricular rhythm (Figure 12-10). As with the other two atrial arrhythmias, in atrial fibrillation, the impulse originates in an atrial ectopic area, thereby creating a chaotic baseline. In fibrillation, the flutter waves are not uniform and vary in shape and width. They can "fire" as high as 500 beats per minute, causing the PR interval to be very irregular.

Premature Atrial Contractions

Premature atrial contractions, or *PACs,* (Figure 12-11) originate from an atrial ectopic focus, thereby producing an abnormal P wave earlier than expected. Because the impulse does not originate in

Figure 12-8
Rhythm strip showing parox-ysmal atrial tachycardia.

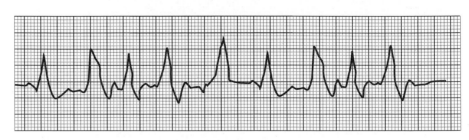

Figure 12-9
Rhythm strip showing atrial flutter.

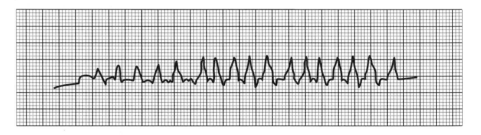

Figure 12-10
Rhythm strip showing atrial fibrillation.

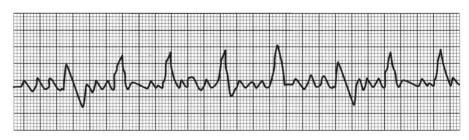

Figure 12-11
Rhythm strip showing a premature atrial contraction.

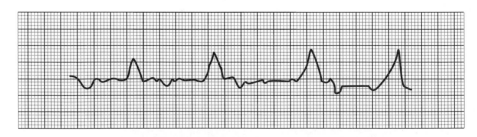

the SA node, this arrhythmia generally appears like other P waves in the same lead. In the ECG, PACs almost always portray an abnormal P-wave configuration, such as being flat, slurred, notched, inverted, or overly widened. The PR interval of the premature beat also appears shorter than normal, depending on the location of the P wave.

Arrhythmias Originating in the Ventricles

Ventricular arrhythmias are almost always considered serious and usually occur quite suddenly, and despite vigorous treatment, often result in rapid death. Arrhythmias classified in this category include premature ventricular contractions (PVCs), ventricular tachycardia, ventricular fibrillation, ventricular flutter, ventricular asystole, right and left bundle branch blocks, and first-, second-, and complete AV blocks.

Premature ventricular contractions (Figure 12-12) are arrhythmias originating in the ectopic focus of the ventricular myocardium. Although they may occur in seemingly healthy persons, they are most often seen when the heart is diseased or injured. During the PVC, the ventricles are stimulated prematurely and therefore will contract before the expected time. Their seriousness is determined not only by how often they occur, but also how close they are to the T wave of the preceding beat.

Ventricular tachycardia (Figure 12-13), as it is seen on the ECG, is easily identified by its wide, uniform QRS complex and its regular rhythm. Since most patients cannot tolerate high ventricular rates for long periods of time, they must be treated immediately with intravenous lidocaine. In some cases, cardioshock can be used in order to revert the heart back to a normal sinus rhythm.

Ventricular fibrillation (Figure 12-14), considered to be a life-threatening emergency, is created by stimuli from many ventricular ectopic foci, causing a chaotic twitching of the ventricles. Because there are so many ectopic foci "firing" at the same time, the result is an ineffective pumping action occurring within the ventricles.

Another arrhythmia originating in the ventricles is called *ventricular flutter* (Figure 12-15). The arrhythmia is preceeded by a single ventricular ectopic focus firing at a rate of 200 to 300 times per minute. The condition is characterized by an extremely fast rate and is considered highly dangerous. It can deteriorate quickly into the patient's death.

Of all the cardiac emergencies, *asystole*, or *ventricular standstill* (Figure 12-16), is considered to strike the greatest fear among nurses and cardiac technicians. It is always life-threatening; however, it does not always have to be fatal.

Asystole means, quite literally, absence of contraction. The heart does not beat and its appearance

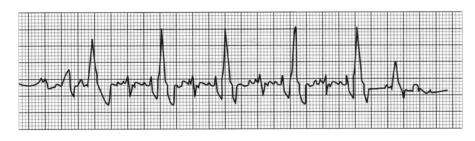

Figure 12-12
Rhythm strip showing a premature ventricular contraction.

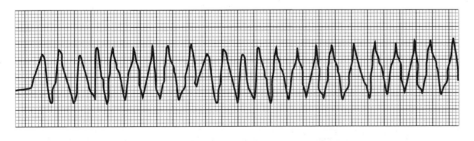

Figure 12-13
Rhythm strip showing ventricular tachycardia.

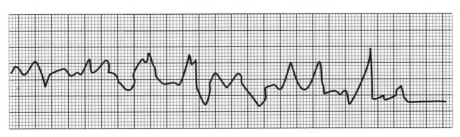

Figure 12-14
Rhythm strip showing ventricular fibrillation.

Figure 12-15
Rhythm strip showing ventricular flutter.

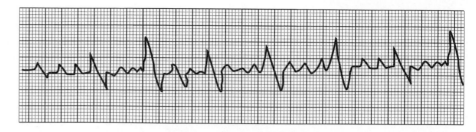

Figure 12-16
Rhythm strip showing ventricular asystole.

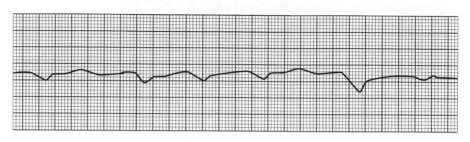

on the ECG is a straight line. It is commonly a direct result of hypoxia, or impaired respiratory functions, however, it can also be caused from a drug overdose.

Bundle branch blocks are classified according to their location and their degree (Figure 12-17A to D). A *right bundle branch block* is usually accompanied by sinus tachycardia. As seen in the ECG, the P wave is not distinct; therefore, it may resemble ventricular tachycardia.

In a *left bundle branch block*, the rhythm may resemble ventricular tachycardia if there is sinus tachycardia, and atrial activity, such as when the P wave precedes a QRS complex, a situation that rarely occurs.

A *first-degree heart block* is defined as a complete heart block, in which case both the atria and the ventricles are beating independently and there is no apparent relationship between the P waves and the QRS

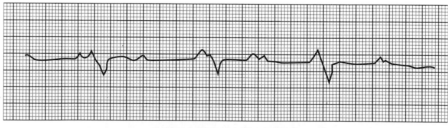

A. First-Degree Heart Block

Figure 12-17
Rhythm strips showing heart blocks.

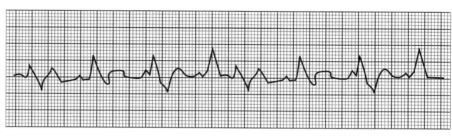

B. Second-Degree Heart Block

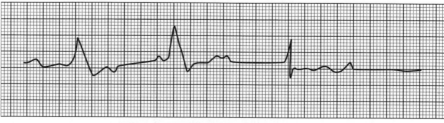

C. Complete Heart Block

complex. In *second-degree heart block*, the P wave is not followed by the QRS complex. In some cases, as in the *Wenkebach phenomenon*, there is a progressive prolongation of the PR interval until a P wave finally fails to conduct to the ventricles.

Summary

In this chapter, we discussed the skills involved in basic arrhythmia recognition and interpretation, including a discussion on the various components of the cardiac cycle, how to recognize an abnormal ECG, and how to identify and interpret arrhythmias of the SA node, sinus tachycardia, sinus arrest, a wandering pacemaker, and sinus bradycardia. We also talked about how to recognize and identify many of the more commonly seen arrhythmias, such as atrial tachycardias, atril flutter and atrial fibrillation, premature atrial and ventricular contractions, ventricular fibrillation and ventricular flutter, and ventricular asystole. Finally, we discussed the differences between right and left bundle branch blocks and first- and second-degree heart blocks.

Review Questions

1. Briefly define the following terms:

   a. bradycardia _____

   b. tachycardia _____

2. Briefly define the following terms related to the heartbeat and pulse:

   a. rate _____

   b. rhythm _____

3. What is a medical term used to describe an abnormal heartbeat?

4. The four elements we look for in basic interpretation of ECGs include:

   a. _____

   b. _____

   c. _____

   d. _____

5. Briefly explain what is meant by the *cardiac cycle*.

6. Briefly explain what is meant by the *QRS duration* and *QRS complex*.

7. What structure within the heart is considered the *pacemaker*?

8. Identify at least three arrhythmias that might be seen on the ECG:

   a. _____

   b. _____

   c. _____

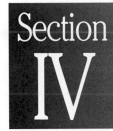
Echocardiography: Basic Concepts and Applications

Author's Disclaimer Regarding Section on Echocardiography

The following chapters dealing with the study of medical ultrasound and echocardiography are being provided to the reader as informational, and in no way are representative of the many aspects and skills involved in studying to become a Licensed Cardiac Echocardiographic Technician. If you are interested in seeking a career in medical sonography, echocardiography, or becoming licensed, the author recommends that you contact the American Registry for Diagnostic Medical Sonography. They will provide you with an updated list of schools and institutions that offer career programs in these fields.

13

Introduction to Medical Ultrasound

Performance Objectives

Upon completion of this chapter, you will be able to:

1. Identify four variables used to determine how sound is transmitted through a medium.
2. Briefly explain acoustic velocity as it relates to how sound travels in air, muscle, and bone.
3. List the major components of an ultrasound machine.
4. Briefly explain why a gel is applied to a patient's skin for an ultrasound examination.
5. Name three ways to record ultrasound examinations for documentation.
6. Identify four different organ systems in the body that can be imaged by ultrasound.
7. Describe the role and the responsibilities of the ultrasound technologist.

Terms and Abbreviations

Acoustic velocity   the calculated speed at which sound waves travel through a given medium, such as a solid, liquid, or gas.

Artifact   the production of normal echoes from the sound beam found on an ultrasound image.

Echo   the sound that bounces back to the transducer after a pulse of sound has been transmitted into the body.

Echocardiography   the study of the heart using ultrasound to document motion and internal structures of the heart.

Frequency   the number of cycles per second.

Real-time scanner   an ultrasound machine that records simulta-

neously as the event occurs, e.g., recording a tracing of how a person's heart is beating.

Transducer   a device used to transform energy from one form to another, e.g., electrical energy into sound energy.

Transmission   the transfer of energy from one molecule to another without the energy changing form.

Ultrasound   any sound wave having a frequency greater than 20,000 hertz; when used for medical imaging, ultrasound is also referred to as diagnostic medical sonography.

While the concept of ultrasound technology was originally developed for industrial and military use, it has also proven to be very successful in medical applications. The use of diagnostic ultrasound in the clinical area was first introduced back in the late 1950s and early 1960s. At that time, it was determined that such a device could be used to record the heart sounds as well as provide the clinician with an image of the pregnant uterus. However, in the first two decades such a technology was not very widely accepted. Then came the 1970s, when the use of ultrasound as a tool for diagnosing proliferated the medical world. All of a sudden the device was considered a "miracle machine" because of its capabilities in distinguishing normal from abnormal tissues in various parts of the body. Currently, high-speed, real-time scanners are used that allow rapid visualization and interpretation of scans. Diagnostic ultrasound continues to advance with the ever-increasing ability to use computer technology to store data that can give the physician more information and improve the overall standard of health care.

How Ultrasound Works

Ultrasound, which is also known as *sonography*, is based on the concept of using sound waves that occur at frequencies much higher than the human ear can detect, to record an image of a specific structure. Humans generally hear sound within a 20 to 20,000 hertz (Hz, cycles per second) range, so ultrasound is considered anything greater than 20,000 Hz. When used for imaging purposes, ultrasound is able to generate frequencies between 1 million and 12 million Hz.

The sound waves carry energy from one place to another. The speed depends upon variables in the medium being used. These variables include pressure, density, temperature, and particle motion. Sound waves need gas, liquid, or solid media to transmit energy from one particle to the next. In a gas, sound travels relatively slowly because the molecules are spaced farther apart, while in a liquid or solid, the molecules are closer together and more rigid, thus resulting in a faster transmission of the sound waves. The rate at which sound passes through any given substance can be measured and is known as *acoustic* or *sound velocity*. Table 13-1 lists some of the velocities of sound traveling through different parts of the body. Ultrasound machines are programed to generate images using the average velocity of soft tissue, which is 1540 meters/second (m/s). Currently, ultrasound machines are unable to scan areas that have significantly higher or lower velocities than 1540 m/s. Therefore, ultrasound examinations cannot include lung, intestine, or bone structures, because these body parts have velocities that are beyond the capabilities of the machines.

The Ultrasound Machine

Typically, the ultrasound machine consists of a computer that contains various hand-operated knobs for manipulating the images. These images are seen on the CRT, which is a viewing monitor much like a

Table 13-1
Acoustic Velocity in Body Parts

Tissue or Material	Acoustic Velocity (m/s)
Air	331
Fat	1450
Water	1495
Soft tissue	1540
Kidney	1561
Muscle	1585
Bone	4080

television screen. The machine also contains devices for both photographing and probing the images being scanned (Figure 13-1).

A typical ultrasound machine will have from 3 to 10 probes, which are also known as *transducers*, each of which is designed for a specific purpose. One probe, for example, would be used for the pregnant uterus, while another would be used for the heart, another for the thyroid gland, and so on. Each probe contains crystals, usually made of a quartz or ceramic material, that when electronically stimulated, produce ultrasound waves. The probes are called transducers because they are able to change energy from one form to another; in this case, an electric pulse is changed to a sound pulse. These sonic waves are transmitted into the body through a water-soluble gel that is applied to the patient's skin. The gel eliminates air particles between the probe and the skin, which helps the sound beam penetrate farther into the body. The probe also emits a very short pulse of ultrasound, then "waits" for the second waves to interact with the tissues, and then bounce or reflect back to the probe. The probe is in this waiting mode about 99 percent of the time, during which it is gathering information from the reflected sound. The machine can then calculate whether the waves traveled through a liquid, solid, soft tissue, or a gas.

Recording the Ultrasound Examination

There are several different ways to photograph the ultrasound examination. Most commonly, hard-copy film, which is the same as x-ray film, or black-and-white Polaroid film is used for documentation. For very complete recordings, the examination can also be put on videotape, which is a great deal more useful for documenting the entire examination than selecting and freeze-framing a picture to photograph on hard copy. In comparing the methods used for photographing, during a 20 minute examination, a hard copy would provide approximately 30 images, while a video would indicate about 1800 images. The ultrasound machine produces about 30 frames per second, which is about the same rate as for video equipment. Thus, ultrasound machines show a full range of motion, such as blood particles swirling through a vein, without visual delay.

Using Ultrasound as a Tool in Diagnosing Cardiovascular Disease

The list of examinations that can be done by ultrasound is quite extensive. It includes such structures as the heart, the pelvis, the uterus, the abdomen, the

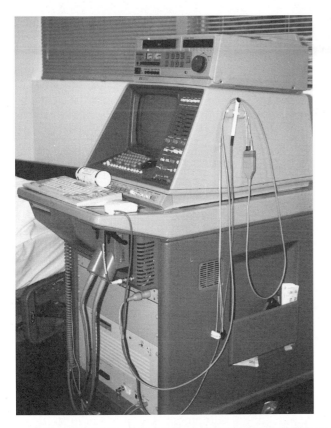

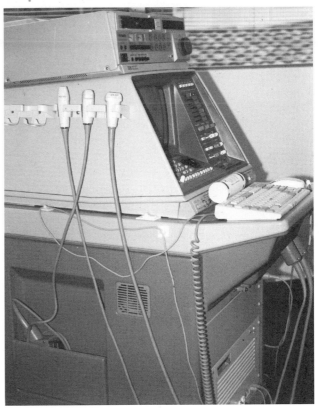

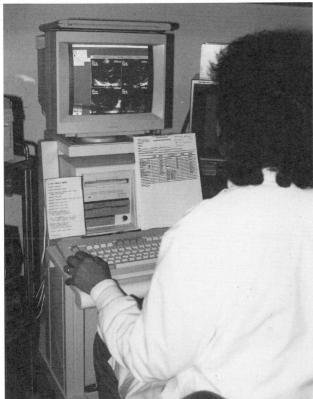

Figure 13-1
The ultrasound machine.

gallbladder, and the kidney. The machine can also examine very minute structures such as blood clots in arteries and veins.

When the heart is being imaged, the examination is known as *echocardiography*, which literally means studying the heart with sound waves. This imaging can provide the physician with valuable information on how well the heart muscles and valves are working. In patients with heart disease, this test can record abnormal movement of blood through the heart, as well as reveal areas in the heart wall where the muscle has been replaced with scar tissue from a previous heart attack. Or this test could show that a virus has made it difficult for the heart to pump adequately. In severe cases, where a patient has received a heart transplant, the ultrasound examination can also provide close monitoring of potential complications. This test can also be performed to evaluate for birth defects, some of which may be surgically corrected. More rarely, tumors that have originated from the heart muscle can also be detected.

In some cases, the physician may want to use ultrasound to detect abnormal blood flow patterns. By using an examination known as *Doppler* ultrasound, the examination is able to both distinguish between normal and abnormal blood flow patterns, as well as measure the velocity of the blood flowing through the arteries and veins. Doppler is particularly useful in measuring blood flow in transplanted organs, and in the evaluation of the blood's circulation in artherosclerotic arteries.

Role of the Ultrasound Technologist

In no other imaging modality is the role of the technician who performs the examination as crucial in assisting the physician as it is in ultrasound. Also known as a sonographer, this person must not only choose which image to photograph, but also is responsible for incorporating clinical and technical knowledge in order to obtain pertinent information. To be able to integrate both the patient's history with the information seen on the images, this person must be familiar with many different aspects of clinical medicine. Working together with the physician, the sonographer provides maximum diagnostic information about each patient.

During the ultrasound examination, the technician's role is comparable to that of a detective solving a mystery. For example, a patient checks into the hospital emergency room because she is having pain on the right side of her abdomen. An abdominal ultrasound examination is ordered to try to determine the source of pain. It is the responsibility of the sonographer to gather as many "clues" as she can from interviewing the patient. The interview would include such questions as "Where do you hurt? How long have you had the pain? Does food upset your stomach? Have you had a fever? Have you ever had this pain before?" and so on. What the patient relates to the technician in terms of his or her history must also be correlated with other tests, such as blood tests or x-rays. By the end of the ultrasound scan, the technician will have thoroughly studied the images and put the facts together to form an opinion on the patient's diagnosis. The next step is to present such findings to the doctor for interpretation. Based upon an accurate and complete examination, it is the doctor who is ultimately responsible for making the diagnosis. In some very rare cases, the technician and the physician may need to consult with various textbooks or other physicians in order to gain an understanding of how the disease would appear on the ultrasound images.

In addition to being well-versed in anatomy, physiology, and pathology, the ultrasound technician must also know how to use the equipment effectively. Modern machines have many different features that allow the operator to change the way in which the information can be displayed. Skillful interaction with the equipment is required both to recognize created artifacts that may be mistaken for pathology and to avoid missing pertinent diagnostic information. *Artifacts* can be created by the production of nonreal echoes from the sound beam on the ultrasound image. An echo is the sound wave that is reflected back from the patient's anatomy. Reflected sound waves that give a distorted, inaccurate image are called *nonreal echoes*. The ability to distinguish nonreal echoes from real ones is a skill that can only be achieved through experience and a knowledge of the physics involved in transmitting sound waves through the human body.

The ultrasound technician is also expected to recognize emergency conditions in a patient and be able to perform or assist with basic life-support procedures. Some examinations are ordered because a life-threatening situation exists. Also, like all health care professionals, sonographers must be equiped with the skills to exercise proper judgment in their interactions with the patient and his or her family. It is of great importance to respect and honor the patient's or the family's right to choose an appropriate level of treatment.

The sonographer may elect to work in any number of settings. Since most hospitals require 24-hour coverage, the technologist may have to carry a beeper to cover the hospital after a regular work shift. Most hospitals also have set protocols on handling specific medical conditions, such as handling patients with communicable diseases, that are designed to protect both the patient and the health care worker.

Careers in Medical Ultrasound

Working in the field of medical ultraound is very challenging. Students entering this area of health care must acquire clear communication skills and problem-solving techniques, as well as have the ability to address both ethical and legal questions. They must also have the insight to address actual life-altering decisions. Ultrasound is an expanding field, and in the future, even more exciting technological breakthroughs can be expected.

Currently, throughout the United States, there are not enough qualified technologists to fill the job market for skilled medical ultraound technicians. To ensure the highest degree of technical competence, most health care facilities required the sonographer to have passed a national examination given by the American Registry for Diagnostic Medical Sonography. Graduation with a Bachelor of Science or a Bachelor of Arts degree automatically qualifies the sonographer for higher paying positions and faster promotions.

There are a variety of programs that exist for training ultrasound technicians. Most states have at least one formal program in diagnostic medical sonography. Some larger medical schools accept a few students to train along with medical residents and interns who are training in radiology. About half of the training schools require applicants to have previous training in an allied health field so that they will already have successfully completed basic generalized courses, such as anatomy and mathematics, and can focus only on ultrasound. These schools may also offer a certificate upon completion. Other schools might require two years of general college courses for admission into their ultrasound technology program.

Summary

In this chapter, we looked at the study of diagnostic medical ultrasound, which is also known as sonography. We identified four variables that determine how sound is transmitted through a medium, as well as discussed the speed of sound transmitted as it relates to how sound travels in air, muscle, or bone. We also talked about the ultrasound machine, and briefly described three ways we use the machine to record ultrasound examinations for documentation on different organ systems. Finally, we discussed the role and responsibilities of the ultrasound technician, determining that such a position requires that the student be a clear communicator and problem-solver, and have the ability to address both ethical and legal questions and make life-altering decisions.

Review Questions

1. Define the following terms as they relate to the study of medical ultrasound:
   a. acoustic velocity _____
   b. frequency _____
   c. artifact _____
   d. transmission _____

2. What is the name of the device used in medical ultrasound that transforms energy from one form to another?

3. The study of the heart using ultrasound to document motion and internal structures is called _____.
   a. electrocardiography
   b. echocardiography

4. The acoustic velocity is lowest in which of the following:
   a. air
   b. water
   c. bone

5. The acoustic velocity is highest in which of the following:
   a. air
   b. water
   c. bone

6. The acoustic velocity (in m/s) of soft tissue is:
   a. 1585
   b. 1540
   c. 1450

7. How are artifacts created on the ultrasound image?

8. Briefly explain the role of the *American Registry for Diagnostic Medical Sonography* as it relates to the training and certification of the echocardiographic technician.

14

Doppler Principles and Hemodynamics in Echocardiography

Performance Objectives

Upon completion of this chapter, you will be able to:

1. Define the purpose and function of Doppler echocardiography.
2. Discuss Doppler systems.
3. Briefly explain the use of continuous-wave, pulsed-wave, and high-PRF Doppler.
4. Briefly explain the use of color flow Doppler.
5. Discuss hemodynamics as it relates to echocardiography.

Terms and Abbreviations

Cardiac catheterization   a procedure to record the hemodynamic data in specific chambers and the great vessels of the heart.

Color flow Doppler   a form of pulsed Doppler that displays flow data directly onto a two-dimensional image.

Continuous-wave Doppler   the arranging of two ultrasound crystals within the same transducer.

Doppler Principle   a principle used in echocardiography to determine the direction and velocity of moving blood.

Hemodynamics   the branch of medicine dealing with the forces and mechanicsms involved in the circulation of blood throughout the body.

Pulsed-wave Doppler   integrates one spot for abnormal flow within a two-dimensional array.

Doppler echocardiography has been around for more than 25 years. The relatively recent explosion in the interest and use of Doppler occurred when the technique was combined with two-dimensional echocardiography. Knowing the direction of the Doppler beam and where the Doppler sample is placed has allowed the technician to acquire an easier understanding of spectral traces. Today, Doppler echocardiography is used expressly for determining the direction and velocity of moving blood, the estimation of valvular gradients, and in the detection of turbulent blood flow.

The very first description of the physical principles of Doppler echocardiography was attributed to a scientist and mathematician by the name of Johanna Christian Doppler. In his initial writings he described the Doppler principle as having to to do with changes in the wavelength of light from the stars. In 1842, he presented a paper entitled "On the Colored Light of Double Stars and Some Other Heavenly Bodies." In this paper, he suggested that the color of some stars was caused by their motion relative to the earth. Blue stars, he said, "were moving towards the earth and the red stars were moving away." We now know that his descriptions of the changes in wavelength of light was wrong and that blue stars are actually moving away from the earth and red ones, moving towards us.

Although Dr. Doppler never extrapolated his theory to include sound waves, others who came after him tried to prove his theory wrong by testing it using a change in pitch of sound. This change in pitch is familiar to anyone who has heard an ambulance siren. As the ambulance moves toward you, the compression of sound waves results in a higher pitch being heard. As the siren is moving away from you, it has a lower pitch to it. This change in pitch or frequency is the basis for what is now known as Doppler echocardiography.

Understanding Doppler Ultrasound

Doppler ultrasound measures the difference between the transmitted and returned frequencies of sound waves. The change in frequency occurs when the ultrasound wave hits a moving target. In Doppler, the moving targets are the red blood cells. The faster the red blood cells are traveling in relationship to the stationary transducer, the greater the change in frequency. When the flow moves away from the transducer, the frequency changes to a lower frequency than the one transmitted. Flow moving toward the transducer results in an increase in the returned frequency.

Normal blood flow is laminar, meaning that the direction and velocity of the red blood cells are approximately the same. When there is a disturbance to this blood flow, there is a disruption to the normal laminar flow pattern. Most of the time turbulent blood flow indicates underlying pathology. For example, aortic stenosis has both an increased turbulence and a marked rise in the blood flow velocity.

Most Doppler systems display velocity information utilizing spectral analysis. Flow toward the transducer results in a positive deflection above the baseline on the spectral display, while flow away from the transducer results in a negative deflection. The faster the velocity in either direction, the greater the deflection. When most of the red blood cells are moving together, a narrow band of spectral data is displayed. This is the laminar flow. When flow is turbulent, there are many different velocities that are being detected at the same time. Thus a wide spectrum of velocities is displayed. Because spectral analysis records not only peak velocity but also the distribution of velocities, both the *mean* and the *maximum velocity* can be derived.

Doppler Systems

Continuous-wave Doppler

Of the various Doppler systems currently in use, continuous-wave Doppler is the oldest and easiest form to understand. It involves the arranging of two ultrasound crystals within the same transducer. One crystal is used to constantly emit sound waves, while the other crystal is used to constantly receive the returning signals. The advantage of continuous-wave Doppler lies in its ability to record high velocities accurately. Many of the Doppler machines being used today can record velocities of up to 15 m/s. This is twice what is normally considered to be the peak velocity found in the human body. The main disadvantage of using continuous-wave Doppler is that it lacks depth discrimination; that is, the technician does not know where along the ultrasound beam this high velocity is occurring. A 5-m turbulent jet may be just as likely to be located at a depth of 3 cm as it is at a depth of 15 cm. Moreover, the Doppler shift is recorded from all moving red blood cells along this Doppler beam. Therefore, a possibility exists that more than one abnormal jet is being studied at any one time.

True continuous-wave Doppler is a technique without any imaging capabilities. There are machines that rapidly switch between imaging and Doppler modes using pulsed ultrasound and continous wave Doppler. In these time-sharing systems, there is some loss of signal-to-noise ratio of the Doppler and some degradation in the two-dimensional image. The advantage is that the ultrasound technician can see precisely where the Doppler beam is directed.

Pulsed-wave Doppler

Pulsed-wave systems allow the technician to selectively study one spot for abnormal flow within the two-dimensional array, thus allowing the sampling depth to be selected by the ultrasound technician. The size of the sample volume may be variable depending on the machine used and the depth at which you are trying to sample. Like all other ultrasound beams, the further away from the transducer, the more the beam diverges and the larger the sample volume becomes.

The main disadvantage to using the pulsed-wave Doppler is that there is a technical limitation to the peak velocity which can be accurately displayed. This limitation is known as the *Nyquist* limit, at which point *aliasing* occurs. Aliasing is represented on the spectral trace as a cutoff or limiting of the velocity in any one direction. Velocities that exceed this aliasing point or Nyquist limit are still maintained on the spectral trace and appear to be going in the same direction but in the opposite channel.

Most pathological states result in an increase in the velocity beyond which a pulsed Doppler system can accurately record. The detection of peak velocity must be left up to continuous-wave Doppler. Pulsed-wave systems are useful for determining the exact location of abnormal flow and for looking at timing sequences.

High-PRF Doppler

Some ultrasound systems increase their pulsed repetition frequency (PRF), so that they operate between a pulsed and continuous mode. The Doppler machine sends out sequential pulses at known intervals, thus increasing the pulse repetition frequency and allowing the Nyquist limit to increase. The trade-off of high-PRF Doppler is that the velocity information is also recorded from other depths, thus causing the range selectivity to be lost. Table 14-1 shows the normal flow velocities for various flows.

Color Flow Doppler

Doppler color flow imaging is a form of pulsed Doppler that displays flow data directly onto the two-dimensional image. There is no spectral tracing and no audio signal available using this modality. This, however, allows excellent spatial information to exist between the anatomy and blood flow. This color display allows the inexperienced Doppler technician to understand more readily the size, direction, and the velocity of the blood flow. It also significantly reduces the examination time for regurgitant flows.

In color flow Doppler, flow toward the transducer is assigned a red color and flow away from the transducer is blue. All color flow machines have some type of a reference bar that shows these colors displayed on the Doppler screen. The center of the color bar is usually black and is representative of zero flow. Velocity is displayed as an increase in brightness going from a deep red toward a bright red in the forward direction and a dark blue to a lighter blue for flow moving away from the transducer.

Because color flow systems utilize the same principles as pulsed Doppler, there is a limitation to the velocity that can be recorded in any one direction based on the pulsed repetition rate. Aliasing in a color flow system results in a color shift when the mean velocity exceeds the Nyquist limit. Aliasing is easily seen because the shift that occurs across the

baseline would be from dark blue to dark red or vice versa.

Besides direction and velocity information, color flow systems can also detect the presence of turbulent flow. These systems detect when there is a large variation of velocity between adjacent flow areas and then adds shades of green into the display. When turbulence is detected and variance is added to the display, a multitude of colors, including a mosiac of red, blue, yellow, and cyan, is seen in the area of the abnormal flow.

Hemodynamics, Doppler, and Echocardiography

Hemodynamics is the branch of physiology that deals with the forces and mechanisms involved in the circulation of the blood. Although most cardiac sonographers are quite proficient in their knowledge of cardiac anatomy and echocardiographic appearance of pathology, they have little or no knowledge and understanding of cardiac pressure relationships.

With the advent of Doppler echocardiography, there is a need for the cardiac Doppler technician to have a sound understanding of normal and abnormal hemodynamics. Therefore, it is important that you fully familiarize yourself with basic pressure relationships in both the normal and the diseased heart.

Blood flows from an area of higher pressure to one of lower pressure. Figure 14-1 shows the normal timing and pressure differences between the various cardiac chambers and great vessels. Notice that the mitral valve closes (M1) when the left ventricular pressure exceeds the left atrial pressure. There is a time delay while the pressure builds high enough within the left ventricle to exceed the pressure in the aorta and open the aortic valve. This shaded area on the figure represents the isovolumic contraction time. At end-systole, there is another corresponding shaded area representing the isovolumic relaxation period after the aortic valve closes and before the mitral valve opens (OM). In normal healthy patients, the systolic pressure in the aorta and left ventricle are essentially the same.

Measuring Normal Pressures

The diagram of the heart shown in Figure 14-2 depicts the normal pressures for the various cardiac chambers and great vessels. Systolic pressures on the right side are four to five times lower than systolic pressures on the left.

When the physician wants to record the hemodynamic data in specific chambers and the great ves-

Table 14-1
Normal Doppler Flow Velocities

Flow	Children (m/s)	Adults (m/s)
Mitral diastolic	1.00 (0.7–1.4)	0.92 (0.6–1.4)
Tricuspid diastolic	0.62 (0.5–0.9)	0.58 (0.4–0.8)
Pulmonary systolic	0.84 (0.6–1.2)	0.72 (0.5–0.9)
Aortic systolic	1.52 (1.2–1.7)	1.40 (0.9–1.8)

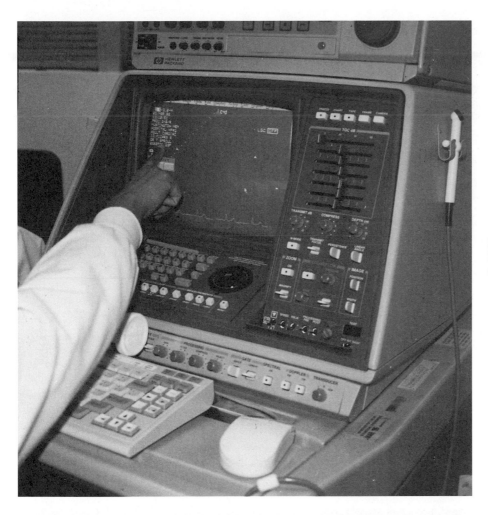

Figure 14-1
Normal timing and pressure differences.

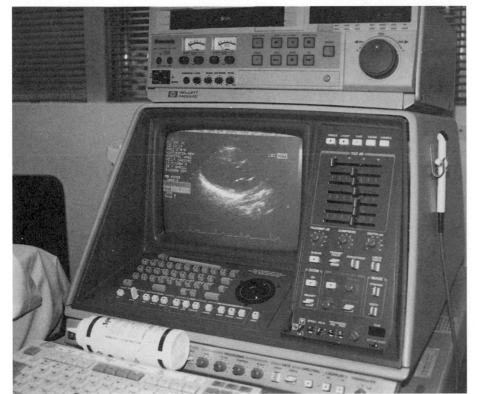

Figure 14-2
Heart showing normal pressures.

120

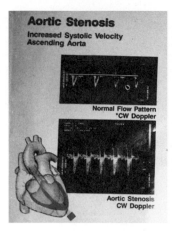

Figure 14-3
Pressure tracing seen in aortic stenosis.

sels, he or she uses a procedure known as *cardiac catheterization.* Figure 14-3 shows a pressure tracing from a patient with an aortic stenosis. A catheter within the left ventricle recorded a systolic pressure of approximately 140 mmHg. Another catheter is placed in the right femoral artery, which records a pressure of just over 110 mmHg. Normally, the systolic pressure in the left ventricle and aorta are equal.

The peak-to-peak difference or gradient between the left ventricle and aorta is quickly seen to be 30 mmHg. Since there is a time delay for the pressure to

be transmitted from the proximal aorta to the right femoral artery, the pressure waveform for the aortic pressure is delayed in relationship to the left ventricular pressure. It is much easier to calculate a peak-to-peak gradient in this patient than a peak instantaneous gradient that would necessitate moving the aortic pressure tracing to the left in order to correspond with the timing of the left ventricular systole.

Most catheterization laboratories report a peak-to-peak and a mean aortic gradient but not the peak instantaneous gradient. Doppler echocardiography records the peak instantaneous gradient and problems that may arise concerning the differences between gradients obtained with Doppler and catheterization methods. Many gradients obtained at catheterization and with Doppler techniques, correlate well.

Summary

In this chapter, we discussed the purpose and function of Doppler echocardiography. We also talked about the various types of Doppler systems currently in use, including continuous-wave, pulsed-wave, high-PRF, and color flow Doppler. Finally, we discussed hemodynamics and its relationship to echocardiography.

Review Questions

1. What is the name of the procedure used to record the hemodynamic data in specific chambers and blood vessels of the heart?

2. Briefly explain the difference between *color flow Doppler* and *continuous-wave Doppler.*

3. What is the name of the branch of medicine that deals with

the forces and mechanisms involved in the circulation of blood throughout the body?

4. What purpose does *pulsed-wave Doppler* provide?

5. What is the difference between *systolic pressure* and *diastolic pressure*?

15

Patient Echocardiographic Examinations

Performance Objectives

Upon completion of this chapter, you will be able to:

1. Define what is involved in determining patient echocardiographic examinations.
2. Identify initial control settings for patient examinations.
3. Discuss transducer positioning and angulation.
4. Discuss echocardiographic examination of infants and children.
5. Briefly explain contrast echocardiography.
6. Discuss two-dimensional echocardiography.
7. Explain how the echocardiographic technician overcomes difficulties in obtaining the echocardiograph tracing.

Terms and Abbreviations

ASE abbreviation for the American Society of Echocardiographers, a national organization established to set the standards for licensed echocardiographers.

Contrast echocardiography technique in which some type of ultrasonic contrast agent is introduced into the heart in order to study its anatomy and function.

M-mode echocardiography system of echocardiography in which moving structures within the heart are recorded as wavy lines moving across an oscilloscope.

Parasternal border area that refers to the left sternal border.

Two-dimensional echocardiography system of echocardioigraphy in which the ultrasonic beam is electronically or mechanically moved through a sector over a specific area of the heart.

Patient examination in echocardiography involves locating various intracardiac structures and then obtaining the very best possible recording of them so that their movements can be evaluated and adequately measured. The technique requires that the technician become very familiar with cardiac anatomy and physiology, rapid recognition of valve structures and motion patterns, and thoroughly understands all of the individual controls found on the echocardiographic machine.

Before beginning an echocardiographic examination, it is extremely helpful to have any available and relevant clinical information regarding the patient. This may include a cardiac history, a chest x-ray report, an ECG interpretation, a listing of the patient's medications, and the physician's clinical diagnosis. These will aid the technician in obtaining a better tracing and ultimately will help the cardiologist in interpreting it.

During the examination, the patient should be comfortably lying on a bed or examination table. Initially, the patient should be supine, although this probably will be changed as the test progresses. Most often the patient must be turned to a left lateral position in order to provide for an optimum recording of all pertinent structures, particularly the interventricular septum. A small pillow, or foam rubber wedge, may be placed against the patient's back, which will provide for a comfortable position at a desired angle. All clothing from the patient's waist up should also be removed prior to beginning the examination.

Although it is possible to peform an echocardiographic examination at a patient's bedside, better results are usually obtained in the echo laboratory. For example, at bedside the space may be cramped, the bed and other furniture may have to be moved, and the lighting may be too intense for adequate visualization of the oscilloscope, or CRT, part of the machine. In the laboratory, however, light levels can be controlled, the equipment can be arranged to your best advantage, and the patient can be made more comfortable.

An important first step in patient examination consists of relating a little about the test and reassuring the patient that it is a completely painless and harmless, yet somewhat tedious, procedure. The patient may be afraid that the transducer will emit an electric current or otherwise harmful beam. Explain briefly and simply what will happen and that it will in no way cause the patient any harm.

Since most patients have absolutely no idea what an echocardiogram is and what the test accomplishes, explaining it in simple, understandable terms will ease the patient's worries. Also be sure to mention that the examination cannot be completed in 5 or 10 minutes, and that one-half hour or longer is not unusual for an echocardiogram. This is important, because many patients equate any heart examination with an ECG and therefore presume it will be finished within a very few minutes. When it is not, they become increasingly nervous and apprehensive, fearing that something is radically wrong. Always remember, that a patient who knows what to expect and how to cooperate to facilitate the test will help the examination progress much faster, provide better results, and make the technician's job much easier.

The importance of being relaxed and comfortable applies to the technician as well as to the patient. Because the examination may be lengthy, and because the tiniest of transducer movements could result in losing a much-sought-after echo, your instrument should be positioned so that you can easily reach the controls without stretching or bending or moving the transducer. It does not matter if you use your right hand to manipulate the transducer and your left to adjust the instrument controls or vice versa. This is simply a matter of preference. What matters is that both you and the patient are as comfortable as possible.

Once the preliminaries are over, attach the ECG limb electrodes in the same standard manner as though you were going to run an ECG. Next, squeeze a generous portion of transmission gel onto the patient's chest at the chosen site and place the transducer in that area. Once you have started the procedure, it is important that you remember not to press too hard, since pressing will not bring in valve echoes; only proper angulation and instrument control will do that. Exert only enough pressure to maintain an airtight contact between the transducer and the skin and to keep the transducer from sliding. Steady your own hand by letting the palm rest lightly on the patient's chest.

Setting Initial Controls

If your echocardiograph machine is not equipped with simultaneous A-mode and M-mode display screens, you will have to start the examination with the oscilloscope in the A-mode in order to ensure that all controls are properly adjusted. Set them in the following manner:

- *Start delay*. At minimum. If an ECG is run at the top, be sure that the start delay is low enough so that the QRS complexes are not lost.
- *Depth*. 15 cm. You should see echoes from the posterior wall, plus a few centimeters beyond.
- *Coarse gain*. Set at midrange. Use just enough coarse gain to provide adequate visualization of valve structures.
- *Near gain*. Set at approximately one third of available gain. You will need only enough near gain to "fill in" the anterior display with adequate echo signals.
- *Depth compression*. For routine purposes, set at the level of the interventricular septum. The purpose of this control is to compensate for the amount of body tissue the ultrasound waves must penetrate. Therefore, if your patient is thin, the initial depth compression should be set closer to the chest wall than in obese patients.
- *Damp*. In those machines with a five-position control, set on 1, or at approximately 20 percent of available damping power. Excessive damping will affect the amplitude of echoes displayed.
- *Reject*. In machines with a five-position control, set on 2; otherwise set it at the approximate midrange.
- *ECG*. Lead II should be positioned at the top or bottom of the display.
- *Paper speed*. Set at 25 mm/s. Always remember to advance the paper speed to 50 mm/s to facilitate the measurement of valve slopes.
- *Time marker*. Should be set at 0.5 s. When 50 mm/s recording speed is used, set the timing markers to 0.1 or 0.2 s.

It is important that you remember that the controls, as they are initially set, must be constantly adjusted in order to obtain an optimum tracing. It is of primary importance, then, to become thoroughly familiar with every control and to be able to use them to their, and your, best advantage.

Transducer Positioning and Angulation

The mitral valve is an excellent landmark for beginning the echocardiographic examination. It is best recorded with the transducer placed along the *parasternal border* in either the third or fourth intercostal space. From this position, the transducer can be swept in an arc from the apex to the base of the heart, thus permitting excellent visualization of all four valve structures.

The areas of transducer placement, however, are limited, and herein lies much of the difficulty in the echocardiographic technique. Medially, placement is bounded by the sternum; laterally, by the edges of the lungs; inferiorly, by the boundaries of the heart itself and the diaphragm; and superiorly, by the lungs again. The ribs, too, limit transducer placement, because ultrasound is absorbed by bone. It must be placed in the spaces between the ribs, which are referred to as "acoustic windows" (Figure 15-1).

A good place to begin is in the fourth intercostal space, along the parasternal border. Bear in mind also that no single transducer placement is standard for every patient. In some patients, particularly those who are obese, the transducer may have to be placed in the third interspace and a little further to the left of the sternum. Angulation when going from one structure to another is also more lateral, because obese patients tend to have more horizontal hearts.

In tall, thin persons, a lower placement, such as

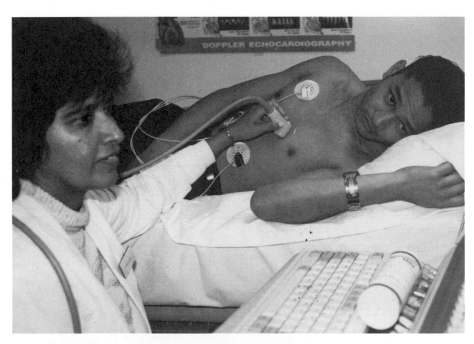

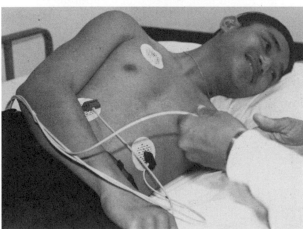

Figure 15-1
Transducer positioning and angulation.

perhaps the fifth interspace, will allow better visualization of the mitral valve. In these cases, the heart is more vertical; therefore, angulation of the transducer also is more vertical.

If your patient has a barrel chest, such as those suffering with certain lung diseases, the mitral valve may be best recorded from the fourth, fifth, or even the sixth intercostal space. The best method to follow at the onset of the examination is to try each interspace, then determine which window allows you the best visualization of the mitral valve and which permits a clean scan from the apex to the base of the heart. This window will provide the most accurate results.

Once you have placed the transducer in an appropriate interspace and have located a valve, you must obtain the best possible display of it. This is easily accomplished first by proper transducer angulation and, second by correct adjustment of the instrument controls.

Bring in the best echo signal by slowly rotating the transducer in a tiny circle, or by gently rocking it from side to side or up and down, all the while maintaining contact between the transducer and the skin. This will help you to change the direction of the beam until you "hit" the desired structure as close as possible to a 90 degree angle. When that happens, the strongest echo signal will be reflected. Remember always to move the transducer slowly and minutely, and always to maintain a mental image of where the best position previously was. If returning signals appear as broken lines, this means that the beam is not hitting the structure perpendicularly, and either the transducer angle or its position on the chest, or both, must be changed.

When going from one structure to another, it is equally important to move the transducer slowly and carefully and to always remember where the previous position was. Then, if you completely lose the echo signal, you can backtrack to the original position, and, if necessary, you can start again at a slightly different angle.

One final point must be emphasized. Severe transducer angulation can result in errors on the echocardiogram. It is of extreme importance, therefore, to position the transducer as close as possible to a perpendicular angle when recording any intracardiac structure, not only to obtain the strongest echo but, more importantly, to obtain the most accurate one.

Examination of Infants and Children

In general, the echocardiographic examination in infants and children does not differ appreciably from adults. It offers the advantage of fewer bony struc-

tures to impede the echo beam. Therefore, the transducer can usually be placed anywhere on the precordium with good results. Angulation, however, must be extremely minute because of the small heart size.

The transducer that is used for children and infants should be of a higher frequency than that used in adults. This is because there is less tissue to be penetrated. In infants, 5 to 7 mHz is satisfactory, while in younger children, 3.5 to 4.5 mHz provide good results.

Difficulties in examining children lies mainly in their fear and consequent lack of cooperation. It may help to relax a young child by having a parent stay in the room or even sit on the bed during the examination. Also, permitting the child to hold the transducer briefly may help prove that the device will not hurt.

If possible, infants should be fed prior to the examination so that they are more content and, hopefully, asleep. A pacifier may also help to quiet the baby. If excessive moving, struggling, or crying cannot be controlled, the examination should be postponed until the young patient can be sedated. Of course, this can be done only by the doctor.

In order for the cardiologist to interpret a pediatric echocardiogram accurately, it is necessary for you to record all the valves and the chambers. This is because their motion patterns and appearances are the same in youngsters as in adults, with only a few significant differences. And just as normal structures in infants and children exhibit the same appearance as in adults, the features of cardiac abnormalities are also identical. There are some congenital abnormalities, however, that are extremely complicated and difficult to evaluate. Therefore, it is obvious that in order to perform a pediatric study adequately and allow for an accurate interpretation, it is necessary for the technician to have a thorough understanding of adult echocardiography. Conversely, adults sometimes are found to have previously undiagnosed congenital heart disease, so that an awareness of congenital malformations also is of prime importance to any well-rounded and skilled professional echocardiographer.

Understanding Contrast Echocardiography

Contrast echocardiography is a technique in which some type of ultrasonic contrast agent is introduced into the heart in order to study its anatomy and function. It is a fairly new technique, and in fact was first used by Claude Joyner in the 1960s to study the mitral valve. Other early contrast studies were performed by Raymond Gramiak and Navin Nanda, who are credited with using injections of indocyanine green to identify intracardiac structures. Their original work, which was completed in 1976, identified the aortic root and aortic valve cusps. Although indocyanine green is still regarded as a safe and effective contrast agent, it is not the only one that can be used. Isotonic saline, D5W, and even the patient's own blood, can also be used to provide satisfactory results.

During the contrast study, rapid injections of the desired agent are made into either a peripheral arm or leg vein through an indwelling 18- to 20-gauge catheter. Since normal blood flow carries this agent into the right heart, its passage through the right heart can be visualized on the oscilloscope and recorded. The "contrast effect" appears as either a cloud of echoes, or numerous small individual reflectors, and is caused by the formation of microbubbles from the rapid injection and consequent high rate of flow across the narrow catheter tip.

Contrast studies can be used to identify intracardiac structures, demonstrate valvular insufficiency, or establish the presence of a right to left shunt. They are not particularly helpful in demonstrating left to right shunts, because the contrast effect is lost during passage of the agent through the pulmonary capillary beds before entering the left side of the heart.

Understanding Two-Dimensional Echocardiography

Until now, we have discussed what is specifically known as *M-mode* echocardiography. In this system, moving structures within the heart are recorded as wavy lines moving across an oscilloscope. Recordings obtained with this type of echocardiogram, however, do not resemble the actual configuration of the heart and thus can be confusing and somewhat difficult for the technician to decipher. Additionally, the M-mode echocardiogram provides no exact spatial orientation, because only those structures in the direct path of a narrow ultrasonic beam are recorded. Both these drawbacks have been overcome by the two-dimensional echocardiogram, which is also referred to as the *sector scan*, *real-time echo*, or *cross-sectional* echocardiogram. In this system, the ultrasonic beam is electronically or mechanically moved through a sector over a specific area of the heart.

In addition to producing an image that more closely resembles the heart and providing a better spatial orientation, the two-dimensional echocardiogram offers the physician several diagnostic advantages over the one-dimensional M-mode echo. In valvular heart disease, for example, it provides more information regarding valve thickening and rigidity. In mitral valve prolapse, it sometimes demonstrates

the systolic bowings of the redundant valve leaflets more clearly. In chordal rupture or vegetations, the erratic valve motion can be better appreciated. In coronary artery disease, it offers better definition of segmental wall motion abnormalities. In cardiomyopathy, it enables one to visualize the global nature of the dysfunctioning left ventricle. In infants and children, the two-dimensional echocardiogram provides excellent and immediate demonstrations of anatomical relationships. In fact, the use of this type of echocardiography in congenital heart disease may prove to be its most valuable asset.

Although the images displayed in a two-dimensional echocardiogram are much different from those obtained in the M-mode study, the method of performing the examination is basically the same. As in the M-mode echo, the patient is in either a supine or left lateral position. The transducer is placed along the parasternal border, and the best acoustic window is found. The heart is first examined in a *long-axis plane*, which follows a path parallel to the long axis of the heart. The transducer is then rotated 90 degrees to intersect the heart at an angle that is perpendicular to its long axis. This is referred to as the *short-axis*, or *cross-sectional view*. An apical four-chambered view, in which the transducer is placed directly over the cardiac apex and rotated in order to visualize all four cardiac chambers simultaneously, should also be included in the examination.

Overcoming Difficulties

You may encounter many difficulties in performing echocardiographic examinations, even if you know the basic transducer positions and methods of angulation, recognize every intracardiac structure, and are thoroughly familiar with the echoscope controls.

A frequent problem is caused by one of the properties of ultrasound itself; it does not pass through a gaseous medium such as air. Therefore, it may be extremely difficult and sometimes impossible to perform an adequate examination on patients with emphysema or other types of chronic lung disorders.

Another obstacle to a satisfactory examination is bone. Ultrasound waves are absorbed by the bones; consequently, structures behind them are "unsounded," meaning that there are no ultrasonic vibrations capable of reaching these structures; therefore, no echoes can be reflected. On the oscilloscope, there is a complete absence of all echo signals when the beam hits bone.

Women who have undergone a radical mastectomy also pose a problem in obtaining the echocardiogram. This is because the complete absence of soft tissue prevents an airtight coupling between the transducer and the skin. In these cases, the examination may be impossible.

In obese patients there is so much absorption and scattering of the ultrasonic waves before the beam even reaches a structure that the returning echoes are very weak. This is especially troublesome when trying to record adequate posterior wall echoes. Posterior wall structures reflect an even smaller proportion of echoes even in individuals of average weight. In the obese patient, the percentage of echo signals reflected is greatly reduced, therefore resulting in an extremely difficult examination.

In dealing with the obese patient, it may help to raise the patient's head to approximately a 30 degree angle, position the transducer one interspace higher and a little more laterally on the chest, and scan in a more lateral angle. Another possibility is to raise the patient's head and have him or her lie on the left side in order to drop the heart closer to the chest wall.

Summary

In this chapter, we defined what was involved in determining patient echocardiographic examination for adults, children, and infants. We identified initial control settings for this examinations, as well as defined the importance and function of transducer positioning and angulation. We also briefly discussed contrast and two-dimensional echocardiography. Finally, we identified and explained various types of difficulties the echocardiographic technician may encounter in obtaining the examination, as well as how to overcome these difficulties.

Review Questions

1. What is the name of the organization responsible for setting the standards for licensed echocardiographers?

2. Briefly explain the concept of *contrast echocardiography*.

3. Briefly explain the concept of *M-mode echocardiography*.

4. Briefly explain the concept of *two-dimensional echocardiography*.

5. Briefly explain the concept and importance of *transducer positioning* and *angulation*.

16

Cardiac Pathology and Abnormalities

_____
_____
_____

_____

_____

Performance Objectives

Upon completion of this chapter, you will be able to:

1. Explain the pathophysiology seen in aortic and pulmonic valvular abnormalities as each relates to echocardiographic findings.
2. Explain the pathophysiology seen in mitral and triscupid valvular abnormalities as each relates to echocardiographic findings.
3. Explain the pathophysiology seen in valvular regurgitation abnormalities as each relates to echocardiographic findings.
4. Explain the pathophysiology seen in pulmonic insufficiency and endocarditis as each relates to echocardiographic findings.
5. Explain the pathophysiology seen in prosthetic valve and cardiomyopathy abnormalities as each relates to echocardiographic findings.
6. Identify septal abnormalities and briefly discuss the echocardiographic patterns of each.
7. Explain the pathophysiology seen in pericardial effusion as each relates to echocardiographic findings.
8. Explain the pathophysiology seen in ischemic heart disease, myocardial infarction, congenital heart diseases in an adult, and foreign bodies, masses, and myxomas as each relates to echocardiographic findings.

Terms and Abbreviations

Aortic stenosis a disease of the aortic valve that ultimately reduces the opening of the valve and changes it from a mobile structure into a rigid and calcified mass.

Bacterial endocarditis a bacterial infection of the endocardium that can affect either the inner lining of a cardiac chamber, the intima of a great vessel, or most commonly, one or more of the heart valves.

Cardiac tamponade the accumulation of enough pericardial fluid to impede cardiac filling; severe tamponade most often occurs when a small volume of fluid rapidly enters the pericardial sac.

Cardiomyopathy diseased heart muscle; also used to describe rare, specific heart muscle disease that may arise secondary to disease elsewhere in the body.

Ebstein's anomaly a relatively rare congenital disorder in which all or part of a malformed tricuspid valve is posteriorly displaced within the right ventricle.

IHSS abbreviation for idiopathic hypertrophic subaortic stenosis, which is an obstructive cardiomyopathy characterized by gross hy-

pertrophy of the interventricular septum resulting in a narrowing and obstruction of the left ventricular outflow tract.

Mitral stenosis a common lesion associated with rheumatic fever that is caused by the tissues of the mitral valve developing an inflammatory reaction resulting in a fibrotic thickening and calcification of the valve cusps, adhesions between the cusps, and a shortening and thickening of the mitral valve chordae.

Pericarditis a term used to describe any alteration of the pericardium, whether or not it is an inflammatory or infectious process.

Pulsus paradoxus a physical finding of a dramatic fall in blood pressure and pulse volume during inspiration.

Sonolucent an echo-free space representing pericardial fluid.

Vegetations thick, friable lesions that can totally destroy the valve leaflets or any part of the valve apparatus.

VSD abbreviation for ventricular septal defect, which is a congenital anomaly chracterized by an anatomical defect in the septum.

127

There are many disorders and abnormalities of the heart that can be determined by the performance of the echocardiographic examination. These disorders include abnormalities of the aortic, pulmonary, mitral, and tricuspid valves, as well as complications seen in valvular regurgitation and cardiac and prosthetic valvular insufficiency. The use of echocardiographic examination is also helpful in recognizing cardiomyopathies, septal abnormalities, pericardial effusion, and other diseases of the heart, including ischemic heart disease, myocardial infarction, congenital heart diseases in adults, and foreign bodies, masses, and myxomas.

Abnormalities of the Mitral Valve

Mitral Stenosis

Mitral stenosis is a common lesion that is associated with rheumatic fever. In this abnormality, the valve tissues develop an inflammatory reaction resulting in fibrotic thickening and subsequent calcification of the valve cusps, adhesions between the cusps and their commissures, and shortening as well as thickening of the mitral valve chordae. The mitral valve apparatus therefore becomes scarred, deformed, and obstructed.

Mitral stenosis can be readily diagnosed on the echocardiographic examination. The graph will show a reduced diastolic closing, a reduced opening amplitude of the anterior leaflet, anterior movement of the posterior leaflet during diastole, and a thickening of the valve leaflets. Secondary findings on the examination may also include an enlarged left atrium and pulmonary hypertension. In addition, because prolonged diastolic flow keeps the valve in an open position longer, there is also a diminished reopening when atrial contraction occurs. Therefore, when mitral stenosis is present, there may be no "A" wave on the anterior leaflet or it may be very diminutive.

Mitral Regurgitation

The mitral valve apparatus is composed of four main parts: the annulus, the leaflets, the chordae, and the papillary muscle. In order for the valve to function properly, there must be normal and coordinated functioning of all these parts. In addition, the left ventricular wall must function properly, because the papillary muscles insert directly into the left ventricular myocardium. If any of these structures becomes diseased or dysfunctional, mitral regurgitation or mitral insufficiency may result. Valve regurgitation produces a backward flow of blood in the heart. It may affect any valve but is most often seen with left heart structures: the mitral and aortic valves.

Chronic mitral regurgitation can have several devastating results. (1) The backward flow adds volume to the left atrium, which is the chamber behind the incompetent valve, and causes left atrial dilatation. (2) Normal forward flow, plus the regurgitant fraction, adds volume to the left ventricle so that it, too, becomes dilated. (3) The left ventricle eventually hypertrophies, because the chamber must contract more forcefully in order to eject its added blood volume.

Echocardiographic studies that may indicate the presence of mitral regurgitation include a dilated left atrium and left ventricle, an exaggerated septal motion and left atrial wall motion, particularly at the atrioventricular junction, and a decreased aortic valve ejection time. Examining the echocardiogram for these signs, together with the specific criteria for isolated causes of mitral regurgitation, might provide the physician with a more diagnostic echocardiogram.

Mitral Valve Prolapse

The most frequent cause of mitral regurgitation, and in fact the most prevalent of all cardiac valvular abnormalities, is mitral valve prolapse. In this lesion, there appears to be myxomatous degeneration of the valve. This refers to a process in which the collagenous supporting tissue is replaced by loose, myxomatous tissue, thus permitting stretching and redundancy of the valve. Normal coaptation of the anterior and posterior leaflets is therefore disrupted, the valve balloons back into the left atrium rather than closing tightly during systole, and regurgitation may occur. However, there can be a mitral valve prolapse present without this backward flow.

Mitral valve prolapse is referred to by several other names, including *Barlowe's syndrome*, *floppy valve syndrome*, *mitral click and murmur syndrome*, and *ballooning mitral valve*. They all refer to the condition in which one or both of the mitral valve leaflets balloons or buckles back into the left atrium during systole. It is a very common disorder, affecting as much as 10 to 15 percent of the population, and is seen more frequently in women. Mounting evidence also indicates that it may run in families.

Diagnosing mitral valve prolapse is clinically important because of the significantly increased incidence of bacterial endocarditis, mitral valve dysfunction, coronarylike pain, and arrhythmias associated with it. Its secondary effects also are significant. Left atrial enlargement, left ventricular enlargement and hypertrophy, pulmonary hypertension, and congestive heart failure (CHF) all may develop in advanced cases of mitral valve prolapse. There have even been cases of sudden death reported among patients afflicted with the syndrome, although the actual number of reported cases is quite small.

Rheumatic Mitral Regurgitation

In true rheumatic mitral regurgitation, there appears to be a thickening and calcification at the edge of the leaflets that distort the valve and roughen its surface, so that tight closure cannot be achieved. However, when rheumatic heart disease is found to be the cause of the mitral regurgitation, it is highly uncommon for the lesion to be purely regurgitant, with no evidence of mitral stenosis. Varying degrees of mitral stenosis almost always are present with rheumatic mitral regurgitation. If the leaflets themselves are uncalcified and pliable, it may be the chordae that are heavily thickened and shortened, thus preventing complete closure.

Echocardiographically, it is impossible to distinguish between rheumatic mitral regurgitation and mild mitral stenosis. Similarly, mixed mitral valve disease, that is, combined mitral stenosis and mitral regurgitation, cannot be distinguished from true or pure mitral stenosis on the echocardiogram.

Idiopathic Hypertrophic Subaortic Stenosis

Idiopathic hypertrophic subaortic stenosis (IHSS) is a condition that may be present with or without mitral regurgitation, and when regurgitation is present, it is usually of a minimal degree. The diagnosis of IHSS is clinically important, however, because with it cardiac arrhythmias and even sudden death, may occur.

The M-mode echocardiogram is a highly reliable noninvasive method of diagnosing IHSS. Its principal echocardiographic features include a grossly thickened, relatively immobile septum, a narrowed left ventricular outflow tract, and an abrupt anterior motion of the anterior mitral valve leaflet during systole, generally referred to as a *SAM movement*. It is extremely important to remember that not one of these findings is specific for IHSS, but that all three must be present before a positive echocardiographic diagnosis can be made.

Congestive Cardiomyopathy

Congestive cardiomyopathy is a primary disease of the myocardium in which the heart walls exhibit poor motion and the cardiac chambers, particularly the left ventricle, become dilated. Mitral regurgitation

occurs when the dilated annular ring prevents complete closure of the mitral valve.

Although the mitral valve itself may be structurally normal in the presence of congestive cardiomyopathy, its appearance does show findings typical of this disease. The entire valve seems to float in a dilated, poorly contracting left ventricle, and the distance from the mitral valve to the left side of the septum is often increased from its normal range of 2.5 mm to greater than 21 mm. In diastole, the anterior and posterior leaflets form what is almost a diamond-shaped appearance and both leaflets are diminished because of reduced flow through the valve because of a poorly contracting heart.

Aortic Regurgitation

Because blood flows from the left ventricle into the aorta and then through the aortic valve before entering the systemic circulation, regurgitation from the aortic valve will affect the appearance of the mitral valve. Aortic regurgitation may occur with dilatation of the aortic valve ring, so that the margins of the valve cusps fail to meet and seal the valve shut. It also can be the result of rheumatic fever, in which the valve cusps become thickened and scarred. It can occur with congenital heart disease, such as bicuspid aortic valve, or as the result of bacterial infection, traumatic rupture, or perforation of the valve cusps. Regardless of the cause, the principal findings in aortic regurgitation is a fine fluttering of the anterior mitral valve leaflet during diastole, which is caused by the backward surge of blood from the regurgitant aortic valve striking the mitral valve leaflet and then mixing with the normal inflow from the left atrium. So much turbulence is created that the mitral valve exhibits its rapid diastolic fluttering.

Left Atrial Myxoma

Although it is a rare condition, left atrial myxoma is regarded as the most common type of intracardiac tumor. It is usually found in the atria, with the left atrium involved three times as often as the right. Also, it is almost always pedunculated, that is, attached to a stalk arising from the rim of the interatrial septum.

Clinically, the diagnosis of left atrial myxoma may be difficult because its symptoms greatly resemble those of mitral stenosis. Detection is vital, however, because surgical removal can result in a complete cure, while lack of detection is fatal.

Echocardiography provides the physician with an excellent noninvasive method of diagnosing left atrial myxoma. Its predominant findings include a flattened diastolic slope on the anterior mitral valve leaflet, resembling that of mitral stenosis, a cluster of echoes located behind the anterior mitral valve leaflet during diastole, and echoes in the left atrial cavity during systole.

Bacterial Endocarditis

Bacterial endocarditis (BE) is a bacterial infection of the endocardium that can affect either the inner lining of a cardiac chamber, the intima of a great vessel, or most commonly one or more of the heart valves. In order for bacterial endocarditis to occur, there must be a portal of entry for the offending organism to enter the bloodstream and a site susceptible for the infection to develop. The most common portal of entry is the mouth. Others include the skin, the genitourinary tract, the gastrointestinal tract, and the respiratory system. A susceptible site of infection is a valve that has already been affected by a prior lesion, such as a rheumatic mitral valve or a prolapsed mitral valve. When extremely virulent bacteria are present, however, even a normal valve can be affected.

When bacterial endocarditis occurs and the offending organisms settle on a heart valve, they produce thick, friable lesions called *vegetations* that can totally destroy the valve leaflets or any part of the valve apparatus. With BE, therefore, ruptured chordae tendineae or a flail mitral valve leaflet is quite common.

Abnormalities of the Aortic Valve

Aortic Stenosis

Aortic stenosis is responsible for approximately 25 percent of all chronic valvular lesions. Initially it is not significant, but as the disease progresses, it reduces the opening of the valve and changes it from a mobile structure into one that is an extremely rigid and calcified mass. This acts to increase left ventricular workload and results in left ventricular hypertrophy. As the disease progresses, the patient may develop angina, heart failure, syncope, or sudden death.

The most common cause of aortic stenosis in the adult is a congenital bicuspid aortic valve. It may also occur as a result of rheumatic fever, or it may simply be a part of the aging process, wherein the valve becomes rigid and calcified. The echocardiographic findings in aortic stenosis include multiple echoes within the aortic root during diastole and a decrease in the aortic valve opening during systole.

The echocardiographic picture presented by aortic stenosis varies. At times the reduced valve opening can be cearly demonstrated, while at other times, the aortic valve is heavily calcified, making it ex-

tremely difficult to do so. In still other cases, there is simply a mass of echoes filling the lumen, with only a brief systolic break where the valve opening should be, yet with no leaflets visible.

Bicuspid Aortic Valve

Bicuspid aortic valve is regarded as one of the most common congenital malformations within the heart, appearing in up to 50 percent of all cases involving aortic valve disease. Diagnosis is clinically important because patients with bicuspid aortic valve are quite susceptible to BE, are prone to aortic insufficiency, and in later life may develop fibrosis and calcification of the valve, resulting in aortic stenosis.

A normal aortic valve has three cusps that are situated at equal distances of one-third the circumference of the tubelike aortic ring. In a bicuspid aortic valve, however, there are only two functional cusps, and these are usually unequal in size. Young patients with supposedly innocent functional systolic murmurs, and patients with aortic ejection clicks who may exhibit no other signs of aortic valve disease, may indeed have bicuspid aortic valves. Their presence or absence can be determined on the echocardiogram by an eccentric position of the closed valve in diastole. Eccentricity means an inequality in the distance of the cusp echoes to the aortic root walls during diastole. The transducer position and angulation is an important point in this finding, because the diastolic closure can appear normal from one angle and eccentric from another. At times, multiple linear echoes can be seen emanating from the valve during diastole, making it quite difficult for the physician to determine the true closure point, and thus be able to assess the presence or absence of a bicuspid aortic valve.

Abnormalities of the Tricuspid and Pulmonary Valves

Since complete visualization of the tricuspid and pulmonary valves cannot always be obtained, it may sometimes be difficult to assess abnormalities involving these structures. But just as the normal tricuspid valve waveform is similar to that of the mitral valve, the tricuspid valve abnormalities are similar to those involving the mitral valve.

Tricuspid Prolapse

Tricuspid valve prolapse is an abnormality that tends to exhibit either a hammocking appearance throughout systole or a midsystolic posterior displacement of the valve leaflet. Although this condition often exists with mitral valve prolapse, it may also be seen as an isolated finding on the echocardiograph.

The M-mode echocardiogram is not highly reliable in the diagnosis of tricuspid valve prolapse. This is because in most cases the entire valve is not visualized, particularly the systolic segment. Also, the M-mode does not allow the valve to be examined from different transducer positions, and at times the transducer angle needed to visualize the valve may artifactually produce a pseudo, or false, prolapse pattern.

Tricuspid Stenosis

Tricuspid stenosis is a relatively rare occurence, and when present, it usually coexists with mitral stenosis. Its key echocardiographic findings are the same as in mitral stenosis, meaning that there is a reduced diastolic slope and a posterior leaflet that moves anteriorly during diastole. The difficulty in making a diagnosis of tricuspid stenosis, however, is that the posterior tricuspid valve leaflet is usually not recorded and a decreased diastolic slope may just simply indicate that there is a decreased compliance of the right ventricle with a structurally normal tricuspid valve.

Ebstein's Anomaly

Ebstein's anomaly is another relatively rare congenital disorder in which all or part of a malformed tricuspid valve is posteriorly displaced within the right ventricle. In the newborn, Ebstein's anomaly is often accompanied by cyanosis and heart failure, and must be differentiated from other forms of cyanotic heart disease. In milder cases the patient may be asymptomatic, even into adulthood.

In Ebstein's anomaly the posteriorly displaced tricuspid valve divides the right ventricle into two parts: the functional right ventricle, which lies apically or inferiorly to the displaced valve, and the "atrialized" right ventricle, which lies between the normal tricuspid valve annulus and the abnormal valve origin. The most specific echocardiographic finding shows a delayed closure of the tricuspid valve. Normally the tricuspid valve closes in less than 30 ms after the mitral valve. If this interval extends to at least 50 ms or more, the physician must consider the diagnosis of Ebstein's anomaly.

Pulmonary Hypertension

Pulmonary hypertension may be the result of an increase in the pulmonary blood flow, as with a left-to-right shunt, or it may be retrograde in nature, that is, resulting from an increase in the left atrial pressure being transmitted back to the pulmonary vasculature, as in the case of mitral stenosis. It may also be a primary condition, in which case the cause is unknown. Regardless of the cause, the echocardiographic findings in pulmonary hypertension are the same. They include an absence A wave on the pulmonary valve and a fluttering and/or notching of the pulmonary valve during systole.

In pulmonary hypertension, the pulmonary artery pressure is increased, and the difference between right ventricular and pulmonary artery pressure is much greater. Atrial contraction, therefore, is not sufficient enough to overcome the increased pulmonary artery pressure, and consequently no A dip is seen.

Recording the pulmonary valve to show a demonstration of the systolic fluttering or notching during systole is important when examining a patient for pulmonary hypertension. This is especially true when the patient is in atrial fibrillation, because there is never an A wave present then. The only method of diagnosing pulmonary hypertension in the presence of atrial fibrillation, therefore, is by demonstrating the midsystolic notching or fluttering.

Pulmonic Stenosis

Pulmonic stenosis is a congenital disease that occurs in approximately 10 percent of all reported cases of congenital heart disease. It may occur as a result of either a condition known as *valvular pulmonic stenosis*, in which there is a narrowing of the valve orifice, or opening, itself, or *infundibular pulmonic stenosis*, in which there is a narrowing of the outflow portion of the right ventricle just below the pulmonary valve. Because echocardiographic findings in infundibular pulmonic stenosis are not specific, for our purposes we will only be discussing valvular pulmonic stenosis.

In valvular pulmonic stenosis, the pulmonary valve is deformed and domes when it opens. Right ventricular, and consequently right atrial pressure, must be high in order to propel blood through the narrowed valve opening into the pulmonary artery. Pulmonary artery pressure, meanwhile, remains normal. Extreme care must be taken in interpreting pulmonic stenosis on an M-mode echocardiogram, because a variation in the pulmonary valve A dip is a normal finding associated with respiration. However, if the A dip is exaggerated during expiration and inspiration, and particularly if secondary findings such as ventricular enlargement or right ventricular hypertrophy, are present, the diagnosis of pulmonic stenosis should be suspected. The two-dimensional echocardiograph, with its long axis views of the pulmonic valve, may demonstrate the doming nature of the stenotic valve and thus provide the physician with a more reliable diagnosis.

Septal Abnormalities

The interventricular septum responds to changes in the volume and direction of the blood, to ventricular arrhythmias, to conduction defects, to alterations in intracardiac pressures, and to certain forms of congenital heart disease. Consequently, septal abnormalities can manifest themselves in many ways, including changes in the normal septal thickness, direction of motion, amplitude of motion, and septal-aortic root continuity.

Septal Thickness

A thickened septum is one whose measurement exceeds the upper normal limit of 1.1 cm. When determining the septal thickness, the measurement should be taken at the onset of the QRS complex, at the same point as the left ventricular dimensions, that is, with both sides of the septum together with the posterior left ventricular wall and portions of the mitral valve leaflets visible.

The septum is not easily recorded in all patients, and at times, its right side in particular can be quite difficult to determine. What appears to be the right side of the septum might very well be part of the tricuspid valve or a right ventricular chordal structure. Neither of these will exhibit the slight posterior motion in systole, as does the true septum. In fact, they may even show a slight anterior movement during this phase of the cardiac cycle.

Direction of Motion

Normal septal motion, evaluated in the same area as the septal thickness, means that the structure moves posteriorly in systole and anteriorly in diastole. If it moves in the opposite direction, its motion is said to be *paradoxical.*

Numerous abnormalities, both congential and acquired, are associated with paradoxical septal motion, and the echocardiograph must be interpreted in light of the patient's clinical findings. Congenital abnormalities would include atrial septal defect, total anomalous pulmonary venous drainage, and congenital absence of the pericardium. Acquired abnormalities would include any condition that resulted in a right ventricular volume overload, such as tricuspid or pulmonary regurgitation.

Other conditions that could produce paradoxical septal motion include severe left ventricular dysfunc-

tion, septal ischemia or injury secondary to coronary artery disease, constrictive pericarditis, and pericardial effusion from rocking of the heart in the fluid-filled sac. It may also be a postoperative artifact; therefore, previous cardiac surgery should be noted on the tracing.

Amplitude of Motion

Normal septal amplitude generally falls between 0.3 and 1 cm, with the average being 0.5 cm. When its amplitude exceeds 1 cm, it is said to be exaggerated. When the amplitude is less than 0.3 cm, it is said to be hypokinetic, or even akinetic if the motion is totally flat.

Exaggerated septal motion combined with an exaggerated motion of the posterior left ventricular wall is usually the result of a volume overload in the left ventricle. This is most often seen in either mitral or aortic regurgitation. It can also be seen as a compensatory mechanism in coronary artery disease where there is ischemia or an infarction involving the posterior or inferior walls. In an effort to maintain cardiac output, more of the left ventricular pumping action is undertaken by the interventricular septum. Similarly, a hypokinetic or an akinetic septum compared to a normally moving posterior wall indicates ischemia or injury involving the septal region.

Discontinuity

The normal echocardiogram reflects fibrous continuity between the anterior mitral valve leaflet and the posterior aortic root and between the interventricular septum and the anterior aortic root. Whenever this continuity is absent or interrupted, a discontinuity exists.

The most common cause of interruption in septal-aortic root continuity is a ventricular septal defect (VSD). This is a congenital anomaly that is characterized by an anatomical defect in the septum. The lesion may either be isolated or exist as one component of a combination of congenital anomalies.

Small VSDs are not readily diagnosed through M-mode echocardiography. The reason is that the hole must be large enough for the entire beam to pass through it without hitting any of its sides. This is not, however, usually the case. If the VSD is larger, it is seen as a "dropout" or a loss of septal echoes at the site of the lesion. This is demonstrated by means of the M-mode scan, which may have to be repeated several times and at slightly different angles in order for the dropout to be visualized. Here again, the echocardiogram is not totally reliable, because the loss of septal echoes can be artificially produced by improperly low gain settings or by not having the transducer properly aligned with the septum.

Another type of discontinuity occurs when the septum does not merge with the anterior aortic root. This phenomenon is referred to as an *overriding aorta* and is generally found in a number of congenital abnormalities, including *tetralogy of Fallot* and *truncus arteriosus*. When the scan demonstrates this type of discontinuity, it is extremely important to examine the area again from a lower interspace, since the impression of an overriding aorta can be falsely produced when the transducer is placed too high on the precordium and angled downward.

Pericardial Effusion

The pericardium is a membranous sac that holds the heart and protects it from adjacent disease processes. Normally there is up to 15 mL of fluid between the epicardium, which is the outermost lining of the heart, and the pericardium. Interestingly, during the echocardiographic examination, the two structures appear as a single heavy line referred to as the posterior epipericardium, or simply the posterior pericardium. The same holds true for the anterior right ventricular wall and the inner chest wall; one is flush with the other. When fluid accumulates in the pericardial sac, however, the posterior epicardium separates from the pericardium. If this occurs, it is called *pericardial effusion*. It is seen quite often in patients with congestive heart failure and chronic renal failure. It can also occur in patients diagnosed with pericarditis, cardiac puncture, metabolic disturbances, and those suffering from metastatic carcinomas.

Diagnosing pericardial effusion is one of the most useful applications of echocardiography and was, in fact, the basis for its development and use in this country. During the echocardiographic study, two classical findings are produced. First, there is a flattened posterior pericardial echo. This is followed by an echo-free space located between the nonmoving posterior pericardium and the moving epicardium. The echo-free, or *sonolucent*, space represents the pericardial fluid; the flattened pericardium results from the accumulation of fluid in the sac, which prevents it from moving normally. Anterior fluid may also be demonstrated by a separation between the anterior right ventricular wall and the inner chest wall, but the effusion must be at least a moderate one before this can be seen.

In some instances, a small anterior echo-free space will appear, but with no posterior separation. This does not indicate that a pericardial effusion has occurred. Any tissue between the heart and the chest wall can cause it. Other causes can include connec-

tive tissue within the anterior mediastinum, excess adipose tissue in obese patients, a hernia, and lung tissue in patients suffering from chronic obstructive pulmonary disease. Even the configuration of the chest wall itself, where the right ventricle does not come in direct contact with the chest wall, can cause an anterior separation. Therefore, fluid must be found posteriorly before a diagnosis of pericardial effusion can be made.

Diagnosing Common Cardiac Disorders Using Echocardiography

There are several common cardiac disorders which can recognized and diagnosed through the use of the echocardiographic examination. These include ischemic heart disease, myocardial infarction, coronary artery disease, congenital heart disease, and various types of masses.

Ischemic Heart Disease

Coronary artery disease is the leading cause of death in this country. The major symptom is angina, or chest pain, and death is frequently the first manifestation of this disease. Two-dimensional echocardiography is ideally suited for the noninvasive evaluation of the abnormal wall motion that is associated with ischemic heart disease.

Cardiac ischemia is the physiologic consequence of impaired myocardial perfusion and may result from either severe aortic stenosis or coronary artery disease. The myocardium is very efficient at extracting oxygen, so that increased myocardial oxygen needs must be met by increased blood flow. Profusion of the left ventricle occurs primarily in diastole and is influenced by cardiac output, diastolic pressure, intramyocardial pressure, and coronary arteriolar resistance.

The major determinants of myocardial oxygen consumption are heart rate and myocardial tension developed during the contractile state. Although the exact mechanisms of pain production by myocardial ischemia are unclear, it is thought that the chest pain brought on by ischemia may be transient or prolonged, depending on the effectiveness of physiological compensatory mechanisms or medical interventions.

As long as myocardial oxygen needs are minimized, a significant degree of narrowing of the lumen of a coronary artery may be well tolerated. Chest pain may not be present until there is approximately 80 percent stenosis of a coronary artery.

Myocardial Infarction

The value of echocardiography in patients with myocardial infarctions, or heart attacks, is found in the assessment of the left ventricular function and in the diagnosis of possible complications that may arise in postinfarction patients. Unfortunately, patients with coronary artery disease sometimes have the most technically difficult echoes to perform, since they tend to have large barrel-shaped chests with hyperinflated lungs, thus making it difficult to visualize all of the left ventricular wall segment.

Patients with transmural myocardial infarctions have a characteristic thinning and hypocontractile pattern to the affected wall; therefore, using two-dimensional echocardiography is superior to M-mode echocardiography in the detection and localization of regional wall motion asynergy. In addition to employing the use of two-dimensional echocardiographic examination to diagnose an acute myocardial infarction, it has also proved to be quite helpful in evaluation following surgical repair, or some other reperfusion technique.

Disorders Following Acute Myocardial Infarction

In cases where an acute myocardial infarction has occurred, echocardiographic examination may be used to evaluate the presence of any number of complications. These include the presence of a thrombi, aneurysm, Dressler's syndrome, papillary muscle dysfunction, ventricular septal defect, and coronary artery dysfunction.

Thrombi

The formation of a mural thrombus occurring within a week following a myocardial infarction has been reported to be as high as 25 percent. These thrombi are most commonly found in the apex following an anterior myocardial infarction. A relatively small number of these patients have associated systemic emobilization and anticoagulation therapy as being helpful in decreasing the size of these thrombi.

Aneurysm

The presence of a left ventricular aneurysm occurs in approximately 20 percent of patients suffering from an acute myocardial infarction. The aneurysm can form in either the apical, inferior, or posterior portions of the left ventricle and it is generally characterized by a thinned and dyskinetic portion of the ventricular wall. By definition, an aneurysm refers to a surgically resectable area of dyskinesis. This is different from a generalized cardiiomyopathy in which there is no area of preserved myocardial function.

A rare complication of a transmural myocardial infarction is rupture of the ventricular muscle. The integrity of the myocardium is preserved by the pericardium. Classic echocardiographic signs of what is referred to as a *pseudoaneurysm* are that it usually involves the lateral or posterior wall and there is a small discreet neck, which then balloons out into an area containing clots or fibrous tissue. There is a 30 percent rupture rate on pseudoaneurysms, so surgical intervention is necessary. A large neck pseudoaneurysm may be difficult to distinguish from a true left ventricular aneurysm that involves all the layers of the myocardium.

Dressler's Syndrome

Dressler's syndrome refers to a type of pericarditis that is associated with a myocardial infarction. This syndrome usually manifests itself within 10 days following an acute infarction. There is usually an associated pericardial effusion and chest pain that is aggravated by the patient breathing in, changing position, or coughing. As in other pericardial effusions, echocardiography is an excellent means for detection of this excess fluid around the heart.

Papillary Muscle Dysfunction

A patient who suffers an acute myocardial infarction and then develops a new systolic murmur should be closely examined for the presence of papillary muscle dysfunction, ruptured papillary muscle, or ventricular septal defect.

Papillary muscle dysfunction occurs most often with inferior myocardial infarction. The mitral valve coaptation pattern may appear relatively normal, but there will be Doppler evidence of mitral regurgitation. Patients with extensive inferior myocardial infarctions in which the infarcted area includes one of the papillary muscles may develop a rupture of the papillary muscle that could then result in a flail mitral leaflet. This almost always leads to wide open mitral regurgitation in which a heart murmur may not be heard, but the patient is in shock and heart failure.

Ventricular Septal Defect

Rupture of the ventricular septum also produces a systolic murmur heard near the lower sternal border and at times at the apex. Two-dimensional echocardiography is useful for the location of any large ventricular septal defects. Doppler echocardiography, especially color flow Doppler, is an excellent technique for the identification and localization of traumatic ventricular septal defects.

Coronary Arteries

Because of the increased resolution and scanning abilities of the newer echocardiographic machines, there is a much greater ability to see coronary arteries. With color flow Doppler, it is now possible, in certain select patients, to see flow in the proximal portions of the coronary arteries.

As far as being able to detect the buildup of plaque in the coronary arteries, this is still not feasible by echocardiography. There have been some reported cases of the detection of left main coronary artery disease, but this diagnosis is so beset with technical problems, that using echocardiograhy is almost next to impossible as a means of making an accurate diagnostic assessment. It is useful, however, in detecting coronary artery aneurysms from *Kawasaki's disease*, which is a disease of the coronary arteries usually affecting young children.

Congenital Heart Disease in the Adult

During the past 10 years, the terms and classifications concerning congenital heart diseases have become a great deal more descriptive in nature and easier to understand by nonpediatric cardiologists. The more complex the congenital heart disease, the more necessary it is to use this descriptive nomenclature.

Two-dimensional echocardiography with its ability to provide the physician with spatial information concerning the location of the various cardiac chambers, is an excellent means in determining these abnormal connections.

When faced with an adult patient with corrected congenital heart disease, it is sometimes impossible to figure out what palliative or corrective procedures have been performed. Therefore, the use of Doppler echocardiography helps in determining the presence and direction of blood flow in the various chambers, vessels, and conduits.

The echocardiographic examination for corrected adults should follow the same guidelines as an examination of a child with suspected, undiagnosed congenital heart disease. This sequential approach to congenital heart disease begins with the determination of atrial arrangement. The location of the pulmonary veins and the junction of the inferior vena cava, hepatic vein, and the right atrium should all be identified.

Missiles, Masses, and Myxomas

In echocardiography, the terms *missiles*, *masses*, and *myxomas* are used to describe various foreign bodies, masses, and tumors that may pass through the heart, thereby damaging cardiac structures. They may also be used to refer to an entity that enters the heart and then lodges itself within the myocardium or a cardiac chamber. The foreign bodies may range from a misplaced pacemaker wire to a bullet.

Penetrating wounds to the chest, especially those involving or thought to involve the heart, require careful examination using two-dimensional, Doppler, and contrast techniques. Visualization and localization of bullets and lead fragments can usually be obtained from almost anywhere in the heart. The bright reflections and reverberations from these metal objects make them good targets as they send out a "beacon" of reverberation with their movement.

Masses and Myxomas

Masses within the heart are most commonly the result of thrombus formation or vegetations associated with endocarditis. Two-dimensional echocardiography is much better than M-mode for the detection and locationalization of any intracardiac mass. Thrombus formation is usually associated with an abnormally moving wall. It may be very small and layered, or, in a case of dilated cardiomyopathies, it may be very large and pedunculated.

Of all the cardiac tumors, myxomas are by far the most common. These are usually located in the left atrium and are pedunculated with their attachment to the atrial septum. They may also be found in the right atrium, and there are reported cases of biatrial myxomas where they are found in both the left and the right atria. Their length may range from 2 to 10 cm and occasionally they may show deformation from an impingement upon a valve opening. Often the clinical signs of left atrium myxoma will mimic those of mitral stenosis.

Echocardiography is an excellent technique for the diagnosing of myxomas. The M-mode appearance is similar to mitral stenosis but usually there is an echo free space in early diastole before movement of the tumor into the mitral opening. A Dopper examination is necessary in any patient with a mass lesion in order to rule out either valvular stenosis or regurgitation.

Benign and Malignant Tumors

Rhabdomyomas, especially those seen in children, are considered the most frequently appearing benign ventricular tumors. Most often seen within the ventricular septum, they seem to appear in any wall of the chambers or even in the atrial septum. *Fibromas* and *myxomas*, which seem to occur in a ventricular wall or cavity and almost always produce symptoms, are considered the second and third most common benign tumors found in the ventricles of children.

Rhabdomysosarcomas and *malignant teratomas* are considered the most common primary malignant cardiac tumors and occur most frequently in the right side of the heart, while *carcinoid syndrome*, which sometimes results in cardiac involvement of valve thickening and stenosis that commonly affects the tricuspid and pulmonic valves, seems to be less common. Other tumors that frequently metastasize to the heart include carcinoma of the lung and breast, malignant melanoma, malignant lymphoma, and leukemia.

Summary

In this chapter, we discussed the pathophysiology of various disorders of the mitral, tricuspid, aortic, and pulmonary valves, as each was related to echocardiographic findings. We also talked about many of the disorders of the heart that could easily be recognized through the implementation of M-mode, two-dimensional, and Doppler echocardiography. These included cardiomyopathies, pericardial effusion, ischemic heart disease, myocardial infarction, congenital heart disease, and foreign bodies, masses, myxomas, and tumors.

Review Questions

1. What is the name of the disease of the aortic valve that ultimately reduces the opening of the valve and changes it from a mobile structure into a rigid and calcified mass?

2. A disease that affects the endocardium and can eventually damage the inner lining of the heart is called:

   a. cardiac tamponade

   b. bacterial endocarditis

   c. mitral stenosis

3. What does the abbreviation *IHSS* mean?

4. A disease characterized by an accumulation of pericardial fluid that can ultimately impede cardiac filling is called:

   a. cardiac tamponade

   b. aortic stenosis

   c. pericarditis

5. A disease characterized by diseased heart muscle and can cause secondary muscle diseases elsewhere in the body is called:

   a. pericarditis

   b. bacterial endocarditis

   c. cardiomyopathy

6. A relatively rare congenital disorder in which all or part of a malformed tricuspid valve is posteriorly displaced within the right ventricle is called:

   a. cardiomyopathy

   b. Ebstein's anomaly

   c. pulsus paradoxus

7. What does the abbreviation *VSD* mean?

8. A term used to describe thick, friable lesions that can totally destroy the valve leaflets or any part of the valve apparatus is called _____.

Laboratory Assisting: Basic Concepts and Applications

17

Laboratory Safety and Organization

Performance Objectives

Upon completion of this chapter, you will be able to:

1. Briefly discuss the Occupational Safety and Health Act (OSHA) and the Centers for Disease Control and the relevance of each to the laboratory assistant.
2. Identify and briefly discuss the procedures for fire prevention, reporting, and control in the medical laboratory.
3. Discuss and demonstrate how to dispose of contaminated materials and equipment used in the medical laboratory properly, using universal precautions.
4. Demonstrate how to follow safety procedures in operating laboratory equipment.
5. Identify and discuss safety practices used in the medical laboratory.
6. Explain the proper procedure for reporting accidents in the medical laboratory.
7. Identify the most common hazards indicated by the National Fire Protection Association.
8. Identify and briefly discuss the training and functions of each of the members working in the medical laboratory.
9. Explain how a large medical laboratory is organized.
10. Identify and distinguish work areas in the medical laboratory by name and functions.
11. Explain the use of a computer in a health care facility, and in particular, its application in the medical laboratory.

Terms and Abbreviations

CDC abbreviation for the Centers for Disease Control, a federal public health agency with headquarters in Atlanta, Georgia.

Certification issuance of a certificate by a regulating professional organization verifying that a person has fulfilled standards of education, training, and performance.

Code used to signal an emergency; names of colors may be added to indicate the type of problem.

Computer an electronic device with the ability to develop, store, and transfer data.

Corrosive a chemical that is able to wear away by its action, such as strong acids.

Extinguish to put out or quench; to cease burning.

Flammable easily set on fire.

Ignite to set on fire.

Incident report a report of an unusual event or accident that does not fit into normal procedure.

Incinerate to burn to ashes.

Internist a physician who specializes in internal medicine and who treats illnesses of adults nonsurgically; this person sometimes heads the medical laboratory where no pathologist is available.

Laboratorian pertaining to a laboratory worker.

Legible easy to read.

Liability under legal obligation; responsible for.

Licensure permission to practice awarded by a state or national board to persons who have proved competency for an occupation.

NFPA abbreviation for the National Fire Protection Association.

OSHA abbreviation for the Occupational Safety and Health Act; also, for the Occupational Safety and Health Administration.

Pathologist a specialist responsible for examining cells and tissues in order to aid in the diagnosis and treatment; heads laboratory and performs autopsies.

Registry a list of qualified individuals kept on an official record, indicating satisfactory completion of standards for some profession.

Safety freedom from danger, risk, or injury.

Terminal a workstation for a computer consisting of a video screen and a keyboard.

Before we can begin to discuss your role as a member of the medical laboratory team, it is important to first explain the implications that both safety and organization play in this very technical and hands-on atmosphere.

Safety, as it is most easily defined, refers to something being free from danger, risk, or injury. The clinical or medical laboratory contains many potential hazards and is therefore constantly concerned with safety. Personnel in the laboratory use hazardous substances, such as chemicals, glass, infectious materials, radioactive materials, and compressed gases, in their daily work. They use pipettes for transferring liquids, microtome blades for tissue preparation, needles, and corrosive chemicals. The list of potential dangers is a long one. In order to avoid injury and danger to yourself and to others, it is important to always be aware of hazards and to practice safety methods.

Workers in the medical laboratory are carefully trained to deal with potential hazards. Although incidents do occur, those that cause serious injury are extremely rare. Disease transmission is also minimal.

Regulatory Agencies

In an effort to ensure safe and healthful working conditions for every worker in this country, the federal government has established general safety rules for all employers. These are outlined in the Occupational Safety and Health Act, or OSHA. Under OSHA, all employers must conform to specific safety and health standards that are enforced by the Secretary of Labor. Any worker who feels that conditions on the job are unsafe and do not meet OSHA specifications, may ask the local OSHA office to investigate and make recommendations for improvement.

All health care facilities are responsible for practicing Universal Blood and Body Fluid Precautions. These rules, which are mandated by the Centers for Disease Control, located in Atlanta, Georgia, clearly state that all patients and staff are considered possible carriers of harmful pathogens, and because of that, any employee who works around, or is exposed to, any body fluids, such as blood, sputum, semen,

vaginal secretions, urine, stool, tissues, and drainage from open wounds, must follow universal precautions. In order to decrease the risk of accidental infection, a facility will have strict infection control procedures that must be followed by all staff members when handling any body fluid.

Fire Safety

All laboratory personnel must be responsible for fire prevention and control. Most laboratories have fire doors, fire blankets, and fire extinguishers to control fires. A *fire door* is a heavy, fireproof door located between defined areas of a building. In case of fire, the doors close automatically in order to help contain the fire.

A *fire blanket* is used to put out flash fires of clothing, because chemical extinguishers may be harmful to the skin. To use a fire blanket, you should first grasp the rope handle, then place the right arm through the rope loop, and finally, pull vigorously while turning to the left. This wraps the person in the blanket as it is unrolled and extinguishes the fire.

Since there are three types of fires, there are also three types of *fire extinguishers*. You must be able to operate the correct extinguishers efficiently. This means being alert in order to determine what is burning and which extinguisher must be used.

Class A fires are those in which the fuel is an ordinary combustible, such as wood, paper, or cloth. *Class B* fires are those fueled by flammable liquids. *Class C* fires involve electrical equipment, such as motors and switches. Medical laboratories contain materials that fit into all three categories.

Extinguishers may contain foam, carbon dioxide, soda acid, water, dry chemicals, or may be a multipurpose type. Many institutions provide the multipurpose dry chemical extinguisher for use on any type of combustion. The symbols for the three types of fires have different shapes and are color-coded. The symbol for Class A fires is a green triangle; Class B is a red square, and Class C is a blue circle. These symbols will appear on the side of the extinguisher. You should learn to recognize these symbols and remember what type of fire they indicate in order to select the correct extinguisher.

Flammable Liquids

Flammable liquids require special care. They must be stored in a designated area, preferably in a fire safety cabinet labeled "FLAMMABLE—KEEP FIRE AWAY." To dispose of empty containers of flammable chemicals, first fill to overflowing with tapwater. Repeat this three times. (This is a requirement of the Environmental Protection Agency.) Then drain the containers, and place them in the disposal area as designated by your hospital's policy.

Fire Emergencies and the Lab

If a fire does occur, as a member of the laboratory team, one of your responsibilities may be to alert all personnel. Each worker must know his or her exact responsibility, how to report a fire, and the exit routes from the laboratory. All of these things are included in fire drills, which are generally held at regular intervals in most medical facilities.

Some institutions sound chimes or bells to indicate a specific location of a fire by the number of rings. Others use codes that are announced over the facility's loudspeaker system. *Codes* indicate than an emergency has occurred and what that emergency might be. These codes are designed to prevent frightening patients or visitors in emergencies.

Other emergency situations besides fires are included in the code system. Health care facilities may devise a code for their specific use or they may use the International Code System, which consist of four codes: Code Red, Code Blue, Code Yellow, and Code Green.

A *Code Red* means that there is a fire in the hospital. A *Code Blue* means that someone has stopped breathing, or that their heart has stopped beating, or both. *Code Yellow* means that there is an uncontrolled individual or a threatening situation in the facility. And a *Code Green* means that a special team of people should report to the emergency area. This code would be called when a disaster occurred.

A *disaster*, as it relates to the hospital environment, is a sudden event that causes great damage or loss, such as an airplane crash, a train wreck, or a hurricane or tornado. To prepare for such an event, hospital personnel participate in disaster drills with patients having simulated injuries. Students observing or working in a health care facility must know the meaning of the codes and how to conduct themselves according to the local hospital's policy.

Contaminated Materials and the Medical Laboratory

A serious problem in the medical laboratory is the safe handling of infectious materials. The *universal precautions* assume that all samples are potentially infectious. All specimens that could be contagious are considered to be contagious. All biologically contaminated trash is considered to be infectious. This includes laboratory materials such as sponges, glassware, syringes, and needles, as well as specimens from patients. There is no distinction between the disposal of specimens known to be contaminated with the HIV virus and other samples. All specimens and samples are autoclaved or incinerated. All discarded specimens should be disinfected with sodium hypochlorite (bleach), then autoclaved. Finally, the entire specimen is placed in a heavy plastic bag showing the biohazard symbol and labeled CONTAMINATED, and then incinerated. Large equipment that cannot be autoclaved may be soaked in bleach.

In case of spills of contaminated matter, such as blood, body fluids, or laboratory solutions, the entire area must be covered with paper towels and then flooded with bleach. Wearing gloves, you should then place the soaked towels and spillage into a container for autoclaving. Finally, flood the area again with the bleach, and clean the area as usual.

Other contaminated specimens should be returned to their original container, and then placed in bags labeled CONTAMINATED, BIOHAZARD. They should then be incinerated. Disposable laboratory equipment is treated in a similar manner. Reusable equipment is soaked in a disinfectant and then autoclaved.

All sharps, needles, scalpel blades, and disposable syringes with needles attached should be placed in a puncture-proof container located in the area where they are used. Used needles should not be broken, bent, recapped, or handled with the hands, but rather, placed directly into the container.

Fluorescent orange or orange-red labels bearing the biohazard symbol must be placed on anything containing potentially infectious materials or wastes, such as refrigerators, freezers, medical waste receptacles, and shipping containers. Marked bags may be used instead of labels in some instances.

Equipment, Safety, and the Medical Laboratory

All laboratory equipment in itself may be dangerous. Glassware can be particularly hazardous. Never use broken or chipped glass equipment. Remember, the time you lose to cuts from such equipment may be a lot more costly than replacing it. If glassware is broken, clean up each and every particle. Tongs or forceps should be used to discard pieces in a sharps container.

Any time there is a risk of splashing or aerosol formation when you open a blood collection tube, you must use some type of barrier. This barrier should be placed between yourself and the specimen. Generally, clear transparent plastic screens are used. They come in various sizes, thicknesses, and shapes. The screens also serve to protect you against any unexpected chemical reactions and injury from instrumentation or breakage of equipment.

A *safety shower* is part of the safety equipment used by all laboratories. It should be centrally located and easily accessible to all workers in the lab. It is used to flush corrosives from the skin and clothing. Pulling the handle causes a large amount of water to flood the victim immediately.

An *eyewash station* is another safety device used by all laboratories. It is a small sink that has been designed to direct water into the eyes. It is usually located close to the area where strong chemicals are used. If you should splash any toxic substances into your eyes, go at once to the eyewash station, and flood your eyes with water. Continue to flush the eyes with water for 15 minutes, or until medical treatment is begun. Keep your eyes open while flooding. The first 15 seconds after an accident to the eyes are crucial to the preservation of your sight.

A third safety device used in the medical laboratory is a *ventilation hood*. This is used to carry away any fumes or to trap and contain contaminants. Hoods come in various sizes and are most often found in the chemistry or microbiology sections of the medical laboratory.

Safety Practices in the Medical Laboratory

Following good safety practices is the responsibility of all members of the medical laboratory staff. It involves using common sense, as well as following some sound general guidelines. These guidelines include the following:

- Clean up all spills from the work area and floor immediately.
- Always report any broken or hazardous equipment to your supervisor.
- Never leave storage drawers open or cabinet doors ajar.
- Always use an automatic pipette or a rubber bulb and pipette to transfer materials from one container to another, and never pipette by mouth.

- Whenever you are required to collect a specimen, be sure to check the patient's identification.
- Never use frayed or damaged electrical cords.
- All reagent bottles must be labeled, and the labels must be legible.
- Always read labels three times: as you reach for the bottle, as you pour from the bottle, and as you replace it.
- Never keep food of any kind, such as lunches or cold drinks, in the laboratory refrigerator.
- Never eat, drink, or smoke in the laboratory.
- Always remove contact lenses while working with chemicals.

Protective Clothing in the Medical Laboratory

As a member of the medical laboratory team, you will deal routinely with all types of body fluids. Therefore, it is extremely important that you protect yourself through proper handwashing techniques and the wearing of protective clothing. Protective clothing in the laboratory usually consists of gloves, masks, eyewear, gowns, jackets, and aprons.

You will be expected to wear gloves whenever your work may lead to contamination of your hands. Once you have thoroughly washed your hands, you are ready to glove. First, take a disposable vinyl glove and slip your fingers into it. Then place a second glove on the other hand. Work your fingers into the interdigital spaces so that the gloves fit comfortably on each hand. When you remove them, catch the edge, turn them inside out, and discard them. Figure 17-1 shows the correct procedure for donning and removing gloves. Remember, when you are wearing gloves, you will contaminate whatever your hands touch with the gloves, such as the telephone.

For some procedures, you may need to wear a mask. If you are required to do so, place the mask over your nose and mouth, and pull the elastic over your head to a comfortable position. Discard the mask in the proper container when the procedure is complete.

For some procedures, safety standards may require you to use protective eyewear. Eyewear generally consists of special big-lens glasses or safety goggles. Face shields that will completely protect your face and allow you to wear eyeglasses underneath may also be used.

You must always wear a laboratory jacket or coat when working in the medical laboratory. Remove it when you leave. OSHA mandates that protective clothing be removed before leaving the workplace. Before leaving, however, you must follow the appropriate procedure: first clean and disinfect the work area, then remove your gloves and laboratory coat or jacket; finally, wash your hands.

Procedure for Completing Aseptic Handwashing

As we have already discussed, you must always make sure that you wash your hands before and after a procedure, as well as prior to leaving the medical laboratory. In health care, there is a very exact way of completing this task. Following the proper steps will provide you with the greatest opportunity for maintaining an aseptic environment, as well as keeping yourself free from any potential contamination. To properly wash your hands, you should:

· Never allow your uniform, laboratory jacket or coat, or clothing to touch the sink.
· Use paper towels to turn on warm water.
· Wet your hands, holding them lower than your wrists, and apply soap. If at all possible, use liquid soap.
· Use strong rubbing movements to loosen any bacteria from your hands. Wash between your fingers and thumbs.
· Rinse well, with your hands lower than your wrists. Inspect your hands, and if necessary, repeat the washing.
· Dry your hands and arms well, and use a paper towel to turn off the water.

Exposure Control in the Medical Laboratory

Employers in the health care industry are all required to offer hepatitis B vaccine to any employee who may be exposed to infectious materials. This is always done at the employer's expense. Your employer will evaluate the potential for exposure to any hazardous materials and will then communicate the information to you. You may refuse the vaccine by signing a waiver; however, should you change your mind at a later date, you may still receive the vaccine.

All employees working in the medical laboratory are offered the vaccine. If the vaccine is refused, the employer could refuse to pay for treatment if hepatitis B is contracted. Some employers may also require that you show proof of immune status for measles, mumps, and rubella. If your status is unknown, the immunization is offered. If it is refused and an employee is exposed to measles, mumps, or rubella on the job, the employee is required to stay home until the incubation period is passed, usually without monetary compensation.

Reporting Accidents

In spite of all efforts to practice safety, accidents happen. If so, you must report the accident to your supervisor at once. The victim must be given proper first aid, and prompt corrective action must be taken if needed.

In a hospital, when an unusual event or accident has occurred outside routine procedure, it is called an *incident*, and an *incident report* must be filed with the administration. The incident report must include: (1) a description of the accident; (2) the time, place, and cause of the accident; and (3) the names of any witnesses. The incident report may be used for any future claims for workers' compensation or possible liability lawsuits.

Organization of the Medical Laboratory

The largest number of allied health careers is found in the hospital environment. These facilities generally employ about two-thirds of all health care workers. Other smaller facilities include clinics; nursing homes and extended care facilities; and the offices of doctors, dentists, and veterinarians. Most of these facilities have some type of laboratory. They vary in size from multidepartmental laboratories in larger hospitals and medical centers, to the small one-person laboratory in a doctor's office.

Members of the Laboratory Team

There are several different levels of training for workers in health care facilities. The size and type of facility will generally dictate the skill level of the laboratory practitioner. Personnel in laboratories also have specific titles. In the medical laboratory, the *medical technologist* (MT) is a highly trained professional who is required to carry out the more complex laboratory procedures. This person may also be required to supervise the work of other laboratory workers. Several educational paths can lead to qualification as an MT. The person may have a bachelor's degree and train for one year in a certified hospital; have three years of college, plus one year of hospital training; or two years of college, plus two years at a training hospital. The two latter plans lead to a bachelor's degree in medical technology. With the first plan, the medical technologist's degree may also be in a related field, such as biology or chemistry.

After training has been completed, the person must then successfully pass an examination. The examination is administered by a certifying agency, such as the American Society of Clinical Pathologists (ASCP), the American Medical Technologists (AMT),

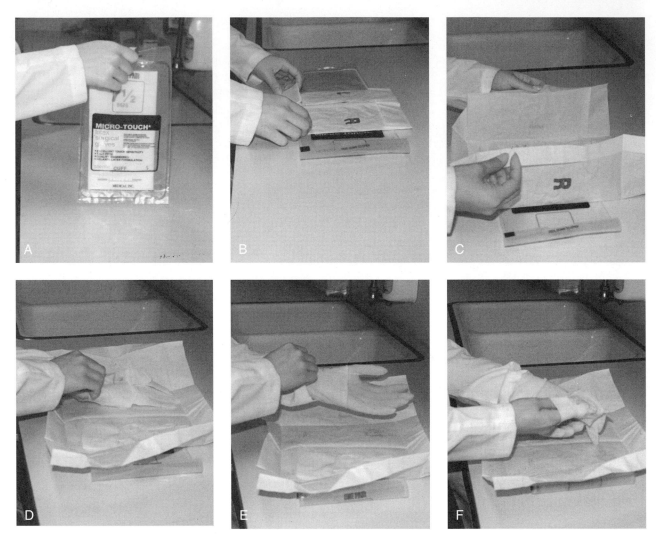

Figure 17-1
Donning (A through G) and removing (H through K) gloves.

the National Certification Agency for Medical Laboratory Personnel (NCAMLP), and the International Society for Clinical Laboratory Technology (ISCLT).

A *medical laboratory technician*, or MLT, is an individual who has completed at least two years of medical laboratory training in a community college and who has successfully passed a national accreditation examination. MLTs are responsible for performing basic laboratory procedures and routine tests.

The *laboratory assistant* may either be trained on the job or may complete a prescribed course of training from an accredited facility. The duties of the laboratory assistant may vary, but in general, their responsibilities range from cleaning laboratory equipment, glassware, and instruments, to preparing and collecting specimens and performing basic and routine laboratory tests. Many laboratory assistants continue their education in order to qualify for more advanced positions.

A *phlebotomist* is a member of the medical labo-

ratory team who is solely responsible for drawing blood samples. He or she may either be trained on the job, or, like the laboratory assistant, may receive formal training from an accredited facility. Some phlebotomists are also laboratory assistants.

The *cytotechnologist*, or CT, is the person responsible for preparing and studying slides of human cells. This person also makes preliminary reports of abnormalities or evidence of disease to the pathologist, in order to indicate whether further study may be needed. The required training for a CT is two years of college, plus another year in a laboratory school. Accreditation is voluntary and is available through registries such as the American Society of Clinical Pathologists.

Tissue samples that are prepared for microscopic examination by a pathologist are done so by the *histotechnologist* (HTL) or the *histologic technician* (HT). These pathology laboratory workers prepare and preserve body tissue for sectioning and staining

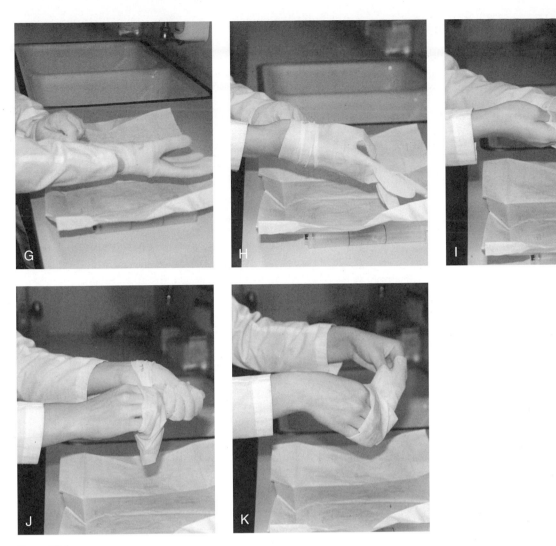

Figure 17-1
Continued.

before placement on slides. The histotechnologist has studied for four years in college plus one year in a laboratory school. The histologic technician has worked and studied for two years in a pathology laboratory or for one year in an accredited program. Certification is offered through the American Society of Clinical Pathologists.

Any member of the medical laboratory team who wishes to continue his or her education may obtain specialty certification in areas such as microbiology, hematology, clinical chemistry, virology, and other related areas.

The Laboratory Physicians

A *physician* is the sole person responsible for diagnosing and ultimately treating the patient. The education and training to become a Doctor of Medicine, or MD, is long and difficult. It requires three to four years of college and then four more years of study in

a medical school. The MD degree is conferred on graduation. The new MD must successfully pass a qualifying examination given by a state board of medical examiners. After this, most states require that the MD work at least one year as an intern before beginning to practice medicine without supervision and consultation. If the doctor wishes to specialize in a particular branch of medicine, he or she will also be required to serve a *residency* by spending an additional two to five years working in a hospital under supervision in order to learn the specialty.

A *pathologist* is a medical specialist who examines body cells and tissues removed during surgery or at autopsy for abnormal conditions. This person is usually responsible for directing medical laboratory activities and consults with other physicians about the results of tests. Small laboratories in clinics, lacking a pathologist, are sometimes headed by an internist, or a physician who specializes in the practice of internal medicine.

The Working Environment

In most large medical laboratories, the working environment or work area, may be a large room or a department with several rooms. In a smaller clinical laboratory, the work area may be limited to a counter or portion of a counter. Not all work areas are represented in every laboratory. The names of areas are based upon the types of tests performed, or the function of the location. Major divisions, or departments of the medical laboratory, include bacteriology, parasitology, pathology, serology, urinalysis, and a section for recordkeeping. Some of these sections may be combined or called by different names.

In addition to growing bacteria in cultures, members of the laboratory working in *bacteriology* stain slides and use special culture media to identify specific types of bacteria. Sensitivity tests are also run in order to determine the medication of choice and the proper dosage of the drug.

Donors are screened and their blood drawn in the *blood bank*. The units of blood are typed, carefully tested for purity, and placed in the bank for future use. Blood will be divided into its components for distribution to more than one person. When a patient needs blood, the blood bank worker will cross match units of blood to determine compatibility with the recipient's blood. Any reaction to a transfusion is investigated, and any unusual types of antibodies are identified.

Laboratory workers in the *chemistry* department are responsible for analyzing the contents of blood, urine, gastric juice, cerebrospinal fluid, and any body fluid, in order to determine whether it is abnormal and how much it deviates from normal.

Cytology and histology are often together. *Cytology* is concerned with cells discarded by the body, while *histology* deals with tissues. Both accept tissues and cells for fixing, sectioning, staining, and mounting on slides. Technicians identify normal and abnormal cell structures, including cancer, during microscopic examination. Pathology usually refers to these sections of the laboratory.

The other departments in the laboratory are called the *clinical laboratory*, or the *medical laboratory*. The morgue in a hospital may be closely associated with the pathology department, since the pathologist is directly involved in all three areas.

In the *hematology* department, blood cells are examined as to number, morphology, type, and proportion to fluid. Abnormal cells are also noted, as is the presence of any infection or other disease process. Cerebrospinal fluid examination and studies on the ability of blood to coagulate are also carried out in the hematology department.

Microscopic organisms that cause disease are isolated and identified in the *microbiology* department of the laboratory. These may be fungi, rickettsiae and other parasites, as well as bacteria. Because of this variety, the term *bacteriology* has been changed to *microbiology department* in most medical laboratories.

Blood and fecal specimens are studied in *parasitology* in order to test for the presence of parasites. Tests for the presence of blood are run on feces.

Phlebotomy may be a section in the blood bank where donor blood is drawn, or it may refer to a section of the laboratory where blood samples are collected for testing.

Workers in the *serology* department use antigens to test for the presence of antibodies in tissue or blood for the purpose of diagnosis of a specific disease, including venereal disease. Pregnancy testing may also be done here or in connection with urinalysis.

Urine is tested and examined in the *urinalysis* department for its physical properties, its chemical content, and microscopic examination.

Finally, one very essential section of the laboratory is the bookkeeping or clerical department. In this department, all requests for tests and reports on the results of testing are collected and recorded. Office supplies and the purchasing of laboratory equipment, are also furnished and conducted through this section.

Communication and the Medical Information System in the Medical Laboratory

The majority of hospitals throughout the United States use some type of computer system as their form of interdepartmental communication. *Computers* are electronic devices with the ability to create, process, retrieve, and store data. They are also, by far, the quickest and most accurate means of communicating information throughout the very busy and high-tech atmosphere of today's hospitals. Computers come in different sizes and have various uses in the health care field. Extensive systems are found in hospitals, nursing homes and extended care facilities, and clinics. With the development of small, less expensive models, computers have also appeared in the private offices of physicians, dentists, chiropractors, and veterinarians. An office may have its own system or a terminal for input into a large processing service at a distant site. Linkage is by telephone. A *terminal* is the workstation for a computer consisting of a video screen and a keyboard. A printer may also be attached if printed reports or a hard copy is needed. A computer workstation is shown in Figure 17-2.

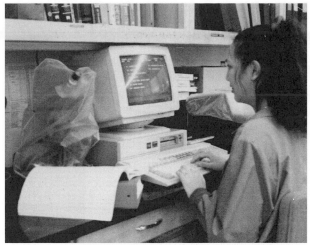

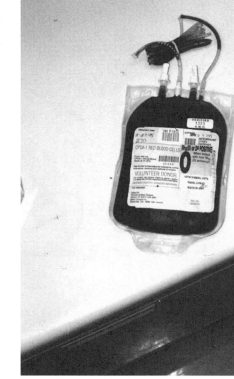

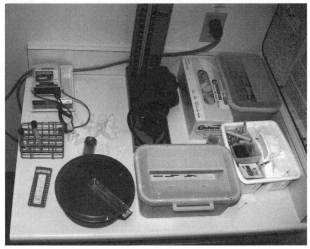

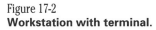

Figure 17-2
Workstation with terminal.

The two major divisions of a medical information system are patient care and business management. Under these divisions are programs that deal with bookkeeping, billing, correspondence, supply inventory and management, patient data, and clinical support. A computer system provides speed, accuracy, and efficiency that are not possible with a manual record entry system.

In most hospital environments, a computer terminal is placed at each nursing station and in each department. The screens should be placed to ensure confidentiality of what appears on the display. Doctor's orders can be put into the computer and transferred to the medical laboratory to order tests. Results can then be reported by the computer printout for inclusion in the patient's chart. An entry is made as the service is provided, together with the cost, and transferred to the business office for billing.

In the record room, a patient's chart is incorporated into a data bank. The present admission, to-

gether with any records of the patient's past admissions, are stored here. This information is also available to authorized personnel in the laboratory.

Within the laboratory, computers have many uses besides receiving and dispensing patient data. Some of these uses include preparing labels for identification of patient and tests, running the automated equipment to test patient samples, evaluating quality control procedures, and preparing reports of test results.

Summary

In this chapter, we discussed two very important aspects of working as a member of the medical laboratory team. These areas include laboratory safety and laboratory organization. The first point we noted is that there are two organizations responsible for enforcing safety regulations in the laboratory setting.

The agencies are OSHA and the Centers for Disease Control. We further stated that fire safety, equipment, codes, plans, and procedures are all part of the laboratory worker's safety, and because of that, all members of the laboratory staff are given proper instruction in procedures for carrying out safety measures in the hospital and medical laboratory environment.

In terms of laboratory organization, we discussed the various titles, educational requirements, and functions of specific members of the medical laboratory team. We also identified and described laboratory work areas, their general location, and the specific purpose and function each plays in the laboraotory. Finally, we discussed communications and information systems used by the medical laboratory, noting that computers are used by most laboratories because of their ability to accurately and readily process, store, and retrieve data.

Review Questions

1. What does the abbreviation *CDC* stand for?

2. What is the purpose of an *incident report*?

3. What branch of the federal government is ultimately responsible for overseeing the health and safety of all employees working in the clinical laboratory?

4. What is the name of the medical doctor responsible for examining cells and tissues in order to determine diseases and possible diagnosis and treatment?

5. When an agent is said to be *corrosive*, what does that mean?

6. When an agent is said to be *flammable*, what does that mean?

7. What does the abbreviation *NFPA* stand for?

8. What does the term *incinerate* mean?

9. What is the name of a physician who specializes in internal medicine and treats adult illness nonsurgically?

18

Laboratory Equipment

Performance Objectives

Upon completion of this chapter, you will be able to:

1. Explain how to store laboratory equipment.
2. Identify and be able to demonstrate how to use graduated cylinders, beakers, flasks, and test tubes.
3. Identify and be able to demonstrate how to use volumetric and serological pipettes.
4. Discuss the purpose and function of centrifuging and describe some of the more commonly used centrifuges in the medical laboratory.
5. Discuss the function of a microscope and be able to identify its various parts.
6. Discuss the function of an autoclave and an oven used in the medical laboratory and be able to demonstrate how each is used.
7. Explain the use of constant temperature appliances in the medical laboratory.

Terms and Abbreviations

Autoclave   an apparatus used for sterilization by steam under pressure.

Calibration   a mark on a piece of glassware or equipment that indicates the amount it will measure.

Centrifuge   a machine that spins at high speed in order to separate materials of different densities.

Graduated cylinder   a straight-sided tube with a base, used for measuring the volume of liquids.

Meniscus   a crescent-shaped curvature found on the upper surface of a liquid as it is measured.

Pipette   a cylindrical glass tube, which may or may not be calibrated, used to measure and to transfer liquids.

rpm   abbreviation for revolutions per minute; unit of measure for the speed of centrifuges.

Serological pipette   a pipette that is graduated to measure various volumes within a given amount.

Sterilization   a process used to make something free of all living organisms.

TC   abbreviation for to contain; marked on pipettes.

TD   abbreviation for to deliver; marked on pipettes.

Thermostat   an automatic device used to regulate or control temperature.

Volumetric pipette   a transfer pipette that measures a single amount.

Every medical facility uses many different types of supplies and equipment. The exact type will depend upon what department within the facility the equipment or supplies are being used. And the method used for storage of the many hundreds of individual pieces of equipment and supplies will generally depend upon the needs of the individual institution. The most important point to remember here, is that all equipment and supplies should be kept where they are most readily accessible, yet are protected from the possiblity of any damage or hazard to others.

Storage and Use of Laboratory Equipment

Storage Areas

Most hospitals have a large storage area. Supplies are ordered in quantity and dispensed as needed. Usually, a written request is required by the department in need of the specific supplies. Some facilities have computer capabilities for ordering supplies. The use of the computer may also facilitate updating of inventory in the supply area.

In small offices, the medical laboratory assistant may be assigned the task of maintaining supplies and equipment. If you are the person who is required to do this, it will be important for you to keep a list of all equipment and supplies. Keeping this list, or a regular inventory, will tell you what has been used and what must be ordered. It is a good idea to keep a pad and pencil close to, or even in, the supply area, in order to record needs as they occur. This will make it much easier to remember to order needed items. A list of suppliers with their names and telephone numbers or the sales representative, should also be prepared and kept up to date.

It is also important to keep and maintain an accurate file of operating manuals, warranties, and service personnel for all equipment. One factor to consider in the purchase of new equipment is the availability of maintenance service.

In order to maximize efficiency in the use of glassware and disposable equipment, it will be necessary to devise some logical method for their storage. Glassware must be easy to find, whether it is stored by size, type, use, or a combination of all three. Pipettes and test tubes are usually stored in drawers built to hold specific sizes. Other glassware is stored on accessible shelves. Glassware that is not used often should be covered in order to keep it free from dust and other airborne particles.

All large pieces of equipment should be stored out of the way. Equipment that is used most often should be the most accessible. Labels can be used to indicate not only the name of the equipment but also what test it is used for and if a hazard is present.

Using Calibrated and Volumetric Glassware

Graduated cylinders are designed to measure various quantities of liquid in graduated amounts. A *calibration* is a mark on the glassware that indicates the amount it will measure. For example, a 100-mL cylinder is graduated from 1 mL through 100 mL. Readings of volume of liquids must always be made at the bottom of the meniscus. A *meniscus* is the crescent-shaped curvature a liquid assumes when it is placed in a slender container. To read a volume of liquid in calibrated or volumetric glassware, the bottom of the meniscus is read against the graduation or calibration. The reading should always be done at eye level (Figure 18-1).

Flasks are a type of glassware used most often in the laboratory to measure volume. The most commonly used flasks include the volumetric, Erlenmeyer, and the Florence flasks. Volumetric flasks are designed to contain a single given quantity. They range in size from 1 mL to 2000 mL, and have one calibration on the neck of the container. They usually have a ground glass stopper and are used primarily to prepare specific volumes of reagents. In using volumetric flasks, always remember to read the bottom of the meniscus against the calibration mark.

Erlenmeyer flasks range in size from 50 mL to 2000 mL in volume. Calibrations extend up the sloping side from a flat bottom. The markings on the side can be used to measure or combine volumes not requiring absolute accuracy.

The Florence flask is similar to the Erlenmeyer, except that the sides are rounded. It is available in the same volume capacities and can be used for purposes similar to the Erlenmeyer. Figure 18-2 shows examples of all three flasks, as well as other types of glassware used in the medical laboratory.

A beaker is a straight-sided container. There is a pouring spout formed by the rim on one side. Beakers may show a volume capacity or have calibrations along the side. These containers are used for holding liquids or for mixing when volume is not critical.

Test tubes come in a variety of sizes and shapes and have varied uses in almost all departments in a medical laboratory.

Using Pipettes

A *pipette* is a calibrated glass tube that is open at both ends and is used to measure small volumes of liquid. Pipettes are also used to transfer liquids from

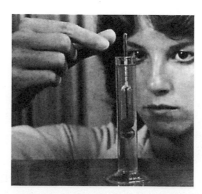

Figure 18-1
Measuring at eye level using calibrated glassware. (Reprinted with permission from Bonewit, K. *Clinical Procedures for Medical Assistants*, 3rd ed. Philadelphia: W. B. Saunders, 1995, p 304.)

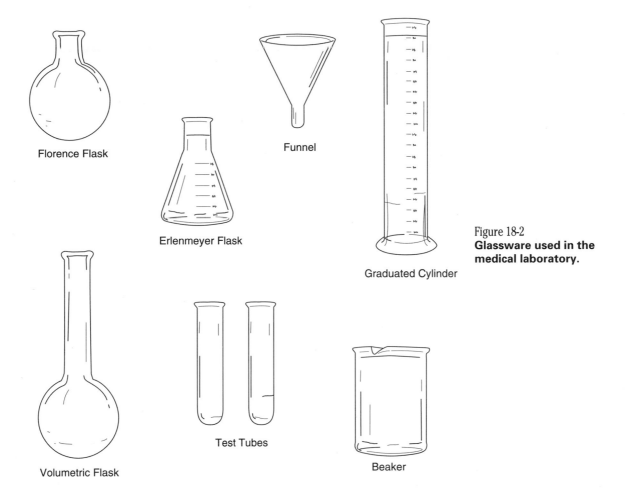

Florence Flask

Erlenmeyer Flask

Funnel

Graduated Cylinder

Figure 18-2
**Glassware used in the
medical laboratory.**

Volumetric Flask

Test Tubes

Beaker

one container to another. These are called *transfer pipettes*. Two examples of transfer pipettes are volumetric pipettes and medicine droppers. Volumetrics are calibrated exactly. Dropper pipettes, which deliver drops, can be used when accuracy is not required. The two general types of calibrated pipettes are serological and volumetric (Figure 18-3).

Serological pipettes are graduated in order to measure various volumes within a given amount. These generally require filling to a calibration mark, then allowing to drain. They are etched at the mouth end and marked TD (to deliver). These pipettes must have the last drop blown out.

Volumetric, or *transfer, pipettes* differ from the serological pipette in that they have only one calibration mark. This pipette is also a TD type. It should be allowed to drain down the side of the vessel. If a volumetric pipette is marked TD, you must allow the pipette to drain, and then rinse with the diluting solution so that the pipette will deliver the exact amount stated.

In order to use a pipette, you will have to first attach a pipette bulb to the mouthpiece, place it into the solution to be measured, and then use suction to draw the solution up to the desired mark. You must

make sure that the meniscus is on the desired calibration mark. Withdraw the pipette, wipe the outside with a tissue in order to dry it, and then place the tip of the pipette against the side of the receiving vessel. Release the suction, and allow the liquid to drain into it. If the top of the pipette is etched, make sure you blow out the last drop. You must also remember to always use a mechanical suction device when pipetting concentrated acids and alkalis, deadly poisons, corrosive substances, and radioactive materials.

Using the Centrifuge

The centrifuge is one of the most commonly used pieces of equipment in the medical laboratory (Figure 18-4). It is a machine that spins at a high speed, creating a centrifugal force that causes substances of different densities to separate, the heavier particles falling to the bottom and lighter particles and fluids rising to the top. Laboratory centrifuges are used most often in the separation of serum or plasma from whole blood, bacteria from liquid media, and to concentrate the sediment in urine for microscopic examination.

Although centrifuges may vary in size, they must

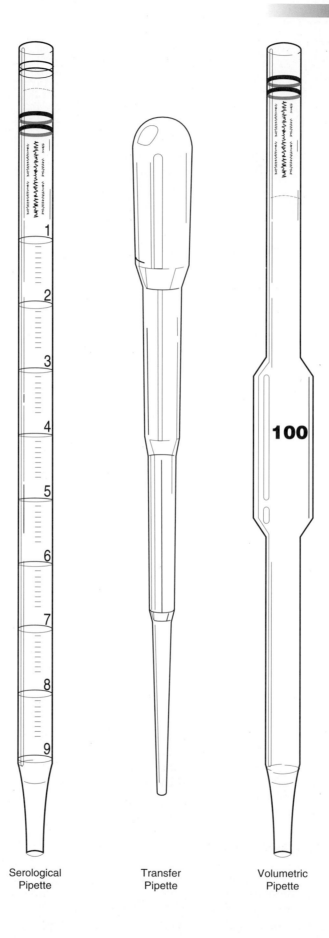

Figure 18-3
Types of pipettes.

Serological
Pipette

Transfer
Pipette

Volumetric
Pipette

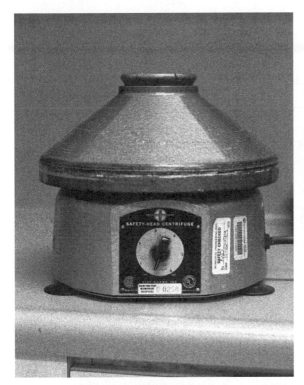

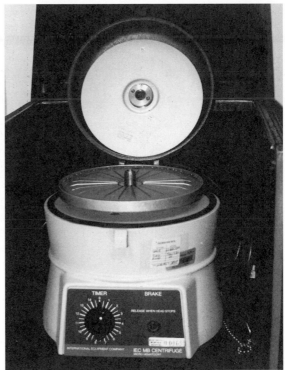

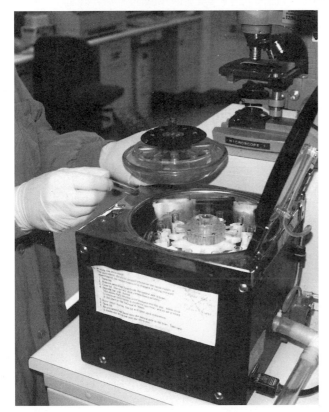

Figure 18-4
Centrifuge.

all be used with great care. Table models, for example, should be placed on a sturdy bench or table where there is plenty of room for the machine to spin. Centrifuges should never be placed near the more delicate or sensitive equipment that might be affected by the vibration of the centrifuge. Larger models of centrifuges are generally bolted into the concrete on the floor.

All items that are placed into the centrifuge must be placed so that they balance each other. For example, if only two test tubes are being used, they must be of the same weight and placed exactly opposite each other. If you are using a large centrifuge, you should make sure that you weigh the specimens to be sure they are properly balanced. This helps to avoid damage to the centrifuge, breakage of the specimen tubes, and danger to yourself. You should also make sure that the lid of the centrifuge is securely closed before you turn the machine on, and remember, speed should be accelerated slowly.

Once the centrifuge has been turned off, it will stop spinning gradually. Most machines have a brake to be used if needed. Never use the brake to stop the machine just because you are in a hurry and do not want to wait until the machine stops spinning. And never try to stop the machine with your hand, since doing so could cause injury to yourself, the specimens, the centrifuge, or all three! If breakage occurs while the machine is running, quickly turn off the power supply, but never open it until it has completely stopped.

Types of Centrifuges

Although there are several types of centrifuges used in the medical laboratory, the types that you will probably encounter most frequently are the microhematocrit centrifuge, the refrigerated centrifuge, tabletop centrifuges, and variable-speed centrifuges. The *microhematocrit* centrifuge is used to perform a microhematocrit test. The machine is specifically designed to hold the capillary tubes required for the test. The purpose of a microhematocrit test is to determine an accurate packed cell volume of red blood cells using small quantities of blood. The centrifuge operates at very high speeds, usually ranging from 11,000 to 15,000 rpm. The machines are usually equipped with an automatic timer because an exact running time is required to produce constant test results. The accuracy of the timer should be checked frequently using a stopwatch or an electric clock.

A *refrigerated* centrifuge is exactly what the name implies. It is a centrifuge cooled by mechanical refrigeration with a thermostat to keep the temperature constant. This protects heat-sensitive specimens from the heat generated by the centrifugal force of the spinning. These are used in some blood banks and in the preparation of biological specimens.

Tabletop centrifuges are used in serological testing in order to improve red blood cell antigen-antibody reaction and also to wash cell suspensions. One type of centrifuge has fixed speed and variable time. The other has both variable speed and variable time. The routine checks of rotation speed and time of centrifugation are absolutely essential for consistent results that meet quality-control standards.

A *variable-speed* centrifuge has a relative setting indicator as part of its speed control. To set the speed control, a tachometer is used to determine the number of revolutions it makes per minute. Then the speed is marked as such. From time to time the laboratory will reverse the procedure. The control is set, and the tachometer is read to see if the specified revolutions are actually being produced. Tachometers may be the strobe or vibrating-reed type.

The Microscope

The *microscope* is used to magnify very small objects. There are many kinds of microscopes, all of which have been designed for different specific uses, and vary in price. A *simple microscope* uses a single lens or magnifying glass. Some simple microscopes can magnify to 200×. A *compound microscope*, which you will probably use most frequently in the medical laboratory, uses a series of lenses to increase magnification and will magnify up to 1000×.

If the microscope has a single eyepiece (ocular), it is called *monocular*. These microscopes are used most commonly to teach students how to use the microscope. *Binocular* microscopes have two eyepieces and are used in most laboratories. *Teaching* microscopes have two sets of eyepieces so that the instructor and the student can see the same field at the same time.

A *darkfield* microscope is used in the identification of some bacteria. In this microscope, a special condenser causes light to reflect from the specimen onto a dark background. Therefore, you are able to see a light object in a dark field.

Finally, the *electron* microscope is used when the greatest magnification is required, such as in the study of viruses. With this type of microscope, magnifications of 400,000× are possible.

Parts of the Microscope

A compound microscope contains many parts. For our purpose, however, we will only discuss the parts shown in Figure 18-5. These parts include the following:

- *Eyepiece (ocular)*. Contains a magnifying lens.
- *Body tube* or *barrel*. Connects the eyepiece to the objectives.
- *Nosepiece*. Supports the objectives.
- *Objectives*. Contain the lenses for magnification. The *oil-immersion objective* is a special objective found on some microscopes. It is designed to be used with a drop of immersion oil between the object and the surface of the lens.
- *Arm*. The support by which the microscope is carried.
- *Stage*. The part of the microscope where the slide is placed.
- *Slide clips*. Hold the glass slide in place on the stage.
- *Substage control*. Moves the stage for focusing but is not found on all microscopes.
- *Diaphragm*. Makes possible the adjustment of the amount of light entering the objectives.
- *Mirror*. Reflects light rays into the objective. Instead of a mirror, most microscopes used in the medical laboratory have a *substage lamp* to provide light.
- *Coarse adjustment wheel (knob)*. Moves either the stage or objective maximally for the first sighting of the object.
- *Fine adjustment wheel (knob)*. Moves either the stage or object minimally for fine focusing.
- *Base*. Supports the body of the microscope.

Procedure for Using the Microscope

One of the most important skills you will ever have to learn is how to use and care for the microscope. Following the steps outlined below will assist you to better understand how these tasks are completed.

1. Turn the eyepiece until the low-power objective is in place. You will feel and hear a "click" when you have reached that point.
2. Adjust the mirror or substage lamp with the eye at the eyepiece (ocular). If you are using a mirror, the flat side should face the stage if a condenser is used. Use the concave side if no condenser is present. Use the diaphragm to control the amount of light present.
3. Place the prepared slide onto the stage. Using the coarse adjustment wheel, move the tube or barrel downward until the low-power objective is close to the slide. Be sure you watch the tube move as you turn the coarse adjustment wheel, and never focus downward with the coarse adjustment wheel while peering through the eye-

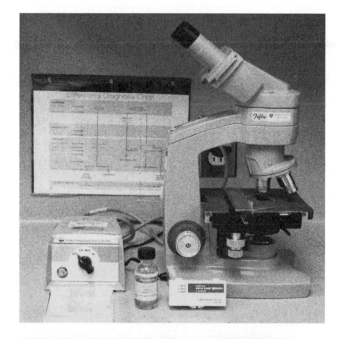

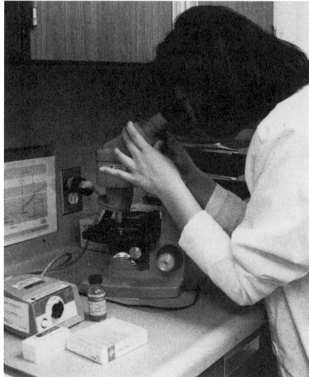

Figure 18-5
Parts of the microscope.

piece. This will help to avoid breaking the slide, cover slips, and even the lenses.
4. Place your eye at the eyepiece, and gradually move the tube upward, using the coarse adjustment wheel, until you see the object on the slide. If you fail to find the object, start over.

Lower the tube again, and gradually raise it. After you have found the object using the coarse adjustment wheel, gradually use the fine adjustment wheel to get a sharper image. You may need to readjust the light source and diaphragm to get the best image.

5. Once you have focused clearly using the low-power objective, you can change to the high-power objective. The image should stay in focus, but you will need to use the fine adjustment wheel in order to maintain a clear image. The magnification of the object viewed is the product of the magnification of the eyepiece multiplied by the magnification of the objective used. For example, if the eyepiece is 10×, and objective is 10×, magnification will be 100×.

6. When you have finished using the microscope, you must first remove the slide. Then clean the eyepiece, objectives, and stage with lens paper. Put the low-power objective in place and focus all the way down with the coarse adjustment wheel. The microscope should be covered or housed in a closed case when not in use.

7. To clean the microscope, you should always use lens paper. Xylol (xylene) can be used to remove oil from the oil-immersion lenses. Since xylol is toxic, it should be used sparingly and in well-ventilated areas.

8. When moving the microscope from one location to another, always make sure you use both hands to carry it. You should put one hand on the carrying arm and the other under the base of the instrument. Never try to carry other objects while carrying the microscope.

The Autoclave and the Hot Air Oven

The two most important pieces of equipment used in the medical laboratory for sterilizing other equipment and supplies, are the hot air oven and the autoclave. The choice of method depends on the type of material to be decontaminated and the equipment that the laboratory has available.

The hot air oven provides dry heat and is used most frequently to sterilize glassware or metal instruments. A temperature of 160°C for 2 hours is usually used.

The autoclave uses steam under pressure to sterilize glassware, sharp-edged or hinged instruments, water, culture media, or linens. Glassware is sterilized at 121°C for 15 to 20 minutes at a pressure of 15

pounds per square inch (lb/in^2). The autoclave is programmed with automatic timed cycles. Time and temperature are set to kill viruses, fungus, and bacteria, including spore forms. Autoclaving is used to decontaminate biohazardous materials such as blood specimens and bacterial cultures before they are finally disposed of.

Constant-Temperature Appliances

Two constant-temperature appliances you may encounter in the medical laboratory include a water bath and a heating block (Figure 18-6). A *water bath* is simply a container of water which is maintained at a constant, fixed temperature. It is used for some laboratory tests in which specimens must be incubated at a given temperature. The temperature of the bath is controlled by a heating device and a thermostat. Some water baths have a pump that is used to circulate the water. Be sure that the pump housing and heater are always immersed in the water.

A *heating block* is a solid metal block on which containers can be set or with holes suitable for holding various sizes of test tubes. It has a heating device with a thermostat so that a constant temperature can be maintained.

All specimens that are incubated in a water bath emerge dripping with water. A heating block eliminates this. However, foreign materials from spillage and breakage tend to accumulate in the test tube holes of the heating block. Some particles may be removed by simply turning the block upside down and shaking or by swabbing the holes. For thorough cleaning, you must remove the top plate.

Summary

In this chapter we discussed several types of equipment used most frequently in the medical laboratory. We also defined the term *calibration*, and discussed its implication to certain types of laboratory equipment, noting that one of the best ways to maintain quality control of test results was through accurate calibration and maintenance. The use of different types of glassware was discussed, including graduated cylinders, pipettes, flasks, beakers, and test tubes. Finally, we talked about the larger pieces of equipment found in the medical laboratory. We identified these pieces as centrifuges, microscopes, ovens, autoclaves, water baths, and heating blocks.

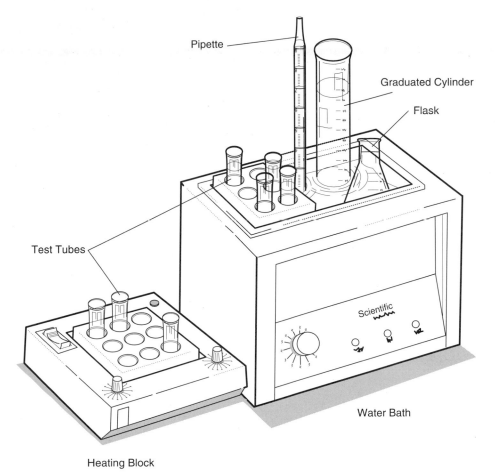

Figure 18-6
Water bath and heating block.

1. What function does an *autoclave* have in the clinical laboratory?

2. What is the name of the machine used to separate materials of different densities?

3. What is the term used to describe making something free from all living organisms?

4. What is the name of a cylindrical glass tube that may or may not be calibrated and that is used to measure and transfer liquids?

5. What does the abbreviation *rpm* mean?

6. When is a *graduated cylinder* used?

7. A _____ is a mark on laboratory glassware that indicates the amount it will measure.

8. A(n) _____ is an instrument used to magnify very small objects.

9. Give examples of at least two types of constant-temperature appliances:

    a. _____

    b. _____

10. Identify at least two types of glassware used in the clinical laboratory.

    a. _____

    b. _____

19

Specimen Collection and Processing

Performance Objectives

Upon completion of this chapter, you will be able to:

1. Discuss how to receive and dismiss a patient properly.
2. Explain how to put a patient at ease during the collection of a specimen.
3. Explain how to protect patient information and maintain confidentiality.
4. Discuss the differences between venipuncture and capillary blood collection.
5. Identify methods for collecting fecal and urine specimens.
6. Describe the types of specimens received in a medical laboratory.
7. Specify how different types of specimens are processed.
8. Explain how specimens are labeled and logged into records.

Terms and Abbreviations

Anticoagulant   a substance that prevents blood from clotting (coagulation).
Bevel   the slanted tip of a needle.
Biopsy   taking out a small piece of tissue for microscopic examination.
Blood plasma   the liquid part of the blood that has been prevented from coagulating.
Blood serum   the clear liquid part of the blood that remains when a clot forms.

Coagulation   clotting of blood.
Hemolysis   rupture of red blood cells with the release of hemoglobin into the plasma or serum.
Lancet   a sharp-pointed, two-edged surgical knife.
Lipemia   pertaining to an abnormal amount of fat appearing in the blood.
Venipuncture   puncture of a vein, usually for withdrawing blood.

Whether you are working or observing in a small clinic or in a large hospital laboratory, you will be required to receive patients. You may be the first professional person the patient sees. It is your responsibility to make the patient feel welcome and to try to establish a comfortable relationship. Every patient, regardless of social or economic status, has a right to expect courteous treatment no matter how busy you may be. All patients' problems are of paramount importance to them, even if they may seem routine or trivial to you. Remember, no one wants to be sick. An attitude of friendliness, concern, and optimism helps patients to cope with their problems. Moreover, you will get great satisfaction from helping patients.

Developing a Good Relationship with the Patient

Rapport is a relationship marked by harmony. It is extremely important that you establish such a harmony with your patients from the very first moments you encounter them. The following suggestions will help you to establish a good relationship leading to rapport with your patients:

- Always use the patient's name. This is important for identification and for indicating interest in the patient as a person. Try to make a real effort to pronounce each name correctly.
- Treat every patient as an important person, and as you would like to be treated. Make the patient aware that you are there to serve. Listen to what the person has to say. A friendly comment will almost always bring about a friendly response.
- Explain the procedure the doctor has ordered. Mention any way in which the patient may assist in the procedure.
- Try to reassure patients if they talk about their fears. Laboratory screening may be the first step of treatment for a frightened person facing a very real problem. Listen carefully and show genuine interest. Some patients can admit fears to you that they feel they must hide from family and friends. Offer sympathy, and never joke or laugh about such fears.
- If a patient is hostile, respond calmly. Hostility is often the expression of fear or worry. It may indicate that the patient is frightened, lonely, feeling helpless, or has the pressure of problems at home or at work added to the anxiety of being sick. Always remain calm and reasonable. If a patient refuses a test or procedure, do not argue. Simply report the refusal to the physician or to your supervisor.
- Since many people are frightened by the very sight of needles and lancets, it is well to remember that such patients may need a little extra reassurance and consideration when blood must be collected.
- Whenever there is a delay in a procedure, explain the reason to the patient. Try to estimate the length of extra time involved. Nothing adds to the fears of patients as much as waiting for appointments. Not only are they apprehensive, but a long wait implies that they are not important, and that you are making them waste their time.

Working with Children

When teenagers and older children are approached for testing, they are treated as adults. Explain what you plan to do, and proceed. Young children and infants, however, do not understand directions and cannot comprehend why they must be "hurt." Immobilize the child if necessary, and proceed with the procedure as rapidly as possible. Sometimes parents may be asked to hold the child. At other times, a disinterested adult should restrain the infant, after the parent has left the room. Never tell a child "this isn't going to hurt."

Dismissing the Patient

When tests and procedures have been completed according to the doctor's orders, courteously instruct patients about the next procedure, or direct them to the next department. You may need to escort them to the next location because the medical facility may seem frightening and confusing to a patient.

Professionalism

As a member of the medical laboratory team, you are considered a professional. Therefore, you are expected to conduct yourself in an ethical manner. One example of required ethical behavior is the privacy of the patient's medical record. The results of testing cannot be given to the patient, family, or friends. Patient information can only be discussed with the health care workers involved directly with the care of the patient.

It is sometimes hard to avoid discussing laboratory results when meeting with a patient for a second time or on a continuing basis. Nevertheless, it is always the responsibility of the doctor to give the patient his or her test results. The laboratory worker never gives test results to the patient.

Collection of Blood Samples by Venipuncture

Blood samples are used for many laboratory investigations. If more than a few drops are needed, blood is generally collected by venipuncture. It is important to establish a good rapport with the patient before you begin this procedure. Always remember to identify yourself, and tell the patient why you are there. Carefully identify the patient, using the name tag, arm band, and bed tag, and call the patient by his or her name. Review the doctor's orders to make sure you are collecting the correct amount of blood and that you have prepared the correct containers to receive the specimen.

You should appear calm, reassuring, and sympathetic to the patient. Remember that although you may collect many blood specimens every day, the procedure is probably new and frightening to the patient.

Always place the patient in a comfortable position. Ambulatory patients should be seated so there is a place to support the arm. Bed patients will need to remain in bed.

Briefly explain the procedure; avoid going into too much detail about the tests to be performed. Your

160

information may confuse the patient. Explain that there is little discomfort and no residual effect from venipuncture.

Venous blood is usually taken from veins in the inner bend of the elbow (Figure 19-1). If for some reason the elbow cannot be used, or if you have difficulty getting blood from these veins, other sites may be used. These include the lower arm, wrist, back of the hand, fingers, lower leg, ankle, or upper surface of the foot. However, these veins are usually very small, although they may appear large. They have a tendency to roll, and they may have toughened walls. Therefore, the veins in the elbow are almost always most satisfactory for venipuncture.

Procedure for Collection of Blood Samples by Venipuncture

To collect blood samples using the syringe method:

1. Assemble the necessary equipment. This will include sponges or cotton balls, alcohol wipes, a tourniquet, a syringe with a needle, test tubes, and slides, if required.
2. Select the site for puncture. Place the tourniquet above the site, and tie it with a slip knot so that it can be easily removed with one hand. Ask the patient to open and close the hand causing the veins to become congested. Then choose a vein that is clearly evident and seems sufficiently well supported by tissue so that it will not roll.
3. Cleanse the area with a sponge and antiseptic such as alcohol, or use an alcohol wipe. Dry with a sterile sponge, or air dry.

4. Insert the needle cleanly and rapidly with the bevel upward. Pull back on the plunger. As blood appears in the barrel of the syringe, you are assured that the needle is in the vein. Then release the tourniquet, and collect the amount of blood required.
5. Place a sponge over the puncture site, but do not apply pressure until the needle is withdrawn. Then apply pressure firmly, and flex the arm until bleeding stops. Caution the patient that a bruise will result if the wound is allowed to bleed.
6. Make blood smears if required. Then remove the needle from the syringe, and carefully distribute the blood to the indicated containers. Do no force blood through the needle, or handle it roughly, since this may cause the red blood cells to rupture, with resulting hemolysis. Label all tubes and slides.
7. Check to be sure that the patient is alright, then dismiss the patient or leave the room, taking all of your equipment with you.

Procedure for Collecting Blood Using the Vacutainer (Vacuum) Method

If you are using the vacutainer method, that is, using a vacuum tube to collect the blood rather than a syringe, the procedure for collection is similar to that of the syringe method.

1. Assemble your equipment. This will include sponges, antiseptic, alcohol wipes, a tourniquet, vacuum tube, and needle. Screw the needle into place on the adapter (Figure 19-2).

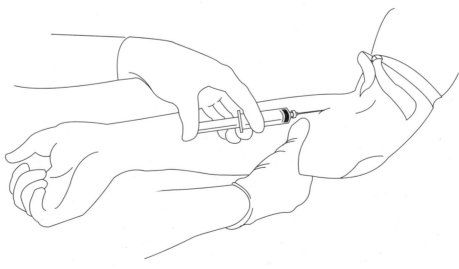

Figure 19-1
Taking venous blood.

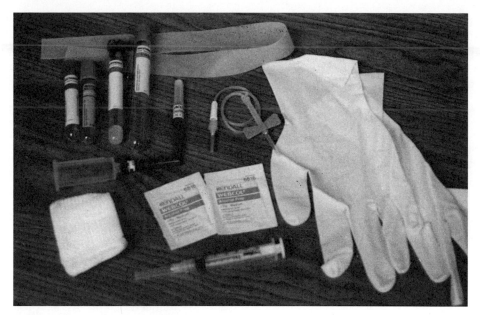

Figure 19-2
Vacuum equipment for collecting blood.

2. Place the tube loosely into the adapter (holder) contacting the double-pointed needle, but not puncturing the stopper. Follow the venipuncture procedure to prepare the patient. Insert the needle into a vein.
3. After the needle end is correctly inserted into the vein, push the stoppered tube firmly onto the adapter. Continue to aspirate until the tube fills to the predetermined amount. Vacuum tubes will not fill completely.
4. If multiple samples are needed, remove the first tube, and rapidly replace it with a second, third, etc. Be careful to keep the needle in place inside the vein as you change tubes.
5. After all specimens have been collected, remove the needle, and care for the patient as previously described. Label all tubes carefully. The label should include the patient's name and hospital number, the doctor's name, the date, and the test required. It may also include the name of the collector, the patient's room number, the time of collection, or any other pertinent information.
6. Dismiss the patient. Remember to always thank the patient for his or her cooperation, and leave with a friendly attitude.

Tips on Venous Blood Collection

For some tests, uncoagulated blood is required. An *anticoagulant* is a substance that prevents clotting of blood. The most popular anticoagulants are oxalate, which is a mixture of ammonium and postassium oxalate; Sequestrene (ethylene diamine tetra-

acetic acid [EDTA]), sodium citrate, and heparin. Be sure to select the correct one for the test to be done. The vacuum tubes are always color-coded so that the stopper indicates which anticoagulant is in the tube. Blood placed in a test tube containing an anticoagulant must be inverted gently to mix. Never shake the tube.

If serum is needed for a test, whole blood is collected in a plain tube. Do not invert or mix, since mixing causes hemolysis of the serum. The blood should be allowed to clot for 30 minutes at room temperature.

Blood placed in a test tube containing thrombin is inverted and can be centrifuged after 5 minutes.

The following tips will be helpful to you in preventing hemolysis of blood during venipuncture:

- Always use a sharp, smooth needle of the appropriate size, usually 20 or 22 gauge.
- Enter the vein as directly as possible.
- Never tie the tourniquet too tightly, and release it before aspirating blood.
- Always remember to remove the needle before distributing blood to the tubes.
- If serum is needed, always allow a clot to form before centrifuging.

Collection of Capillary Blood

Capillary blood is collected when only a few drops are enough for testing. Usually the specimen is collected from the ring finger or middle finger. The earlobe may be used if fingers are thick-skinned, very rough, swollen, scarred, bruised, or if the patient will be handling contaminated materials. The toe can be used if neither a finger nor an earlobe is available. In infants, either the toe or the heel is used.

Procedure for Collecting Capillary Blood

The first steps in collecting capillary blood are the same as those for venipuncture. Establish a rapport with your patient. Identify yourself. Identify the patient by tag and by asking for his or her name. Review the doctor's orders. Once you have completed these steps, follow the procedures identified below:

1. Assemble the necessary equipment. This will include sponges, a sterile lancet, capillary tubes, blood pipettes, and diluting fluid or a diluting unit for the test needed, and slides.
2. Select the site to puncture. Cleanse the area with a disinfectant sponge, and wipe with a dry sponge. If the site is wet, the blood will spread out instead of forming a drop.
3. Grasp the finger firmly across the middle or first joint (Figure 19-3). The patient may involuntarily move if you do not hold the finger securely. Quickly puncture the skin with a sterile, disposable lancet. Wipe off the first drop of blood. To take advantage of gravity, keep the patient's hand conveniently low. Using gentle pressure on the finger, fill containers as ordered. Do no allow air bubbles to form in collection tubes or pipettes. Collect the specimen with a continuous flow of blood. Hold up the distal end of the collection tubes, and then seal the ends of the capillary tubes with clay.
4. If requested, prepare blood smears on microscope slides.
5. Cleanse the finger with a disinfectant sponge, and apply pressure with a dry sponge to stop bleeding.

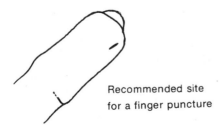

Recommended site for a finger puncture

Figure 19-3
Collecting capillary blood. (Reprinted with permission from Bonewit, K. *Clinical Procedures for Medical Assistants,* 3rd ed. Philadelphia: W. B. Saunders, 1995, p 371.)

6. Make sure that the patient is alright. Thank the patient for cooperating, and then dismiss him or her. If the patient is in the hospital, be sure to collect all your equipment and the specimens before you leave the room.

Collecting Fecal Specimens

Laboratory tests on feces are important in diagnosis, and therefore, are often performed in the medical laboratory. The patient should be carefully instructed in the method of collection in order to ensure a satisfactory specimen. Hospital patients are given a clean, dry bedpan for defecation. Nursing personnel will collect the specimen and send it to the laboratory. If the patient is to collect the specimen, then he or she must fully understand what is to be collected, how it is to be collected, and what container should be used. Whether the patient is in the hospital or is required to bring the specimen into the lab, to ensure that the laboratory receives an appropriate specimen, instruct the patient to follow the guidelines listed below:

1. Never allow the specimen to become contaminated with urine.
2. No laxative should be taken unless it is ordered by the physician.
3. A wide-mouthed container with a tight-fitting lid and a few wooden tongue blades or special collecting spatulas should be provided to the patient for obtaining the specimen.
4. The patient may defecate in a clean, dry bedpan, a disposable paper collection unit, or on a paper plate.
5. Have the patient collect a small amount of feces, about the size of a pecan, place it in the container, and cover the container securely. It is important that the patient take care to avoid contaminating the outside of the container.
6. Finally, remind the patient that it is important to wash his or her hands. Attach the completed label, and return the specimen to the laboratory. The information on the label should include the patient's name, the time and date of collection, the name of the doctor, and any other pertinent information.

There are a variety of tests that may be performed on fecal specimens. Some of these may require very specific instructions for collection. Details such as preservatives, special containers, exact time of collection, or a constant temperature may be important. Such instructions should be made very clear to the patient. Examples of some of the more frequent types of tests performed on fecal specimens include gross examination for consistency, color, mucus, or blood, tests for occult blood, detection of ova and parasites, and viral and bacterial cultures.

Collecting Urine Specimens

Perhaps one of the most common procedures you will be required to perform in the medical laboratory is a series of tests done on urine. The most frequent of these tests, called a *routine urinalysis*, refers to a predetermined series of tests that are performed on most urine specimens. Usually, a routine urinalysis includes a gross examination of appearance, reaction, simple chemical tests, and a microscopic examination of sediment. A *routine specimen*, which is generally used to perform the urinalysis, means any urine specimen collected at any given time during the 24-hour day. Such a specimen may vary in concentration, depending on the patient's liquid intake. Sometimes the first urine specimen collected in the morning is preferred, since it is generally more concentrated. A routine urine specimen is almost always collected upon admission to the hospital or when visiting the doctor's office.

Some tests performed may require that a timed urine specimen be collected. This means that the entire quantity of urine voided for the timed period, usually either during a 12- or 24-hour period, be collected and sent to the laboratory for testing.

Most hospitals use plastic, disposable containers for urine collection. Plastic, glass, or metal containers are commonly used in smaller laboratories, since they can be easily washed, dried, and reused. Occasionally, a patient may be asked to collect a urine specimen at home. If this is the case, you will have to provide the patient with a specimen container. Be sure that the container is clean, dry, and uncontaminated.

Receiving and Logging Specimens in the Medical Laboratory

Many types of specimens are received in the medical laboratory. The purpose of collecting them are threefold. In some cases, these specimens may be used to diagnose a disease. Other instances may require that the specimen be collected in order to determine the proper course of treatment for a specific disease or medical condition. A third reason specimens are obtained is to assist the physician in defining the progress of the prescribed treatment. The amount of specimen that may be needed usually depends on the tests to be performed. Specimens can include any body excretion such as urine, feces, or sputum. Other specimens may be obtained by needle aspiration, such as blood, spinal fluid, pleural fluid, and body cells from the liver, sternum, or kidneys. Tissue obtained from resections or from biopsies can also be sent to the medical laboratory for examination.

Another type of laboratory specimen frequently encountered by the laboratory assistant is a *smear*. This is obtained by touching a body area with a cotton swab, then smearing the swab onto a microscope slide. Such material is most commonly obtained from the patient's nose, throat, or a wound. Many other types of specimens are received in the laboratory, depending on the capability of the laboratory and the need of the patient.

Logging Laboratory Specimens

Most medical laboratories have an established routine for receiving specimens. An area is usually designated where the specimens may be placed when they arrive. As a laboratory assistant, it may be your responsibility to identify incoming specimens and route them to the correct work area.

Some method of *logging* or recording specimens must be used. Such a method will depend greatly on the type of institution, the type of specimen, and the number of specimens handled by the laboratory.

In very large laboratories, numbering systems and color coding may be used. The color coding indicates the various divisions of the laboratory. This makes it much easier to route the specimens in a much quicker and more efficient manner to the appropriate division. Numbers may be used to identify the specimen, the accompanying information, and all the tests required to complete the laboratory examination. A permanent record of the test may also be filed using the same number. There are many types of numbering devices currently on the market and in use by medical facilities. One type involves using numbered adhesive tapes or labels. Labels with bar codes are also available to place on collection tubes and subsequent tests used for that specimen.

In smaller laboratories, where there may be fewer specimens to handle, simpler logging methods may be used. A request form with a single carbon copy may be satisfactory. This form indicates the type of test ordered and all the information needed to identify the patient, including his or her medical record number. This number is affixed to the specimen. When testing is complete, the original request, with the test results, is then returned to the patient's chart, using the number to ensure proper identification. The copy is filed in the laboratory.

In very small laboratories, such as those found in the doctor's office, specimens may be numbered with a marking pencil, and the same number recorded on the accompanying request sheet.

It is important to remember that whatever method of logging is used, mistakes in identification of specimens cannot be tolerated, and all logging methods should be aimed at elmination of any possible errors.

Every means possible should be used to identify a specimen properly with incomplete information. Keep in mind that no laboratory specimen is unimportant, and some may be extremely difficult to collect. Indeed, it is impossible to replace most laboratory specimens. If it is not possible to identify a specimen correctly, it must be discarded.

Preparing Specimens for Testing

Part of your responsibilities as a laboratory assistant may involve processing certain laboratory specimens. *Processing* refers to the preparation of a specimen for the actual analysis after it has been collected. One problem to avoid, if you are asked to process a blood specimen, is hemolysis.

Whole blood should be kept in the original stoppered container until it is ready for analysis. If there is a delay of more than one hour before testing, the specimen should be stored in the refrigerator.

Some blood tests are done using serum. *Serum* is the liquid part of the blood that remains after a clot has formed. To process a blood specimen, you must first allow the blood to clot for 30 minutes. Then, rim the tube with an applicator in order to loosen the clot. Next, centrifuge the specimen, and collect the supernatant serum.

If an anticoagulant is added to whole blood, the liquid part of the blood in which the cells are suspended is the *plasma*. To collect plasma, you must first centrifuge the blood. The cells will then collect at the bottom of the tube. The supernatant fluid is the plasma. Plasma should be refrigerated if there must be a delay between processing and analysis. Both serum and plasma may be frozen if the delay is longer than 4 hours.

Blood that has been collected soon after a patient has eaten a meal may contain neutral fats. These will cause the serum or plasma to have a milky appearance, and will ultimately cause an error in the test results. To avoid this problem, be sure to instruct the patient to fast before the blood is collected.

Other materials for testing may require special processing, but the general rule of thumb to remember is to examine the specimens as quickly as possible after it has been collected. If prompt analysis is impossible, use the appropriate means to preserve the specimen.

Packaging Outgoing Specimens

Few medical laboratories are equipped to conduct every laboratory test that may be required. Some specimens may have to be sent out to other laboratories for testing. Outgoing specimens must be packaged and correctly labeled in their appropriate and suitable containers. The label should include all pertinent information, including the patient's name, address, and medical chart number; the date and hour of collection; the type of specimen; the exact tests ordered; and the name and address of the attending physician. This same information should also be filed in the sending laboratory in order to ensure proper identification of the specimen, verification that it was sent, and for patient billing.

Maintaining Laboratory Files, Records, and Reports

Copies of all laboratory tests performed are always kept in the medical facility, usually as a database in a computer. These records are used to determine charges for laboratory services, to replace reports that may have been lost, and to provide specific information and statistics for research.

Today, modern electronic equipment and computers have made it possible to keep large numbers of laboratory records and reports in small spaces. In some laboratories, however, the laboratory assistant may be required to file laboratory reports by hand.

Reports may be filed under the patient's name, patient's number, type of test, or even the name of the attending physician. Whatever method is used, filing and retrieval should be a relatively easy task.

Summary

In this chapter, we discussed the importance of developing a good relationship between the laboratory worker and the patient, noting that establishing a friendly, caring rapport with your patients will assist you in gaining his or her cooperation, an important step and necessary in obtaining a laboratory specimen. We also identified the various types of specimens that may be tested in the medical laboratory, as well as what the purpose was for their testing. In addition to discussing the different types of specimens tested in the medical laboratory, we talked about what the correct procedures were for properly collecting, processing, labeling, and logging them, noting that proper labeling of specimens was as important as following the correct method for their collection. Finally, we discussed the most common methods for maintaining laboratory files, records, and reports.

Review Questions

1. What is the name of a substance used to prevent blood from clotting?

2. When a red blood cell ruptures and then releases hemoglobin into the plasma or serum, it is called _____ .

3. A procedure that involves the puncture of a vein, usually for the purpose of withdrawing blood, is called _____ .

4. A condition in which there is an abnormally high content of fat appearing in the blood is called _____ .

5. What is the name of the clear liquid portion of the blood that remains after a clot has formed?

   a. blood plasma
   b. blood serum

6. What is the name of the clear liquid portion of the blood that has been prevented from coagulating?

   a. blood plasma
   b. blood serum

7. A procedure that involves taking out a small piece of tissue and examining it under a microscope is called a _____ .

8. A process that involves developing a relationship marked by harmony is called _____ .

9. Give at least two locations in which capillary blood can be obtained:

   a. _____
   b. _____

10. Briefly explain the difference between a *smear* and a *stain.*

20

Urine Testing

Performance Objectives

Upon completion of this chapter, you will be able to:

1. Identify the correct procedures for collecting urine specimens.
2. Explain and demonstrate how to label urine specimens.
3. Describe and demonstrate the correct procedure for performing a microscopic examination on a urine specimen and recording its physical characteristics.
4. Describe and demonstrate the correct procedure for performing specific gravity determinations on a urine specimen.
5. Discuss how to interpret "stix" and record readings of pH, protein, glucose, ketones, bilirubin, urobilinogen, blood, and nitrite on a urine specimen.

Terms and Abbreviations

Amorphous   without a definite shape.
Anuria   the absence of excretion of urine from the body; failure of the kidneys to function.
Casts   cylindrical structures with blunt ends and parallel sides that are composed of mucoprotein.
Convoluted   rolled together or coiled.
Hematuria   the presence of blood in the urine.
Occult blood   a minute amount of blood that is detected by chemical tests or microscopic examination.
Polyuria   excessive urination.

Pyuria   an excessive amount of white blood cells (pus) in the urine.
Quantitative   a test that determines how much of a substance is present as opposed to *qualitative*, which just indicates that a substance is present.
Sediment   substance that separates out of a solution and settles to the bottom.
Specific gravity   the weight of a substance as compared with an equal volume of water at the same temperature.
Void   to urinate.

Urine is a complex aqueous solution made up of several organic and inorganic substances, most of which are either waste products from body metabolism or products formed directly from the foods ingested into the body. The most important organic materials found in urine include urea, uric acid, and creatinine. The chief inorganic substances found are chlorides, phosphate, sulfates, and ammonia.

Whenever disease is present, there are certain materials that may or may not appear in the urine. These substances include proteins, carbohydrates, acetone, bile, and hemoglobin. Examinations should always be carried out on urine specimens that are fresh, since the chemical composition can be altered upon standing. Urine that cannot be examined immediately should be refrigerated.

Collecting the Urine Specimen

Most medical laboratories routinely process urine specimens collected either as the first morning specimen or those which are collected randomly. The *first morning specimen* is preferred because of its concentration. It is generally collected outside the laboratory by the patient or by a member of the nursing staff. A *random specimen* can be collected at any time and has a variable dilution. If the patient is responsible for collecting the specimen at home, you must be sure that the laboratory provides the container. Patients should never be allowed to use dirty receptacles.

In the hospital, the collection of routine urine specimens is the responsibility of the nursing staff. They collect, label, provide the request form, and usually deliver the specimen to the laboratory. The members of the laboratory are then responsible for checking for complete labeling and agreement between the container and the request slip. Then they assign a laboratory number and log the specimen if required.

In some instances, a midstream or "clean-catch" urine specimen may be preferred. This means that the specimen is essentially free of contamination. The patient should be instructed to clean the urethral area if female, or glans if male. In the hospital, nursing personnel will assist the patient. The patient then begins to void in the toilet. This rinses the urethra. The midstream urine is collected in a clean container. The remaining urine is voided into the toilet. If the midstream specimen is to be used for bacteriological studies, a sterile container must be used.

In rare instances, catheterization may be used to obtain a clean urine specimen for bacteriological study. Such procedures are infrequently ordered because the use of the catheter may cause urinary tract infections.

If you are working in a clinic or a physician's office, you may be responsible for urine specimen collection. If you are required to do so, you may use the following procedure to collect the specimen:

1. Provide a clean, dry container.
2. Ask the patient to provide a urine specimen.
3. Tell the patient the location of the restroom and instruct him or her where the collected specimen is to be placed.
4. When the specimen is returned, label it properly, and provide the proper report or requisition form.
5. Perform the tests as soon as possible. If there must be a delay, refrigerate the specimens.

Performing the Urinalysis

Once the urine has been collected, properly labeled, and delivered, you are ready to begin the urinalysis. This is probably the most common laboratory procedure and consists of a series of tests performed on the urine. These tests generally include both macroscopic and microscopic examinations, as well as chemical tests and measurement of specific gravity.

Macroscopic Examination

A macroscopic examination is performed without the aid of a microscope and generally includes color and character. *Color* varies with concentration, urine pigments, and the presence of metabolic products. Terms which are commonly used to describe the color of urine include:

- *Colorless.* Very diluted.
- *Straw.* Almost colorless.
- *Yellow.* More concentrated; medications usually present.
- *Orange.* Very concentrated; carotene, bile, or medications present.
- *Green or blue green.* Dyes or medications.
- *Pink, red, or dark reddish orange.* Blood, hemoglobin, porphyrin, bacteria, vegetables, medicine, or normal pigments after pH change.
- *Black or brown.* Bilirubin, iron, porphyrin, melanin, or medications.

Character refers to the appearance or transparency of the urine and is reported as clear, partly cloudy (due to crystals, white blood cells, or blood), cloudy (many crystals, white blood cells, or blood), or grossly bloody. The odor of the urine is not routinely reported unless it is particularly unusual.

Specific Gravity

The *specific gravity* refers to the weight (mass) of a measured volume of urine compared with the same volume of water at the same temperature. The specific gravity of water is 1.000. Normal ranges of urine specific gravity (sp gr) are 1.010 to 1.020. However, samples of urine taken at random may be far above or below these figures. Generally, the specific gravity is inversely proportional to the quantity of urine. In other words, a large quantity of urine would have a low specific gravity. Variations in specific gravity are of value in detecting whether the kidneys are functioning normally. It may be low in cases of chronic nephrosclerosis, diabetes insipidus, and some functional nervous disorders, while it may be high in cases of fever and functional kidney disease, and is highest in diabetes mellitus. Dehydration and a decreased fluid intake may also yield an increase in the specific gravity.

Measuring Specific Gravity

Specific gravity is conveniently measured by using either a refractometer or a urinometer. The refractometer is a handheld instrument that requires only a drop of urine. It is especially useful when only a small quantity of urine is available for testing. If you are required to use the refractometer to measure the specific gravity, you may follow the steps listed below:

1. Hold the instrument in a horizontal position.
2. Clean the surface of the cover plate and prism with lens paper. Wipe lightly to avoid scratching the soft optical glass.
3. Place a large drop of urine sample on the prism face, and close the cover plate.
4. Hold the instrument so that the prism window faces the light source.
5. Turn the eyepiece to provide a sharp focus of the scale.

The borderline between the light and dark areas indicates the specific gravity of the urine. Always report the answer in four digits, such as 1.009 or 1.020.

If you are required to use the refractometer, always remember to hold the instrument with your fingers close to the eyepiece, and hold the hinged prism cover against the surface with your thumb and forefinger. Never grasp the prism section, since this will raise the temperature, thus resulting in an incorrect reading.

If you are using a *urinometer* to determine the specific gravity of urine, you will need a larger amount of urine to perform the test—usually about 15 mL. The urine should be mixed and then poured into the cylinder (Figure 20-1). Place the urinometer float in the urine, and gently twirl it to be certain that the float is free. It is also important that bubbles be removed from the surface of the urine. These are easily removed with a strip of filter paper. Read the bottom of the meniscus, and report the answer in four digits (e.g., 1.010). Be certain that you make frequent checks with distilled water in order to determine the reliability of the urinometer or refractometer.

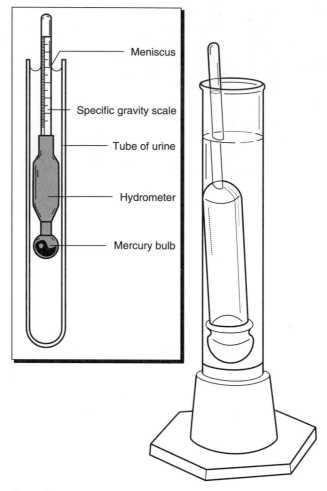

Figure 20-1
Urinometer (float) inside cylinder.

Determining pH

The acidity or alkalinity of the urine sample is referred to as its *pH*. Freshly voided urine is almost always acid, with a pH range of 4.8 to 7.0. Patients who eat foods high in protein may excrete more acid urine than those who consume mainly vegetables. A decreased pH is generally found in patients suffering from diabetic acidosis, fevers, pulmonary emphysema, diarrhea, dehydration, and during the use of some acidifying medications. Alkalinity (increase in pH), is mainly found in patients with chronic cystitis, certain genitourinary tract infections, pyloric obstruction, acute and chronic renal failure, and salicylate intoxication. Normally the urine becomes more acid with high-protein intake and sleep. It becomes more alkaline after collection and delay and usually after meals. The pH of the urine is easily determined by using the commercial "stix" available. These provide a range of pH from 5 to 9, and include a series of distinct color changes from orange to blue. The result is reported as acid, neutral, or alkaline.

Using Reagent Strips

Chemical screening tests using "stix" are comprehensive, convenient, and economical. They give results that are reproducible. The most commonly used commercial multiple reagent strips are manufactured and supplied by Ames, Inc., and called *Multistix*. These strips check the urine for pH, protein, glucose, ketone, bilirubin, blood, and urobilinogen.

Also available commercially are single reagent tests. These include *Clinistix, Diastix,* and *Clinitest,* all of which check for glucose, *Ketostix,* which test for ketones, and *Ictotest,* which may be used to test for the presence of bilirubin. All of these should be negative. Any protein, glucose, ketones, blood, bilirubin, urobilinogen, and nitrites present may indicate a pathological condition.

To use any of the reagent strips, dip the "stix" in the fresh urine. Tap the strip against the container. Observe the specified times, and read accordingly. Compare with the color chart, and record the test results. Remember to test the reagent strips daily in order to be certain that the strips are working. This will ensure accuracy for quality control.

Microscopic Examination

Once you have completed the macroscopic examination and tested the specific gravity and pH of the urine, you are ready to examine the urine microscopically. To complete this task, you must first place 10 to 12 mL of well-mixed urine into a centrifuge tube, and centrifuge at 1500 to 2000 rpm for approximately 5 minutes. Make sure you pour all of the urine out of the tube. Then place the tube in an upright position so that the fluid remaining on the sides flows to the bottom in order to dilute the sediment. Shake the sediment by tapping the tip of the tube on the hand. Place a small amount on a clean slide, and cover it with a cover slip. If too much is poured onto the slide, the elements will be distributed through many layers and may be missed on examination. If too little is poured onto the slide, the sediment may dry before the examination is completed. Some laboratories prefer to use stained sediment. If this is the case, add one drop of crystal-violet safranin stain to the sediment, mix, and allow it to stand for about 3 minutes. Then place a drop on the slide, and cover with a cover slip.

Darken the field of the microscope by almost completely closing the diaphragm just beneath the stage. A well-darkened field is absolutely necessary if hyaline casts are to be found, since they are clear, colorless, and have low refractivity. First examine with the low-power objective, and then with the high-power objective. Be very careful to avoid careless transfer of sediment, use of too much light in the microscopic examination, use of high power only, drying of sediment, dirty equipment, and scratches on the slide.

Using the low-power objective, examine for any casts, epithelial cells, crystals, amorphous material, and mucous threads. Use the high-power objective to examine for erythrocytes, leukocytes, and bacteria. Report all microscopic findings according to the policy your laboratory follows. Some institutions report as *few*, *moderate*, and *many*. Others report in average numbers, which should include 10 fields, per low- or high-power field, such as *6/lpf* or *15/hpf*. Others may report results in pluses, such as "*+*, *++*, *+++*, and *++++*" or *1+*, *2+*, *3+*, and *4+*.

Cellular Structures, Casts, and Crystals

Cellular Structures

There are many microscopic cellular structures found in urinary sediment (Figure 20-2). The most frequently seen include squamous epithelial cells, red blood cells (RBCs), white blood cells (WBCs), bacteria, spermatozoa, trichomonas, yeasts, and casts.

Squamous epithelial cells are made up of large flat cells with small nuclei. Most are found in the urinary system, on the skin, and on the genitalia. Any time *red blood cells* or *white blood cells* are present in the urine, there is usually an indication of some type of infection or inflammation.

Bacteria are not normally found in urine. They multiply rapidly when urine is left at room temperature, and if their presence is significant, it generally means that the specimen has been contaminated. The presence of *spermatozoa* is not abnormal; however, they should be reported. *Trichomonas* is a parasite found in vaginal secretions. Their presence and frequency should also be reported. If *yeast* are detected in the urine, they too should be reported, since they are normally not seen in urine and their presence could be a sign of infection.

Casts

There are several different kinds of *casts* that may be found in urine sediment (Figure 20-3). The number is reported as */lpf*, but identification of type is usually confirmed on high power. Casts are cylindrical structures with blunt ends and parallel sides. They are mostly composed of mucoprotein, and at times various other structures are included. Their presence almost always indicates kidney disease. The type and frequency of casts should be reported. The different kinds of casts most often found in urinary sediment include *hyaline casts*, which are cylindrical and transparent; *finely granular casts*, which contain fine granules; *coarsely granular casts*, containing coarse granules; *red cell casts*, composed of RBCs; and *white cell casts* or *leukocyte casts*, which are composed mainly of leukocytes. Less frequently seen casts that may be visible on microscopic examination include *fatty casts*, containing fat droplets; *waxy casts*, which are similar to hyaline casts, but are opaque and may be convoluted; and *renal failure casts*, which are especially broad, and may be made up of any of the types and may occur in large numbers called "showers."

Crystals

Crystals may be found in urine that is either acidic or alkaline. Those forms of crystals found most frequently in acidic urine include *uric acid crystals*, shaped like plates and generally found in clusters; *amorphous urates*, which appear reddish in color and are often so numerous that they obscure all other structures; *calcium oxalate crystals*, commonly appearing as oval spheres, biconcave disks, dumbbells, or as a crystal with a cross inside; *tyrosine crystals*,

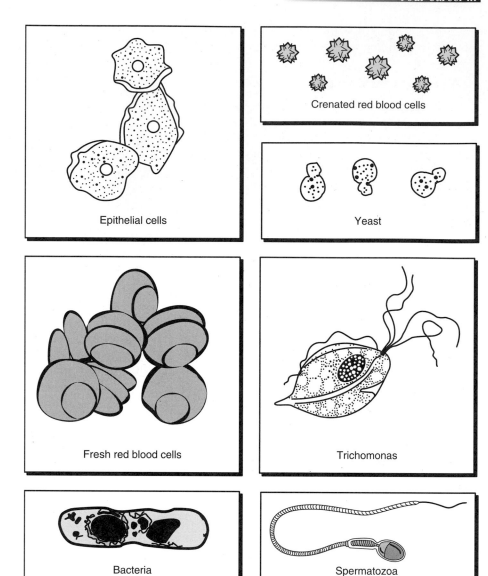

Figure 20-2
Cellular structures found in urine sediment.

which appear as yellowish, oily-looking spheroids; *cystine crystals*, appearing as flat, colorless, hexagonal plates with unequal sides; and *sulfanilamide derivatives*, which may produce crystals that appear as prisms, rhombic plates, or needles in sheaves, but all of which tend to have rounded edges rather than extremely pointed ones (Figure 20-4).

Crystals that are found most frequently in alkaline urine include *triple phosphate* or *ammoniomagnesium phosphate crystals*, which are colorless and usually occur as some modification of a prism with three, four, or six sides; *amorphous phosphates*, appearing as numerous colorless granules similar to amorphous urates found in acidic urine; *calcium phosphate crystals*, which generally appear as long prisms or needles or as large irregular plates; *calcium carbonate crystals*, which may be hidden among

amorphous phosphate granules or may be colorless spheres or dumbbells; and *ammonium biurate crystals*, which appear as yellow spheres covered with spicules and are sometimes called "thorn-apple crystals" (Figure 20-5).

On occassion, additional structures may be present in the urine that may or may not take on the appearance of casts or crystals. Fat globules, for example, may occur in urine that is either acidic or alkaline. They appear as highly refractive globules of various sizes, and if present, will stain black with osmic acid, and orange or red with Sudan III or scarlet red. To the inexperienced eye, other microscopic structures, such as talc and starch granules, may also appear as crystals, and nylon, cotton, or vegetable fibers may be mistaken for casts or mucous threads. Such artificial structures in urine are called *artifacts*.

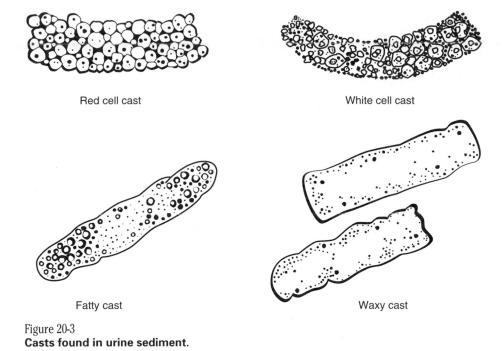

Red cell cast

White cell cast

Fatty cast

Waxy cast

Figure 20-3
Casts found in urine sediment.

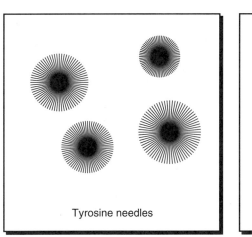

Tyrosine needles

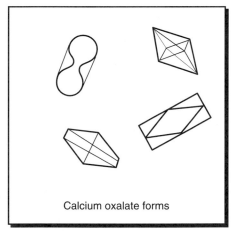

Calcium oxalate forms

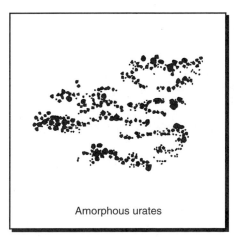

Amorphous urates

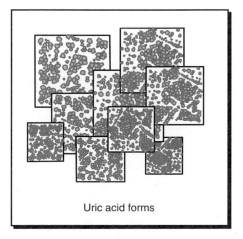

Uric acid forms

Figure 20-4
Crystals found in acidic urine.

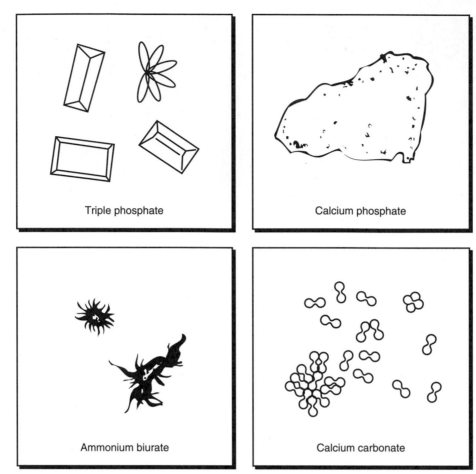

Figure 20-5
Crystals found in alkaline urine.

Summary

In this chapter we discussed how urine specimens are collected and prepared for urinalysis. We discussed both macroscopic and microscopic examina- tions, including how to test for specific gravity using both a refractometer and the urinometer. Finally, we discussed the many cellular structures found in urine, including those identified as cellular structures, casts, and crystals.

Review Questions

1. What does the term *amorphous* mean?

2. A term used to define excessive urination is:

   a. oliguria

   b. polyuria

   c. pyuria

3. What is the term used to describe the presence of blood in the urine?

4. Give three examples of substances that can be found in urine:

   a. _____

   b. _____

   c. _____

5. The _____ _____ pertains to the weight of a substance as compared with an equal volume of water at the same temperature.

6. A term used to describe the absence of the excretion of urine from the body is called:

   a. polyuria

   b. anuria

   c. oliguria

7. A term used to describe a substance that separates out of a solution and settles to the bottom is called:

   a. cast

   b. sediment

   c. soluent

8. What is the name of a specimen that can be collected at any time?

9. The acidity or alkalinity of a urine sample is referred to as its _____ .

10. What is the purpose of a *reagent?*

Hematology

Performance Objectives

Upon completion of this chapter, you will be able to:

1. Identify the various components of a CBC.
2. Explain the correct procedure for performing cell counts using automation.
3. Describe how to set up hemoglobin and hematocrit determinations properly.
4. Discuss how to calculate indices.
5. Demonstrate how to set up an erythrocyte sedimentation rate, and be able to calculate corrections if needed.
6. Discuss how to perform a reticulocyte count.
7. Describe and be able to demonstrate how to prepare, stain, and report blood smears.
8. Explain how to set up platelet counts manually.
9. Describe how specimens are collected for coagulation studies.
10. Identify and be able to explain bleeding and clotting time.
11. Discuss the significance of prothrombin time and the activated partial thromboplastin time.

Terms and Abbreviations

Agranulocytes   white blood cells that have few or no cytoplasmic granules.

Capillary action   the rise of fluid or blood in narrow tubes (capillary tubes).

CBC   abbreviation for complete blood count; a series of separate hematology tests routinely performed at a particular institution.

Differential white count   a report of the percentage and kind of leukocytes present in the blood.

ESR   abbreviation for erythrocyte sedimentation rate; the rate at which red cells settle out in a specified time as a result of changes in the surface charge of red cells.

Granulocytes   white blood cells that have distinct granules in the cytoplasm.

HbS   abbreviation for hemoglobin S; abnormal form of hemoglobin that causes sickling of red cells, thus altering the oxygen-carrying ability.

Hematocrit   measurement of the percentage of the blood that is made up by the red blood cells.

Hematology   the study of blood; the department of the lab-

oratory that concerns itself with blood cells and blood components.

Hemocytometer   a small glass counting chamber with a microscopic ruled area that is placed on the microscope stage and is used for counting blood components.

Hemoglobin   a substance found in red cells that is responsible for transporting oxygen throughout the body.

Heterozygous   a condition in which genes are not identical; for example, HbS and HbA.

Homozygous   a condition in which genes are identical; for example, HbS and HbS.

MCH   abbreviation for mean corpuscular hemoglobin; the average weight of hemoglobin in the red blood cell (RBC).

MCHC   abbreviation for mean corpuscular hemoglobin concentration; the weight of hemoglobin per volume of cells.

MCV   abbreviation for corpuscular volume; the average volume of the red blood cell (RBC).

MPV   abbreviation for mean platelet volume; the average volume of the platelet.

Platelet (thrombocyte) a small piece of cytoplasm that has broken off from a larger mass, and is concerned with the clotting mechanism in the body.

RBC abbreviation for red blood cell or erythrocyte; that part of the blood that contains the hemoglobin.

Reticulocyte a young red blood cell.

WBC abbreviation for white blood cell or leukocyte; that part of the blood that serves as a defense for the body by combating bacteria and viruses.

ematology means, literally, the study of blood. This is a reasonably good, though over-simplified, definition of the work that is performed in the hematology department. *Hematology* is the department within the medical laboratory which concerns itself with blood cells and blood components.

Blood Tests Performed in the Hematology Department

The Complete Blood Cell Count

One of the most frequently ordered tests performed by the hematology department is the *complete blood count*, or *CBC*. The CBC is almost always routinely required on all patients admitted to the hospital. It is actually made up of a group of separate tests, many of which may vary from one institution to another. A typical CBC, however, usually consists of the following tests:

- White blood cell (WBC) count.
- Red blood cell (RBC) count.
- Hemoglobin (Hgb).
- Hematocrit (Hct).
- Red blood cell indices (these include mean corpuscular volume (MCV), mean corpuscular hemoglobin (MCH), and mean corpuscular hemoglobin concentration (MCHC).
- Platelet count.
- Differential white cell count (diff).

Other tests that are frequently part of the CBC include the erythrocyte sedimentation rate (sed rate or ESR), reticulocyte count (retic count), and the sickle-cell tests.

The CBC is a general indicator of a person's state of health. Yet in some cases, a person may still be ill even though all the tests that make up the CBC are within normal ranges. Generally, however, one or more of the tests will be abnormal with results too low or too high. Remember, when working with a living, biological system, the word *always* rarely applies. Keeping that in mind, you should try to understand some of the information provided by some of the tests included in the CBC.

White blood cells combat bacteria when an infection is present in the body. An abnormally high white cell count usually means an infection. An extremely high white cell count might be an indication that a condition such as leukemia is present, while an abnormally low white cell count, known as *leukopenia*, can be caused by viruses, radiation, and even certain drugs.

Red blood cells contain *hemoglobin*, which carries oxygen throughout the body. Persons who have too few red cells or too little hemoglobin inside the red cells are said to be *anemic*. There are many possible causes of anemia. It may be as serious as leukemia or as simple as not getting enough iron in the food eaten. An RBC and an Hgb alone cannot diagnose the cause of anemia. Other tests must be performed in order to determine the actual cause of the anemia. *Erythrocytosis* is an increased RBC. This occurs in people living at high altitudes or who have a disease known as polycythemia vera.

The *hematocrit* (Hct) is a measurement of the percentage of the blood that is made up by the red blood cells. A hematocrit value, for example, of 36% would mean that 36% of the total blood volume consists of red blood cells. A good rule of thumb to remember is that the relationship between the hematocrit and the hemoglobin is that, numerically, the hematocrit value is generally three times the hemoglobin. For example, a hemoglobin of 11.0 grams should have a hematocrit value of 33%.

Thrombocytes or platelets are small pieces of cytoplasm that initiate the clotting process when a person is injured. When the number of platelets in the bloodstream is very low, internal bleeding may occur or the skin may develop severe bruises from only a slight impact with an object. If a person with a very low platelet count does receive a cut or laceration, it may be very difficult to stop the resulting bleeding.

The differential white cell count and blood smear evaluation can provide much valuable information. A thin smear of the blood to be examined is made on a glass slide, stained, and then observed under the microscope. The various types of WBCs seen on the smear are then categorized and tallied until 100 WBCs have been counted. Each cell type counted must be reported as a percentage. For example, if 23 of the 100 WBCs counted were classified as lymphocytes, then 23% lymphocytes would be reported. The size, shape, and appearance of the red blood cells are also observed, and written comments concerning any abnormalities are also included in the report. The approximate number, size, and shape of the platelets are also observed and commented upon if any abnormalities are seen.

Procedure for Performing Blood Cell Counting

The procedures involved in counting both RBCs and WBCs utilizes a system known as the Coulter method. This automated system, first recognized in 1980 by the College of American Pathologists (CAPP), has proved to be the most widely accepted method for counting both RBCs and WBCs throughout the United States. At that time, the CAPP performed a proficiency survey on 3724 laboratories nationwide, to determine how many of them used some type of Coulter instrument. The survey indicated that of that number, 2815 were in fact using the instrument. It was concluded that the number equalled approximately three fourths of those laboratories surveyed. Therefore, based on the information provided in that survey, it is statistically probable that at some point in your career, whether you are working as a student, or as a paid employee of a medical laboratory, you will encounter a Coulter instrument. It is important to note, however, that no recommendation of, or preference for Coulter products, is intended or implied by the author or publisher of this text.

When employing an automated method for counting cells, the blood cells suspended in an electrolytic solution can be sized and counted by passing them through an opening or aperture through which an electric current is flowing. As the cells pass through the aperture and displace an equal volume of electrolyte, the electrical resistance in the path of the current changes. This results in corresponding current and voltage changes. The amount of this change is directly proportional to the size of the cell. As a specific volume of blood sample is drawn through the aperture by vacuum, each voltage change is counted. This count represents the number of cells in the sample.

To perform a WBC and RBC count using an automated Coulter instrument, such as the Model ZF shown in Figure 21-1, you will need the following equipment:

- Isotonic buffered saline solution (diluent).
- Two snap-cap counting vials.
- 20 µL (micro) pipette.
- 10 µL (micro) pipette.
- Lysing reagent.

Pipette 10 mL of diluent into each of the two counting vials. Into one vial, pipette 20 uL of the blood sample. Recap the vial, and mix by slowly inverting it several times. The first vial contains a 1:500 dilution of the blood sample and will be used for the white cell count. The second vial contains a 1:50,000 dilution and will be used for the red cell count.

To the first vial (1:500 dilution), add three drops of lysing reagent to destroy the RBCs. Recap and in-

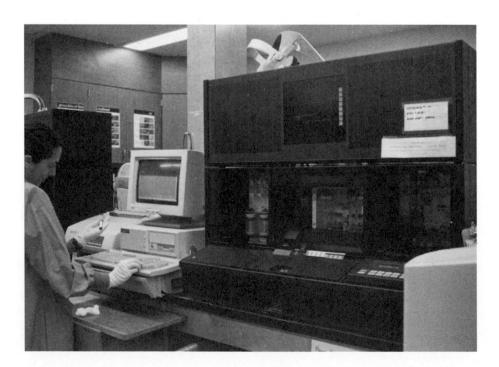

Figure 21-1
Coulter instrument.

vert to mix. To perform the actual counts on the Model ZF, the procedure is the same for both the red count and the white count. To accomplish this, you should:

1. Lower the beaker platform (1), and place the vial to be counted on the platform.
2. Slowly raise the platform, immersing the aperture tube (2) and external electrode (3) into the sample.
3. Position the vial so that the aperture is clearly visible on the debris screen (4).
4. Open the control stopcock (5) to a vertical position.
5. When electrical peaks appear on the sizing screen (6), close the control stopcock (5) to the horizontal position. This will initiate the counting process, and the numbers of the cells being counted will appear on the digital display (7).
6. When the counting stops, observe the final number on the digital display screen (7).

There is a very high probability that two cells may pass through the aperture at exactly the same time. To account for this, the Coulter instrument provides a Coincidence Correction Chart. To correct for coincidence, simply find the number obtained from the digital display screen on the chart, and read the corrected number in the adjacent column. All red cell counts are to be corrected. White cell counts above 10,000 should also be corrected.

When a red count is performed, the digital display result will be in millions of cells per cubic millimeter of blood. This means, for example, that a reading of 4.32 refers to 4.32 million RBCs per cubic millimeter (mm^3). Find 432 on the Coincidence Correction Chart, and read the corrected value (481). Thus, the value reported will be 4.81 million/mm^3.

White counts are displayed in thousands. For example, if the display reads 7482, that means that 7482 WBCs per cubic millimeter. For practical purposes, you would round off the answer to the nearest 100. Thus, 7482 would become 7500/mm^3. Remember, you must correct for coincidence on white counts above 10,000.

Performing Manual Counting

In some instances, a manual cell count may be needed. If this is indeed the case, special equipment will be necessary to complete the testing, and because of this, the medical technologist is usually the person responsible for performing the test.

Determining Hemoglobin

Part of performing a complete blood cell count involves determining the level of hemoglobin, or oxygen-containing element, of the blood. To accomplish this, you may use one of two methods: either using the Coulter Hemoglobinometer, or the cyanmethemoglobin technique. To perform a hemoglobin determination using the Coulter Hemoglobinometer, you will need the following supplies and equipment: a counting vial, isotonic buffered-saline diluent, a 10-mL pipette, a 20-µL pipette, and hemoglobin lysing reagent.

Using the Coulter Hemoglobinometer, follow the steps outlined below:

1. Pipette 20 µL of the blood to be tested into the vial.
2. Add three drops of hemoglobin lysing reagent.
3. Recap the vial, and mix by gently inverting the vial several times.
4. Open the lid of the Hemoglobinometer, and pour the sample into the cuvette until it is completely filled.
5. Wait 5 minutes to allow any bubbles in the specimen to rise to the top of the cuvette.
6. Close the lid.
7. Read the results on the digital display in grams per deciliter (g/dL).

To perform a hemoglobin determination using the cyanmethemoglobin technique, you will need the following supplies and equipment: a spectrophotometer or colorimeter, a 5-mL pipette, a 20-µL pipette, test tubes of greater than 5-mL capacity, optically matched cuvettes for the spectrophotometer or colorimeter, Drabkin's reagent, and cyanmethemoglobin standard of known concentration.

Using the cyanmethemoglobin technique, follow the steps outlined below:

1. Pipette 5 mL of Drabkin's reagent into a test tube.
2. Pipette 20 µL of blood to be tested into the tube with Drabkin's reagent.
3. Mix by gently inverting, and allow the tube to stand for 5 minutes for color development.
4. Set the spectrophotometer at a wavelength of 540 nanometers (nm).
5. Into a matched cuvette, pipette 5 mL of Drabkin's reagent. Place the cuvette into the spectrophotometer, and adjust to 0.0 optical density (OD).
6. In another matched cuvette, pipette 5 mL of standard. Place into the instrument and read the OD of the solution.
7. Pour the prepared specimen, which has been standing for 5 minutes, into a matched cuvette,

and place in the instrument. Read the O.D. of this unknown specimen.

8. Calculate the results according to the following formula:

$$\frac{OD\ unknown}{OD\ standard} \times \frac{Concentration}{of\ standard} = \frac{Hemoglobin}{(g/dL)}$$

Performing the Hematocrit

As was the case with testing the hemoglobin, performing a test to measure the hematocrit of the blood is also part of performing a complete blood cell count. To perform the hematocrit, you will need to gather the following equipment: capillary tubes, sealing clay, a microhematocrit centrifuge, and a microhematocrit reader.

To perform a hematocrit, follow the steps outlined below:

1. By capillary action, fill a capillary tube about three-fourths full of the blood that will be tested. Seal the tube by pressing one end of the capillary tube into the sealing clay.
2. Place the sealed tube into one of the grooved slots in the head of the microhematocrit centrifuge. The sealed end of the tube should rest snugly against the rubber cushion at the outer edge of the centrifuge head. Screw on the cover plate securely.
3. Close the centrifuge lid, and turn the timer on for 3 to 5 minutes, or as the policy your laboratory follows.
4. Remove the spun tube from the centrifuge, and read on any of several commercially available types of microhematocrit readers.

Determining RBC Indices

The RBC indices consist of three calculations that provide the physician with valuable information concerning the size and the hemoglobin content of the red blood cells. The three indices include the *mean corpuscular volume (MCV)*, which expresses the volume of a red cell; the *mean corpuscular hemoglobin (MCH)*, which estimates the weight of hemoglobin in a red cell; and the *mean corpuscular hemoglobin concentration (MNCHC)*, which expresses the concentration of hemoglobin in red blood cells relative to their size. RBC indices are calculated automatically with modern cell counters. If your job requires that they be calculated manually, you can use the following formulas:

$$MCV = \frac{Hematocrit}{RBC} \times 10 \qquad \text{(Normal range: } 82\text{--}92\ \mu^3\text{)}$$

$$MCH = \frac{Hemoglobin}{RBC} \times 10 \qquad \text{(Normal range: } 27\text{--}31\ \mu g\text{)}$$

$$MCHC = \frac{Hemoglobin}{Hct} \times 100 \qquad \text{(Normal range: } 32\text{--}40\%\text{)}$$

Determining Sedimentation Rates (ESR)

This test, commonly referred to as the *sed rate* or *erythrocyte sedimentation rate*, does not yield specific information about a certain disease; however, it is considered to be a general indication of inflammation in the patient. Because variations in the sedimentation rate result from changes in the surface charge of red cells, these changes are related to alterations in the blood's plasma. It is because of these changes that an increased sed rate may very well correlate, in a very general and nonspecific way, to the inflammatory process that may be occurring in the patient's body. Sed rates, or ESRs, at their very best are used to monitor a patient's progress or therapy. One isolated ESR measurement does not really tell the doctor a great deal.

Although there are several ways in which this test is performed, for our purpose we will be discussing the most widely used type, called the Wintrobe method. You should remember, however, that no matter what method is used for determining the sed rate, the basic principle used in all techniques is that red blood cells settle out of plasma at a known rate. In some diseases, this rate is faster than normal, and in others, the rate may be slower than normal.

To perform a Wintrobe method for determining ESR, you will need the following supplies and equipment: A Wintrobe sedimentation tube, a transfer pipette, a Wintrobe sed rate stand, a timer, and a sed rate correction chart. To complete the test, follow the steps outlined below:

1. Using a transfer pipette, fill a Wintrobe tube to the "0" mark with the blood that is to be tested. This is most easily done by placing the tip of the blood-filled transfer pipette all the way to the bottom of the Wintrobe tube, then allowing the blood to flow into the tube out of the pipette.
2. As the tube fills, raise the tip of the pipette so that it is barely submerged in the rising column of blood. Make sure that the Wintrobe tube is free of bubbles.
3. Place the filled tube vertically in a Wintrobe sed rate stand. Set the timer for exactly 60 minutes. Read the level in millimeters to which the red cells have settled after 1 hour. This value is the uncorrected sed rate.

If you find that you have to correct the sed rate, you may use a Wintrobe chart, which is normally provided by the laboratory. Remember also that the hematocrit value for the blood being tested must be known, so be sure to perform a hematocrit.

Determining the Reticulocyte Count

In rare instances, you may be required to perform a test known as a reticulocyte count. Reticulocytes are young RBCs, and in testing are distinguishable by their blue granules located inside the cell when stained with a supravital stain such as methylene blue. Testing of reticulocytes is generally performed to assist the physician in determining whether the appropriate numbers of new RBCs are being produced by the bone marrow.

To perform a reticulocyte count, you will need the following supplies and equipment: a freshly filtered methylene blue N solution, a 12 × 75 mm test tube, a dropper, glass slides, and a microscope. To complete the test, follow the steps outlined below:

1. Using the dropper, place four drops of the filtered blue solution into a 12 × 75 mm test tube. Add four drops of the blood to be tested to the test tube containing the methylene blue solution. Mix the two together by drawing the stain/blood mixture up into the dropper and expelling gently several times.
2. Let the mixture stand for about 10 minutes at room temperature, then mix again in the same manner.
3. Prepare four thin smears on glass slides.
4. Using an oil-immersion lens, count 1000 RBCs. Keep a separate tally of the reticulocytes seen while counting the 1000 RBCs. Count about 250 RBCs on each of the four slides.
5. Divide the number of reticulocytes seen per 1000 RBCs by 10 to determine the percentage of reticulocytes. For example, 18 reticulocytes per 1000 RBCs equals 1.8% reticulocytes.

Determining the Differential Cell Count

A stained blood smear, made from EDTA anticoagulated blood or capillary blood, is the basis for the test called a *leukocyte differential count*, a part of the complete blood cell count. In this test, the five different types of WBCs are identified and counted, and the RBCs and platelets observed and evaluated. A well-made blood smear, stained with Wright's stain, is critical.

As a professional member of the medical laboratory team, chances are that you will continuously be required to make blood smears for differential testing. Proper technique is necessary to prepare a smear that will clearly reveal the cellular elements to be observed.

The technique used to make a good blood smear is called the *two-slide method*. A small drop of blood is placed on one end of a precleaned slide, which is on a flat surface. A second slide is used as a spreader. Figure 21-2 illustrates how the two-slide method is completed.

Since the differential count is almost always performed as part of the CBC, there are some important points to remember about making the slide. First always make sure that the drop of blood you are using on the slide is small. Make the slide as soon as possible after the drop is placed onto the slide. Also, always make sure, that the slides you are using are clean and free of any dust particles. Make sure you use a continuous movement when making the slide, and once you have started, never hesitate or use jerky motions. Finally, always remember that your smears must be completely dry before you begin staining them.

Wright's Stain

If a blood smear is made and directly put under the microscope, the cellular elements will not be readily visible. Staining makes the blood cells easy to see and evaluate. Wright's stain, a staining solution that is used by most hospitals and small laboratories because it is easy to use and readily available, is generally the choice for making differential blood smears. It is called a *polychromatic* or *differential* stain because it stains different cells different shades and colors. Different dyes in the stain migrate to different structures.

There are two techniques used to perform a Wright's stain, including one called the *two-step method*. In this method, the stain is put onto a slide that is then placed on a rack in a sink or a pan (Figure 21-3) for 1 to 3 minutes. A *buffer* is then run over the slide in an amount equal to the amount of stain.

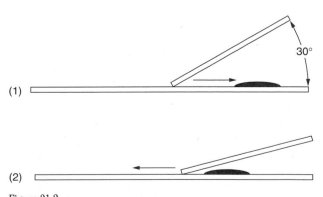

Figure 21-2
The two-slide method of preparing a blood smear.

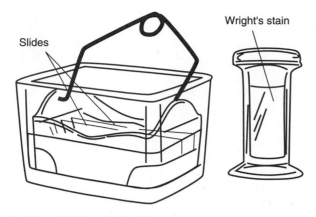

Applying Wright's stain to slides

Figure 21-3
Wright's stain being applied to slides in rack placed over a pan or sink.

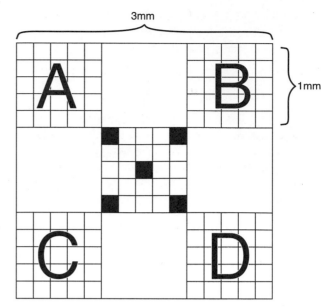

Figure 21-4
Unopette counting chamber.

Buffers prevent changes in the pH of the solution. After you have run the buffer over the slide, gently blow on the slide until a green metallic sheen appears. This usually takes 2 to 4 minutes, and indicates that proper mixing has occurred. The slide is then rinsed with distilled water and allowed to air dry.

Most modern medical laboratories have automatic slide stainers as well as automatic slide makers. In these laboratories, slides are made by hand only when the blood obtained from the patient is minimal, or when the slide maker and stainers are not functioning. Some laboratories also use automated differential counters that do not require slides unless the test is abnormal.

Determining Platelet Counts

The platelet count is used to determine bleeding disorders and clotting ability. Platelets help stop bleeding by forming a "plug" to seal blood vessel walls, assisting in the formation of a clot. Platelets can be counted using many different techniques. If the laboratory you are working in is fully automated, the platelet count is done along with the determinations for WBC, RBC, hemoglobin, and hematocrit. In addition to a count of the number of platelets present, automated hematology departments provide the *mean platelet volume* (MPV), or the average volume of the platelet, on their printouts.

If you are required to perform a manual platelet count, the technique you will probably use is called the *Unopette method*. You will need the following equipment: a Unopette reservoir containing diluent for platelet determination, a Unopette capillary pipette, a microscope, a counting chamber (Figure 21-4), a petri dish, and a counter.

To perform the test, follow the steps outlined below:

1. Pipette 20 µL of blood to be tested into the diluent reservoir according to the technique described by the manufacturer. Let it stand for 10 minutes in order to allow the red cells to hemolyze.
2. Charge the counting chamber.
3. Place the charged counting chamber into a petri dish, cover, and let stand 10 minutes to allow the cells to settle. The bottom of the petri dish should be covered with moistened filter paper to retard evaporation of the specimen.
4. Remove the counting chamber from the petri dish, and place it on the microscope stage.
5. Locate the area to be counted on low power. Then switch to the high-power objective, and count the platelets in all 25 small squares within the large center square. Multiply the number of platelets counted by 1000 to get the total platelet count. If 175 platelets were counted, the total count would be:

$$175 \times 1,000 = 175,000 \text{ platelets/mm}^3$$

Blood Coagulation Studies

Understanding the Coagulation Process

The cessation of bleeding, hemostasis, is a very complex reaction in the human body. Many factors are involved in the body's attempt to repair an injury that is bleeding. Failure of any part of the coagulation process may result in a serious bleeding, hemorrhage, or even death. Since the way in which blood coagulates is very complicated, there are many tests related to the various parts of the entire coagulation system.

When a blood vessel sustains an injury, several factors in the human body come into play immediately, while others take a little longer. Vascular factors are initiated immediately, causing the injured vessel to contract. Platelet factors are initiated causing a plug to form, which is necessary to stop the flow of blood. Platelets also release substances that are necessary in aiding the coagulation process. Clotting factors are the last line of defense. If an injury is slight, vascular factors may be able to take care of the entire problem, perhaps with a bit of aid from the platelets. If the injury is more extensive, clotting factors are summoned, and a substance known as *fibrinogen* is converted to fibrin, helping to secure a blood clot.

Preparing for Coagulation Studies

Much of the coagulation testing done in the medical laboratory requires highly trained technicians. The laboratory assistant is not often involved in the actual testing, but is depended upon to collect the best specimen possible. Some modern hematology laboratories may have sophisticated, fully automated equipment that you may be allowed to operate under strict supervision.

If you are required to obtain the specimen, make sure that you first properly identify your patient for the coagulation study. Then, following the correct procedure for making a quick and accurate venipuncture, using minimal tourniquet pressure, obtain your specimen. Collect the specimen using blue-top (citrate) tubes for the coagulation study after first drawing the EDTA (lavender-top) tubes for cell counts and the red-top (no anticoagulant) tubes for chemistry and serology. These top colors refer to Becton Dickinson Vacutainer tubes.

Types of Coagulation Studies

There are several major tests performed in the coagulation section of the hematology department. These tests include a prothrombin time (PT), an activated partial thrombosplastin time (APTT), fibrinogen, fibrin split product, thrombin time, factor studies, bleeding time, and disseminated intravascular coagulation (DIC) panel. For our purposes, we will only be discussing those studies that are most frequently completed in the medical laboratory. These include prothrombin time, bleeding time, clotting time, and the DIC panel.

The *prothrombin time* is one of the most frequently performed coagulation studies completed in the medical laboratory. It is a measure of the clotting ability of a series of combined coagulation factors in plasma. Prothrombin is a substance produced by the liver and required for the clotting of blood. Although the prothrombin time does not directly measure the amount of prothrombin, the test is a suitable clinical means of determining the presence and functioning ability of prothrombin. When a patient has a prothrombin time drawn frequently, it is likely that this patient has a tendency to form inappropriate blood clots, and is on medication to prevent this problem. This patient may not clot easily, and care must always be taken whenever blood is drawn.

The *bleeding time* is that time between the making of a small incision and the moment bleeding stops. It is a test of platelet function and is frequently used as a presurgical screening test. Many methods have been developed for performing this test. Among the most common are the *Ivy*, the *template*, and the *Duke*, or some modification of each of these. This test is mainly used as a screening procedure in order to identify a patient with bleeding problems. It does not measure all aspects of clotting, but will give the physician a good indication of whether or not the patient's platelets are functioning properly. It is generally performed by a licensed medical technologist, who makes one or two incisions into the forearm and then, using a stopwatch, calculates the length of time it takes for the bleeding to stop. Pressure is always placed on the patient's upper arm while the procedure is being performed in order to avoid any unnecessary bleeding.

Another coagulation study frequently performed in the medical laboratory is a test for *clotting time*. Methods for performing clotting times also vary from laboratory to laboratory. The capillary clotting time is one method that is most widely used. In this method, blood specimens are obtained from the patient's finger, toe, and earlobe, and then placed in three capillary tubes. The blood must be allowed to flow freely from the puncture wound, and not be squeezed or manipulated from the wound. Timing begins with the appearance of the second drop of blood and continues to the formation of a fibrin thread as a capillary tube is broken.

The *disseminated intravascular coagulation (DIC) panel* consists of a series of coagulation tests that are done on a stat basis and handled very carefully. A person suffering from DIC is in great danger, as a trauma has stimulated internal blood clotting throughout the patient's body. Childbirth complications, gunshot wounds, and other traumas can precipitate this life-threatening problem. If you are ever required to complete a DIC panel, it is extremely important that you make sure you know how to handle it!

Summary

In this chapter, we discussed that hematology means the study of blood, and that many tests have been developed to assay the various components and properties of blood. We determined that the complete blood cell count, or CBC, has the widest usage, and includes tests to determine the number and kind of leukocytes and erythrocytes, and the hemoglobin content. We also talked about sedimentation rates, reticulocyte counts, and platelet counts, noting that these tests are generally done to determine abnormal conditions. We discussed differential cell counts and blood smear preparation for completing the differential count. Finally, we described various coagulation studies that are done in hematology, noting that some of the tests are used to determine problems with coagulation are prothombin time, bleeding time, and the DIC panel.

Review Questions

1. Define the following abbreviations:

    a. CBC _____

    b. WBC _____

    c. RBC _____

2. What information is provided in a *differential white count?*

3. What does the term *agranulocyte* mean?

4. Briefly explain what occurs during capillary action.

5. Briefly explain the differences between *heterozygous* and *homozygous.*

6. What does the abbreviation *MPV* mean?

7. What is the name of the instrument used for counting blood components?

8. What is the name of the study of blood?

9. What term is used to describe a young red blood cell?

10. What component of the blood is most concerned with the clotting mechanism in the body?

22

Serology, Microbiology, and Chemistry

Performance Objectives

Upon completion of this chapter, you will be able to:

1. Describe and be able to perform basic serological tests frequently completed in the medical laboratory.
2. Describe and be able to perform pregnancy testing on urine or serum.
3. Discuss tests used to detect AIDS.
4. Discuss the differences between normal body flora and pathogens.
5. Describe the procedure for collection of bacteriological specimens.
6. Describe and be able to demonstrate how to inoculate, streak, and store cultures properly.
7. Explain the use of carbon dioxide (CO_2) atmosphere.
8. Identify and describe the various shapes of bacteria and fungi.
9. Describe and be able to demonstrate how to perform a gram stain and an acid-fast stain.
10. Discuss susceptibility testing.
11. Discuss how to collect properly skin scrapings for fungus study and staining.
12. Discuss methods used for providing reagents and water.
13. Distinguish between manual procedures and automated procedures used in the chemistry department of the medical laboratory.
14. Identify several general categories of test procedures used in chemistry testing.
15. Explain how enzyme assay is used to diagnose abnormal conditions.
16. Discuss the uses of electrophoresis.
17. Identify reasons for therapeutic drug monitoring.

Terms and Abbreviations

Absorbance   The ability of a substance to take in light during photometry.
Aerobic   grows in the presence free of oxygen.
Agar   substance used in culture media.
Agglutination   reaction of antibodies in human blood serum with sheep red blood cells.
Agglutinins   a specific antigen used in agglutination tests.
AIDS   abbreviation for acquired immunodeficiency syndrome.
Anaerobic   grows only if there is no oxygen.

Antibody   protein developed within the body in response to a foreign substance (antigen), often providing immunity to disease.
Antigen   substance that induces the formation of antibodies.
ARC   abbreviation for AIDS-related complex.
Aseptic   free of microorganisms.
Atypical   something irregular or not conforming to type.
Automation   development and use of instruments to complete a testing process without human intervention.
Bacteriology   the study of bacteria.

Broth   a liquid medium for growing microorganisms.

Buffy coat   light-colored layer of blood between the plasma and the RBC; contains mostly WBCs.

Contaminant   a foreign organism developing accidentally in a culture.

Culture   growing microorganisms on artificial media.

Dermatophyte   a fungus parasite on the skin.

ELISA   abbreviation for enzyme-linked immunosorbent assay.

Enzyme   a biochemical catalyst within the body that produces chemical changes without being changed itself.

Fix   to fasten or hold firm and not wash off with water or staining solution.

Febrile   pertaining to a fever.

FUO   abbreviation for fever of unknown origin.

Heterophil antibody test   test for infectious mononucleosis using a series of diluted patient sera and washed sheep red blood cells.

HIV   abbreviation for human immunodeficiency virus.

Human chorionic gonadotropin (HCG)   hormone excreted in the urine of a pregnant woman.

Hydatiform mole   mole formed by rapid multiplication of chorionic villi to form a mass of cysts resembling a bunch of grapes; causes false-positive pregnancy test.

Inactivation   to render inert by use of heat; to destroy biological activities by heat.

Inoculate   the introduction of microorganisms onto culture medium.

Inoculating loop/needle   a handle with a loop of nichrome or platinum wire that is attached to transfer specimens or microorganisms from one medium to another and to streak or spread the material that was transferred.

In vitro   can be observed or demonstrated in a test tube as opposed to in vivo, which occurs within the living organism.

Lysis   destruction of cells by a specific lysin.

Mean   pertaining to something being halfway between two extremes.

Medium   a substance used to provide nutrients for the growth and multiplication of microorganisms; the plural is media.

Microbiology   the study of living organisms that can only be seen under a microscope.

Mycelium   one of the threadlike filaments that constitute the vegetative structure of a fungus.

Mycology   the study of fungi, yeast, and molds.

Normal flora   organisms normally present and for some reason able to resist the defensive mechanisms of the person but at the same time unable to invade body tissues and cause disease unless the person's resistance is lowered.

Opsonin   substance in the blood serum that acts upon microorganisms and other cells, facilitating phagocytosis.

Optimum-growth temperature   the temperature of incubation that gives the most rapid growth during a short period of time (usually 12 to 24 hours).

Pathogenic   capable of producing disease.

Photometer   a device used to measure light.

Precipitation   test reaction during which a deposit falls to the bottom, thereby separating out of the solution.

Range   the difference between the lowest and highest observations.

Reproductibility   the ability to repeat a procedure time after time with exactly the same results.

Rickettsiae   minute rod-shaped or coccobacillary microorganisms that are parasites and cause disease in vertebrates.

Serology   the study of antigen-antibody reactions in vitro.

Serum sickness   a condition that develops following administration of antisera or drug therapy.

Shift   results that are steady but on one side of the mean.

Spectrophotometer   a device used to measure light intensities in different parts of the spectrum.

Spirochete   slender, spiral, motile microorganism.

Standard solution   a solution containing a known amount of substance.

Susceptibility testing   placement of discs containing antibiotics onto culture of microorganisms to determine which antibiotics would prevent or retard growth of that microorganism.

Symbiosis   living together of two or more organisms in a more or less mutually beneficial state.

Titer   highest dilution of serum causing agglutination or strength of serum.

Trends   values that go steadily up or steadily down several days in a row.

Variability   when measurements or results disagree but are still within acceptable range.

T here are three departments within the medical laboratory that generally work together because many of the tests completed in each department usually overlap. These departments are serology, microbiology, and chemistry. The *serology* department performs tests and procedures dealing with the study of antigen-antibody reactions in vitro. *In vitro* means a process can be observed in a test tube or on a glass slide, as opposed to *in vivo*, which occurs within the living organism.

Since most of the reactions observed in the serology department deal with specific microbes and organisms, we cannot discuss serology without also talking about microbiology. *Microbiology*, as it is most simply defined, is the study of living organisms that can only be seen under a microscope. These organisms include bacteria, fungi, yeast and molds, protozoa, and viruses. Some of the larger medical centers may separate their microbiology department into bacteriology, mycology, parasitology, and virology.

In the human body, microorganisms can fester and grow. In some cases, these tiny organisms can make their way into the bloodstream, urine, gastric juices, cerebrospinal fluid, and other body fluids. The department that is responsible for testing and analyzing these fluids is called the *chemistry* department. Much of the procedures performed in chemistry deal with determining whether body fluids are normal or how far they vary from being normal.

Understanding Serology and Serodiagnostics

When a patient has been diagnosed with an infectious disease, certain substances, called *antibodies,* are formed in the tissues that have the ability to destroy or affect the disease-producing agent or *antigen.* These substances are found in the blood, plasma, and lymph, and appear in the serum after the blood coagulates. In most cases, these "antibodies" or "immune bodies" are *specific,* and the demonstration of them indicates the presence of an infectious disease caused by a specific antigen. The antibodies may appear immediately after the onset of the disease, or detection can be delayed until such time as the disease has advanced. The antibodies remain for a variable time after recovery from the infectious disease.

Nonspecific antibodies are antibodies that have formed in response to an agent other than the bacteria that caused the disease. For example, antibodies developed in response to tissue damage in syphilis are considered nonspecific. Their presence can be detected in any number of ways, including agglutination, flocculation, bacteriolysis, precipitation, complement fixation, hemolysis, or the presence of opsonins.

For many years there was a specific serology test available to test for the presence of syphilis. However, now this area has been expanded to include tests for many other pathological conditions that are characterized by a rise in antibodies.

Testing for Syphilis and Other Specific and Nonspecific Antibodies

Syphilis is caused by the spirochete *Treponema pallidum.* In response to this disease process, two antibodies develop. The treponemal antibodies are specific and are developed against the spirochete. The nonspecific antibodies are developed in response to tissue damage by the spirochetes and are called nontreponemal antibodies.

The three most commonly used tests for syphilis

include the FTA-ABS (fluorescent treponemal antibody-absorption) test, the VDRL (Venereal Disease Research Laboratory), test and the RPR (rapid plasma reagin) test. The FTA-ABS test is specific and is performed to confirm reactive sera. This test is performed in large laboratories, reference laboratories, and in state facilities. The VDRL test is nonspecific, requires inactivated serum, and can be done easily in most laboratories. The RPR test is also nonspecific, and can be performed on plasma, because it is more sensitive but less specific than the VDRL. The RPR does not require inactivation of serum and can be done quite easily and rapidly in any laboratory.

The less frequently used tests for syphilis include the Wasserman, Kahn, colloidal gold, TPI (Treponema Pallidum Immobilization), Plasmacrit, and the dark field microscopy.

Procedure for Performing the RPR Test

To perform the RPR test to determine the presence of syphilis, follow the steps outlined below:

1. Place a drop of plasma or serum onto the circle on the RPR card using a capillary tube and a rubber bulb (Figure 22-1A).
2. Carefully spread the drop throughout the circle with the stirrer (Figure 22-1B).
3. Treat the control sera the same as the patient serum.
4. Add one drop of well-shaken antigen from the antigen dispensing bottle (Figure 22-1C).
5. Place on the mechanical rotor, and cover with a humidifying cover.
6. Rotate eight times.
7. Read macroscopically, and report your findings as either reactive or nonreactive (Figure 22-1D). Report as reactive large clumps that are visible to the naked eye to small clumbs that are weakly reactive. Nonreactive means that no clumping is present.

C-Reactive Protein Test

The C-reactive protein (CRP) is an abnormal protein that is found in persons suffering from infectious and inflammatory conditions. The CRP test is nonspecific. The abnormal protein appears within 12 to 24 hours after the onset of the condition, and subsides when the inflammation disappears. A positive CRP may be present in any number of disorders, including pneumococcal pneumonia, streptococcal infections, rheumatic fever, lupus erythematosus, myocardial infarctions, and some kinds of carcinoma. It may also be present during sinusitis, pregnancy, use of oral

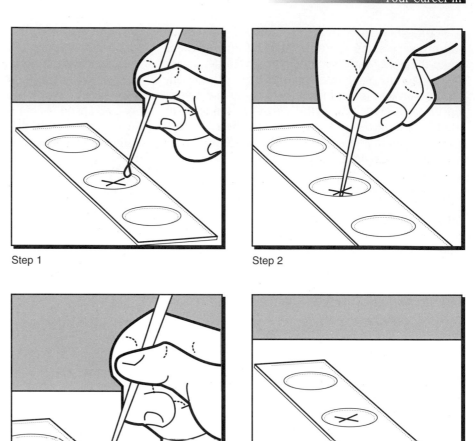

Step 1

Step 2

Step 3

Step 4

Figure 22-1
Procedure for completing RPR test.

contraceptives, and in some women with an IUD in place. It is sometimes found in normal healthy persons past the age of 70.

Rheumatoid Arthritis Tests

The serum of patients with rheumatoid arthritis may contain a macroglobin (protein) antibody called rheumatoid factor, or RF. This RF may be detected by its ability to agglutinate RBCs or latex particles during rapid slide testing. This is a nonspecific test that may also be positive during any number of conditions, including lupus erythematosus, bacterial endocarditis, cirrhosis of the liver, viral hepatitis, and in some forms of leukemia. Many different commercial kits are available for the detection of RF. If any of these are used, always remember to follow the manufacturer's directions carefully. Additional testing, such as serial dilutions or ANA (antinuclear antibodies), may also be required to aid in differentiating specific diseases.

Testing for Infectious Mononucleosis

Infectious mononucleosis is a disease characterized by fever and an enlargement of the lymph nodes and spleen. Atypical lymphocytes and heterophil antibodies are also found in the blood. In the laboratory, the medical technologist is responsible for testing the blood in order to distinguish the atypical lymphocytes from the normal lymphocytes and monocytes, and then recording the percentage of atypical cells as the differential cell count is done.

Heterophil antibodies differ from other antibodies in that they are nonspecific. For example, these antibodies in human blood serum may react with the RBCs of sheep, thus causing them to agglutinate.

There are various types of tests for heterophil antibodies. A tube test consists of a series of dilutions of the patient's serum, which is mixed in the test tubes and then incubated with washed sheep cells. Agglutination of the sheep cells indicates the presence of the heterophil antibodies. The greatest dilution that reacts is reported.

This is a nonspecific test and therefore considered *presumptive*. The increase in serum agglutinins may be either from infectious mononucleosis or from serum sickness. Further tests that are specific for infectious mononucleosis should be done for absolute differentiation.

The spot *Mono-Test* is one example of a modified rapid differential test for infectious mononucleosis. It uses a slide instead of test tubes. To complete this, follow the steps outlined below:

1. Gather all of your necessary supplies and equipment. This will include a centrifuge, control sera, calibrated capillary tubes and bulbs, glass slide or disposable card slide, stirrers, and Mono-Test reagent.
2. Centrifuge the patient's specimen. Do not use heparin during collection of the blood.
3. Fill the capillary tube up to the mark with the patient's serum.
4. Empty the contents of the tube into the center of the middle section of the slide.
5. Place one drop of positive control serum on the left section of the slide, and one drop of negative control serum on the right section of the slide.
6. Using a separate stirrer for each section, mix the serum and the reagent.
7. Spread over an area approximately 1 inch in diameter.
8. Observe for agglutination.

Use a high-intensity lamp for lateral illumination, and observe against a dark background. If you are using disposable cards, remember to:

· Rock gently for 1 minute.
· Leave undisturbed for another minute.
· Observe immediately for agglutination.

After you have completed the procedure, report it as positive if agglutination of the Mono-Test reagent occurs, and negative if there is no agglutination or if the agglutination is of a finely granular pattern.

Testing for Febrile Agglutinations

Whenever a patient continues to exhibit signs of a fever for an unknown reason, a battery of tests known as *febrile agglutinations* may be ordered in order to determine the cause of the fever. This test battery is used to differentiate among typhoid fever, paratyphoid fever, tularemia, undulant fever, and the rickettsial diseases, which include typhus fever, trench fever, and Rocky Mountain spotted fever. The test detects antibodies in the patient's serum. The antigens used in testing are prepared from the specific bacteria that cause the various diseases. For example, the antigen used to test for typhoid fever is prepared from *B. typhi O* or *B. typhi H. B. paratyphoid (A, B,* or *C)* is used to test for paratyphoid fever. *F. tularensis* is used to test for undulant fever, or brucellosis. A nonspecific antigen using *Proteus OX-19, OX-K,* and *OS-2* is used for the rickettsial diseases. These antigens are all available commercially.

To test for febrile agglutinations, follow the steps outlined below:

1. Gather all of the necessary supplies and equipment. This will include a centrifuge; pipettes to deliver serum; febrile-type, glass-ringed slides with five rings across and six rings down; stirrers; commercial antigens; and control sera.
2. Centrifuge the blood in order to separate the serum from the cells.
3. Using special febrile pipette, deliver 0.08, 0.04, 0.02, 0.01, and 0.005 mL of serum to the top row of rings across the slide.
4. Repeat the procedure to the second row and each subsequent row, until all six rows have serum. Be certain to prepare the control serum in the same manner.
5. Add a drop of the commercially prepared antigen to each amount of serum all the way across the slide. Start at the right side of the slide. Use the stirrer to thoroughly mix each ring, and use a different antigen for each cross row.
6. When all rings are mixed, rotate the slide 20 times by hand. Read immediately for agglutination.
7. Report any agglutinations of 2++.
8. Dilutions for the rings are 1:10, 1:20, 1:40, 1:80, and 1:160. If the last ring is positive (1:160), you must make further dilutions and repeat the entire procedure.

Testing for Streptococcal Infections: The Antistreptolysin O (ASO) Test

In more than 90 percent of all streptococcal infections, the body produces specific antibodies that respond to some type of extracellular product of Group A streptococcus. One such type is the streptolysin O antigen. In the body, streptolysin O antigen produces lysis of red bood cells.

Since there are several modifications of the ASO test, you should follow the manufacturer's instructions for the test used in your laboratory. An elevated ASO titer is helpful in diagnosis of recent Group A streptococcal infections, acute rheumatic fever, and in acute glomerular nephritis.

Antinuclear Antibody Test (ANA)

Antinuclear antibodies are produced in serum in response to the nuclei of white blood cells. The ANA test is used to determine the presence of factors associated with autoimmune diseases where the body actually attacks itself. Damage to such organs as the heart, kidneys, and liver can result. Systemic lupus erythematosus (SLE) has a certain antibody that can be detected by this test.

Pregnancy Testing

Pregnancy tests are often performed on urine specimens. In the serology department, they may also be performed on serum specimens. These are either test-tube tests or slide tests. The results of the test-tube tests are usually available in 2 hours, whereas tests completed on slides are generally much quicker and are most often available within minutes.

Most pregnancy screening tests are qualitative, and many types are now commercially available. These are easy to perform and may be purchased over the counter and run by the patient at home. Most of these tests measure the level of human chorionic gonadotropin, or HCG, a hormone excreted in the urine. The HCG hormone is generally found in the urine about 1 week after the first missed menstrual period.

For testing in the laboratory, the patient should be instructed to collect the first morning specimen in a clean container, since the hormone is more concentrated at that time. It is important to note that there are some conditions that can interfere in the results of the test. Some of these include the presence of detergent residue in the collection container, medications taken by the patient, certain pathological conditions, menopause, and the presence of an ectopic pregnancy.

Some tests may require that the urine be filtered. If the urine is turbid, centrifugation may also be required with testing performed on the supernatant. Some tests may also show hemagglutination while others may demonstrate precipitation of latex particles in the test tubes. Therefore, adequate controls must be prepared according to the manufacturer's directions, and the proper time period must be observed. A negative test result may occur in cases of very early pregnancy or if there is a low concentration of HCG. Negative tests should be repeated in 7 to 10 days as specified by the manufacturer. Quantitative tests may also be performed on 24-hour specimens in order to determine any abnormal conditions such as threatened abortion, hydatiform mole, ectopic pregnancy, or fetal death.

AIDS Testing

The transmission of AIDS, or acquired immunodeficiency syndrome, is believed to occur by way of four routes. These include unprotected sexual intercourse with an HIV-infected partner, sharing a hypodermic needle that has been contaminated with the virus, infection transmitted from mother to baby during gestation or birthing, and transfusion of contaminated blood or blood products. According to information from the Centers for Disease Control, HIV has been isolated from blood, cerebrospinal fluid, saliva, semen, vaginal secretions, breast milk, and amniotic fluid. HIV has not been isolated from other body fluids, such as nasal secretions, sputum, sweat, tears, feces, urine, or vomitus unless the body fluid was contaminated with blood.

Because of the question of confidentiality in the identification of persons found to test positive for the antibodies associated with HIV, most medical laboratories use a strict system of identification by number only. Actual patient names are restricted to a limited number of people.

The demonstration of antibodies to HIV is used to diagnose AIDS and ARC (AIDS-related complex). Two types of tests currently in use include the ELISA (enzyme-linked immunosorbent assay) and the Western-blot test. The ELISA is used for screening. A positive ELISA can be confirmed with the more specific Western-blot test, because false-positive ELISA tests do often occur.

For ELISA testing, patient serum is placed in a microtiter plate well or exposed to beads coated with inactivated HIV antigens and immunoglobulin linked with an enzyme. After inoculation and incubation, a color change occurs.

The Western-blot test is used to identify proteins of a specific molecular weight; in this case, HIV. This test is an immunoelectrophoretic procedure.

Understanding Microbiology

As we discussed earlier, whenever we talk about the study of serology and the role it plays in testing for specific antibodies, we must also look at the microbes or organisms that those antibodies are trying to fight. The study that deals with these microscopic living organisms is called *microbiology*. All of these organisms are classified according to their cellular and molecular makeup. They include bacteria, fungi, yeast and molds, protozoa, and viruses. Since many of the tests that you will be observing, or in some cases, performing, in the microbiology department will be limited to those specimens in which bacteria are being identified, for our purposes, we will limit our discussion of microbiology as it relates to the study of bacteriology.

Normal Flora and Pathogens

Microorganisms are found in large numbers on and in the human body. Under normal conditions, these microorganisms are harmless. They are called part of our *normal flora*. Organisms that are part of the normal flora are those that are normally present and for some reason able to resist the defensive mechanisms of the person. At the same time, they are unable to invade the body tissues, unless the person's resistance is lowered. Therefore, the person and the microorganisms exist in *symbiosis*, or in living together in a mutually beneficial state. Normal flora of one part of the body differ greatly from the normal flora of another part. But as long as the person's resistance is maintained at a sufficiently high level, the bacteria that make up the normal flora do no harm. However, from time to time, organisms invade tissues and become pathogenic, or disease-producing. In the medical laboratory, it is the responsibility of the microbiology department to grow, isolate, and identify the microorganism that is causing the disease condition.

Collecting Microbial Specimens

Materials most commonly cultured in the microbiology laboratory include urine, spinal fluid, tissue fluids, stools, specimens collected from the nose, throat, wounds, abscesses, or genitalia, and materials suspected of containing fungi or acid-fast organisms. Since microorganisms tend to grow at a very fast rate, following the correct procedures for collecting them is extremely important.

Generally, there is a joint effort by the nursing staff and the members of the medical laboratory to obtain the proper specimen for analysis. In hospitals, nursing usually has the responsibility of collecting the specimen, labeling it properly, and sending it to the lab. In the clinic or physician's office, the laboratory assistant is often part of the collection team. But no matter who the collection agent is, the specimens submitted for examination must be collected by aseptic technique into the appropriate sterile containers. The specimens must then be carried immediately to the appropriate department of the medical laboratory.

It is extremely important that specimens never be left sitting around the nursing station or the laboratory because the pathogenic microorganisms may be-

come overgrown by contaminants. It is the responsibility of the laboratory personnel to see that the specimen is inoculated as quickly as possible onto the correct medium. Usually, if a specimen cannot be processed within an hour or less after it has been collected, it should be refrigerated to prevent contaminant overgrowth. However, if the specimen is collected in transport medium, it can wait.

Quality Control in Specimen Collection

Quality control in microbiology begins with specimen collection. It then continues through logging, processing, cultivating, isolation and identification, susceptibility testing, and reporting of findings. In order to ensure that proper quality control methods are followed, you should follow the general guidelines listed below whenever you are required to collect specimens for microbiology testing:

- Rectal swabs should always be placed in GN broth.
- Swabs used for collection of *Neisseria gonorrhoeae* should be inoculated on Thayer-Martin or Transgrow at the time of collection.
- Aspirates and washing should be collected into sterile containers and promptly delivered to the laboratory. They should then be processed immediately to ensure recovery of the pathogens and prevent overgrowth of contaminants.
- Cerebrospinal fluid (CSF) must be collected into a sterile screw cap tube and then immediately sent to the lab. This is already an excellent medium for bacterial growth, and it should not be refrigerated.
- Blood specimens should be collected from a venipuncture site that has been properly disinfected with alcohol and iodine. The blood should be collected into a medium that has an anaerobic atmosphere. Some blood should also be collected into one bottle of SPS medium that has an aerobic atmosphere.
- Urine should be either catheterized or a midstream, clean-catch specimen collected after proper cleansing of the genital area. A sterile, wide-mouth container should be used. Specimens should be processed within 2 hours after collection.
- Swabs from wounds and abscesses suspected of having anaerobes should be placed in an anaerobic transport unit.
- A swab of a body part for aerobes and yeast should be placed in a sterile transport medium and then immediately delivered to the lab.
- Biopsy specimens should be collected

aseptically in a sterile container with sterile saline or phosphate buffer added to prevent drying.

- Skin, hair, or nail clippings should be collected in sterile petri dishes or tubes.
- Stool specimens should be collected in clean cartons and immediately carried to the lab for culture and/or ova and parasite examination. If a delay is necessary, a preservative such as 0.033 M phosphate buffer and glycerol should be added to ensure survival of *Shigella* and *Salmonella* bacteria.

Types of Media

Because of convenience, availability, and economics, most medical laboratories no longer routinely prepare their own media. Media are purchased prepared, wrapped, labeled, and packaged, ready to be stored in a variety of positions. The quality of the commercially prepared media is always the same when stored properly.

All biological systems, from bacteria and viruses to humans, have certain nutritional requirements. In order to survive, bacteria require such things as energy source, carbon, nitrogen, several metallic elements, certain vitamins and vitamin-like compounds, and water.

To positively identify bacteria, several different types of media may be required. Some of the more commonly used include liquid media, or *broths*; *differential media*, which give an organism a characteristic growth or reaction; and *enrichment media*, which are used to enhance the growth of a specific bacteria while inhibiting the growth of normal flora or other bacteria that could obscure it or even inhibit its growth.

It is most important that specimens for culture are inoculated onto the correct media. Most laboratories have a chart posted that lists the various sources of specimens and the different media to be inoculated. A limited list of media most often found in laboratories includes blood agar, nutrient agar, eosin methylene blue agar (EMB), thioglycollate broth, Biggy agar slants, chocolate agar, Thayer-Martin agar, McConkey agar, Salmonella-Shigella agar (S.S.) azide, Loefler's, Border-Gengou, Sabouraud, and Petragnani.

Test procedures are available in order to identify bacteria without resorting to differential media. Identification is based on an antigen-antibody reaction for a specific bacterium. The presence of the bacteria in a specimen will produce either agglutination or a color change depending on whether the test uses latex particle agglutination or is based on the principles of enzyme immunoassay (EIA).

Processing Specimens

Once the medium has been properly prepared, you are now ready to process the specimen. Each specimen must be properly labeled with the patient's name, room number, identification number, physician's name, date and time of collection, and the exact source of the specimen. "Wound," "abscess," etc., are not complete and sufficient sources. If the wound is located on the "right side of the head," that is what should be reported as the "source."

After specimen identification is certain, the specimen information should be written into the log book or entered into the computer. A lab number for identification purposes is given to each specimen. Select the media that are appropriate for the type of specimen, streak the petri dishes of media, and prepare smears for staining. Then place the inoculated plates into the incubator upside down to prevent the accumulation of moisture on the surface of the agar.

Procedure for Using Swabs to Streak Plates

The streak plate technique is for specimens that reach the laboratory on swabs and for urine sent for culture. It is importuant to use the entire plate of medium. Remember, the entire procedure must be performed using aseptic technique.

When using a swab to streak the plate, you must always heat the inoculating loop/needle before and after using it, between streaks of a different direction, and, of course, between specimens. This will prevent contamination. The inoculating loop or needle should also be heated before introducing it into any container and after the specimen has been obtained. In the past, many labortories used a Bunsen burner for flaming the loop. Now, most labs use an electric burner device to prevent any potential hazards or problems with an open flame.

Remove the container top, and quickly pass the mouth of the container over the heating device to destroy an contaminants on the outside of the container. Then remove the swab, and inoculate the medium by rolling the swab along one edge of the petri dish (Figure 22-2A). Place the swab back into the container again, and replace the lid. Heat an inoculating needle. Touch to the side of the medium to cool, and then streak across the area where you inoculated the medium (Figure 22-2B). Heat the needle again, and streak across the tip (Figure 22-2C) that you just finished streaking. Heat and repeat (Figure 22-2D). Close the petri dish, heat the needle, and return it to the usual storage place. Be certain that the petri plates are labeled. Place in an incubator at the proper temperature and carbon dioxide atmosphere.

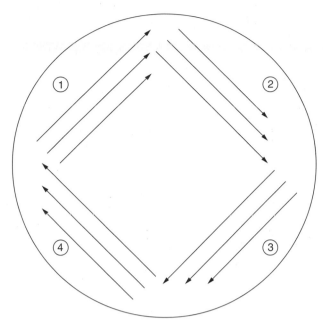

Figure 22-2
Streak plate technique using a swab.

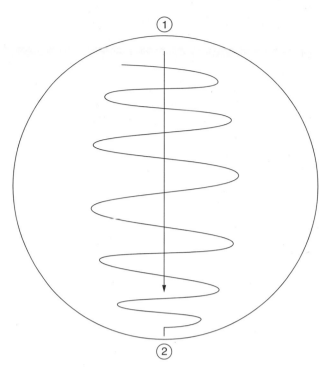

Figure 22-3
Streak plate technique using an inoculating loop.

Using a Loop to Transfer a Specimen

If the specimen is urine or some other liquid, use an inoculating loop to streak plates. Most loops are calibrated to contain a certain amount. Other loops may not be calibrated. Make sure you follow the correct procedure that your facility uses.

Heat the mouth of the container to destroy any contaminants on the outside. Heat the loop to redness, touch the loop at the top of the liquid to cool, and then on the liquid to be transferred. Transfer the loopful to the medium, and streak the loop down the center of the petri dish (Figure 22-3). Heat the loop, touch it to the medium to cool, and then streak across the entire top half of the plate. Turn the plate around, and repeat until the entire plate is streaked.

An inoculating loop may also be used to transfer a specimen to an agar slant A *slant* is a tube containing agar that was tilted before it hardened to form a slanted surface. Follow the same technique for sterilizing the loop and outside of all containers. To inoculate, drag the loop across the surface of the slant with a side-to-side motion, as shown in Figure 22-4.

Be sure that the culture is properly labeled, and then place it on the incubator shelves in oxygen, or under reduced or no oxygen to obtain optimum growth.

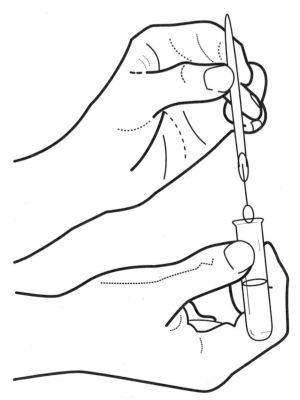

Figure 22-4
Streak technique for a slant tube.

Factors Affecting Growth of Bacteria

Almost every type of bacteria falls into one of four categories according to its individual requirement for growth. *Aerobic* bacteria must have oxygen present in order to grow, while bacteria that are *anaerobic* can only grow if no oxygen is present. Bacteria that fall into the category of *facultative anaerobes* can grow in either the absence or presence of oxygen. And *microaerophilic* bacteria can only grow if there are very small amounts of oxygen present.

Another factor that influences the growth of bacteria is temperature. Most pathogenic microorganisms grow well at body temperature, or 35°C. The optimum-growth temperature is the temperature of incubation that gives the most rapid growth during a short period of time, usually 12 to 24 hours. If the temperature rises too high, the organisms die. If the temperature drops too low, all growth ceases.

Shapes and Sizes of Bacteria

Bacteria have many varied shapes and sizes (Figure 22-5). Each species has its own characteristic shape and range of sizes. However, all can be grouped into three basic categories. The first, called *coccus*, or *cocci*, if more than one exist, are round. They generally appear in grapelike clusters and are termed staphylococci. Cocci that are linked in chains are called streptococci. Pairs of cocci are called diplococci, and small, single cocci are called micrococci.

The second group of bacteria are called *bacillus*, or *bacilli* if there is more than one. These are rod-shaped or fusiform, and may have spores located at one end or in the middle.

The third type of bacteria are curved or spiral forms that vary in shape. They are made up of *spirochetes*, *vibrios*, and *spirilla*. Spirochetes are flexible and cork-screw-shaped bacteria, while vibrios have the appearance of commas. Spirilla are rigid spirals.

Susceptibility Testing of Bacteria

Susceptibility or *sensitivity testing* is a procedure used to test several kinds of antibiotics against a culture of bacteria. If a susceptibility report is requested, further growth is necessary. If this is the case, isolated colonies are transferred to a large petri dish of nutrient agar. The entire plate is streaked heavily. Antibiotic discs are then placed onto the surface of the streaked agar plate. Most medical laboratories use commercial dispensers for the antibiotic discs. The discs must be so firmly placed that they will not fall off when the petri dish is incubated upside down. All cultures on petri dishes are incubated upside down so that the moisture that forms inside the plate will not fall onto the surface of the culture.

Although susceptibility testing of bacteria is not usually a task required of the laboratory assistant, if you are working in a small laboratory, you may have to perform the procedure. If that is indeed the case, follow the steps outlined below:

1. Select four or five colonies of the organism to be tested. Transfer these colonies by touching the top of each colony successively with the same loop to a tube containing 3 to 5 mL of Mueller-Hinton or trypticase soy broth.
2. Incubate the tube at 35°C for at least 2 to 8 hours, long enough to produce an organism suspension with moderate cloudiness.
3. Dilute the broth culture with sterile saline or broth to obtain a turbidity that matches a prepared standard.
4. Dip a sterile cotton swab into the adjusted inoculum.
5. Carefully lift the swab above the fluid level, and gently rotate the swab against the inside of the tube to remove as much excess inoculum as possible.
6. Streak the entire agar surface with the swab evenly in three directions.
7. Allow the inoculated plate to dry for 3 to 5 minutes with the plate closed.
8. Using a dispenser or sterile forceps, place the discs on the agar. With sterile forceps, gently press down on the discs to ensure even contact.
9. Incubate the plates immediately.
10. Read the plates after 16 to 24 hours of incubation.

Report as sensitive or resistant. *Sensitive* means that the bacteria were killed or had growth inhibited by the antibiotic. This is indicated by a clear zone around the disc. *Resistant* indicates that the antibiotic had no effect on the bacteria, which grew to the edges of the disc.

Preparing a Bacteriological Smear

One way to identify bacteria is to make a smear on a slide, stain the slide, and study the organism under the microscope. A smear can be made directly from a swab or from a culture with the aid of a loop. Frequently, two swabs are taken, with one set aside for use as a smear and the other for a culture. The swab for the smear is rolled along the slide leaving a film.

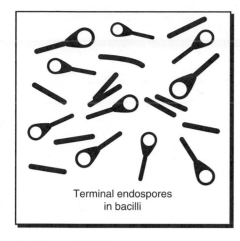

Terminal endospores
in bacilli

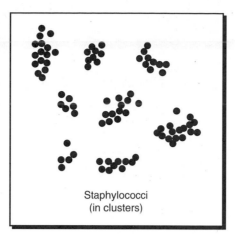

Staphylococci
(in clusters)

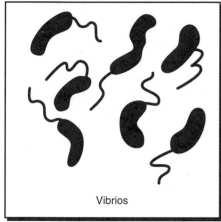

Vibrios

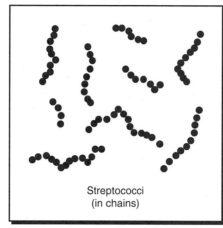

Streptococci
(in chains)

Figure 22-5
Types of bacteria.

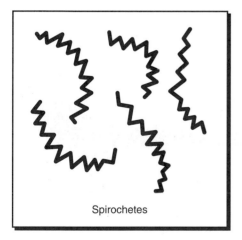

Spirochetes

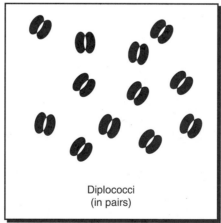

Diplococci
(in pairs)

The slide is then air-dried and heat-fixed before stain-ing.

If you are required to prepare a smear from a cul-ture, use the steps outlined below and shown in Fig-ure 22-6:

1. Place a drop of sterile water on a slide.
2. Heat a wire inoculating needle to redness, and then let it cool.
3. Lift the petri dish lid with one hand, and remove a sample of the organisms with the loop held in the other hand. Close the lid.
4. Add the sample to the water on the slide and mix, spreading thin, to form a 1-inch circle. Be sure you heat the loop before setting it aside.
5. Air-dry the slide.
6. Fix the organisms to the slide by heating rapidly about three times. Make sure you use tongs to hold the slide. Avoid overheating and cracking the slide.

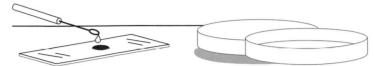

Step 1: Transferring bacteria growing on culture medium in a petri dish.

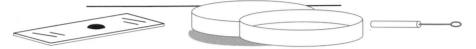

Step 2: Mix with one drop of water.

Figure 22-6
Preparing a bacteriological smear.

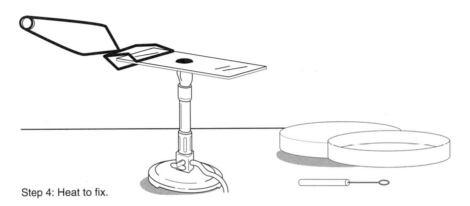

Step 3: Air dry.

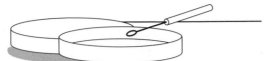

Step 4: Heat to fix.

Gram Staining for Bacteria

One of the most important tasks performed in the study of bacteriology is the Gram's stain. Bacteria are differentiated according to whether they are gram-positive, which stains blue, or gram-negative, which stains red. Examination of smears stained by this technique reveals both the morphology and the Gram's reaction of the bacteria. In the staining technique, the bacteria are treated with the following solutions: crystal violet, iodine solution, alcohol (decolorizing solution), and safranin or some other red counterstain. All bacteria take up the crystal violet. The iodine fixes the stain to the gram-positive bacteria. This keeps the stain from washing off when the decolorizing solution is added. When the counterstain is added, the gram-positive organisms do not stain red since they are already stained. The gram-negative bacteria lose the blue color during the decolorization process, so they stain red. The procedure, usually performed by the technologist, is outlined in the steps listed below:

1. Prepare the slide with the smear, and allow to air-dry. Then fix the smear to the slide by heat. Do not overheat.

2. Cover the smear with crystal violet for 1 minute, then wash it with tapwater for approximately 5 seconds and drain.
3. Pour the iodine solution onto the smear and leave it on for approximately 1 minute. After it has been allowed to stay in place, rinse it with tapwater for approximately 5 seconds, then drain or dry by blotting.
4. Decolorize for 30 seconds with alcohol, then blot dry.
5. Counterstain with safranin for about 10 seconds.
6. Wash with tap water, and blot dry.

Times may vary slightly, but the order is always the same. Observe the slides using the oil-immersion objective of the microscope after locating the stained area using the low power. Note the appearance of the gram-negative and the gram-positive organisms.

Acid-Fast Staining for Bacteria

Another staining procedure that you might encounter because of its wide use by most medical laboratories is the acid-fast stain, which classifies bacteria as either acid-fast or non-acid-fast. Acid-fast organisms contain a large amount of fatty and waxy substances in the cell. Once the dye penetrates the cell, which has been assisted by heating, it is not easily removed by the decolorizing agent. All acid-fast bacteria are also gram-positive. If you are required to perform this procedure, follow the steps outlined below:

1. Cover the fixed smear with carbol fuchsin, and gently heat the slide for approximately 3 to 5 minutes, then wash it with tapwater.
2. Decolorize with acid-alcohol until only a small amount of red dye remains.
3. Wash with tapwater.
4. Counterstain the slide with methylene blue for approximately 30 seconds. After the counterstain has been applied, the acid-fast bacteria will appear red, while the non–acid-fast bacteria will appear blue.

Using Chemicals and Reagents in the Medical Laboratory

The department that works closely with both the serology and the microbiology sections of the medical laboratory is the chemistry department. This is the part of the laboratory responsible for analyzing the specimens that have been collected, in order to determine whether they are normal or how far they vary from being normal.

In order to perform the very specialized procedures needed to analyze the contents of such specimens as blood, urine, gastric juices, cerebrospinal fluid, and other body fluids, the members of the chemistry department must use certain agents to mix the specimens with. These chemicals are called *reagents*. Most clinical laboratory reagents are purchased already prepared and ready to use. However, in some cases, you may be responsible for manually preparing reagents. If this is the case, there are certain precautions that must be taken. For example, when working with acids, always remember to add acid to water in small amounts with mixing until the proper concentration has been reached. And never add water to acid. Some acids, such as concentrated sulfuric acid, can release large quantities of heat when diluted. Adding water to this acid can release enough heat to cause the water to boil and splatter and perhaps splash the acid on the person making the dilution.

Most reagents are supplied as a dry powder or in crystalline powder form. Each of these must be diluted in water. Generally, solutions are prepared by adding the required quantity of powdered reagent to a small amount of water. They are then carefully mixed to dissolve. Finally, enough water is added to bring the mixture to the required volume and mixed. Remember, it is always important to follow the manufacturer's directions on the original label for making solutions.

All prepared reagents including acids should be stored in their original container. Every bottle must have a legible label. It is best to keep the original label, but replacement labels must be an accurate, identical copy of the original.

Water Usage in the Medical Laboratory

All medical laboratories need a source of pure water. Usually, water is supplied by commercial companies who sell bottled water. Two methods of purifying the water are presently used by most facilities. These include *distillation* and *deionization*.

Whenever water is to be distilled, the tapwater that is originally used, must first be heated to its boiling point, eventually forming steam. Steam is condensed to water and collected in another vessel. Impurities are left behind in the boiling vessel.

For deionization, tapwater is passed through a cylinder or a series of cylinders containing tiny beads. The beads are mixtures of resins containing both negatively and positively charged ions. This resin exchange capacity is limited. A dye may be present in the resin column to indicate when its exchange capacity is exhausted. Therefore, a special cylinder may be added in order to trap particulate matter and bacteria.

In some cases purification methods are combined. Distilled water is passed through a deionization column to remove any materials that have been condensed with the water. Deionized water is distilled to remove any un-ionized impurities and to destroy pathogens with heat.

Containers must have a label, since saline and other solutions cannot otherwise be differentiated. All water containers must also be capped in order to prevent dust, contaminants, and atmospheric gases from entering the water. The use of plastic container prevents impurities from glass from dissolving in the water.

Procedures Performed in the Chemistry Department

In the medical laboratory, there are many different tests and procedures that are not only performed in the chemistry department but also in all of the individual sections of the laboratory. Because of this fact, some of the procedures discussed in this text may not be exactly like those in the laboratory where you are ultimately employed. For example, blood analyses may be done manually or with the multisample analyzers (SMA). It is important that while you are a student that you consult with your instructor or supervisor in order to find out which laboratory procedures or tests you may actually be responsible for performing. For our purposes, we will only be discussing those tests and procedures that you, as a laboratory assistant, will be most concerned with, and that you may have to perform as part of your responsibilities as a member of the medical laboratory team.

Manual Testing vs. Automation

Because of the number of procedures and tests performed on laboratory samples, particularly those tested in the chemistry department, as well as the number of patients that may be seen in the laboratory, many facilities have switched over to using automation as a means of analyzing and testing specimens. *Automation* is defined as the development and use of instruments to complete a testing process without human intervention. The automated system must include some kind of sampling device, a means to add the needed reagents and sample, incubating modules, modules to measure, and a recording device. The measuring module is usually a colorimeter. These sample steps are followed in analyzing a specimen using manual technology. In fact, almost any

manual method can be adapted to an automated system.

The human element is still a vital part of laboratory testing, even though automation may seem to diminish the importance of the laboratory person. Whether it is the technologist or the assistant, that person must still prepare the appropriate serum, load sample cups, and most important of all, be constantly aware of the validity of the automated system.

Factors that determine the extent to which a given laboratory uses automated procedures include the size of the laboratory, economic feasibility, the number of tests performed, and the training and preference of the members of the medical laboratory team.

Using the Spectrophotometer

An instrument that is used a great deal in the chemistry department is the spectrophotometer (Figure 22-7). These devices measure light. The two basic types, the photometer and the spectrophotometer, are used in determining the presence and quantity of chemical substances in the blood. The substances in the blood can be treated in such a manner as to yield a color that can be measured quantitatively. Visible light is a result of energy changes of electrons in the outer shell of atoms. Infrared radiation is caused by vibrations of the molecules, and ultraviolet radiation is produced by energy changes of the electrons in the inner shells of the atoms.

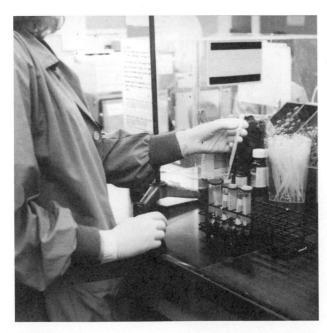
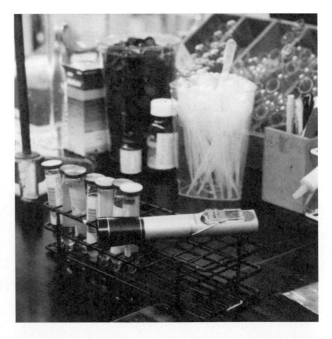

Figure 22-7
Using a photometer.

To use photometry, a reaction must take place between the substance to be measured and a reagent, producing a color change. The determination of the concentration of the substance is based on a concept known as *Beer's law.* Beer's law states that the color intensity is directly proportional to the density. When a reagent or chemical is added to a substance to produce a color reaction, the intensity of the color is proportional to the amount or concentration of the substance present. The portion of the light passing through the substance is called the *percentage of transmittance.* The rest of the beam of light is absorbed by the substance. This amount is measured as *absorbance* or *optical density.* Transmittance decreases as the concentration of the substance rises. Absorbance tends to increase with concentration. A photometer can read either of these. In either case, the unknown substance must be compared with a standard solution. A *standard solution* is defined as a solution containing a known amount of substance.

Spectrophotometers can be a separate instrument used for manual procedures in physician's offices or smaller clinics. They can also be incorporated into an automated system in a large laboratory. All photometers should be protected with a dust cover when not in use. Cuvettes for manual procedures should be absolutely clean and free from scratches. Their outside should be wiped clean after a sample is poured in, and they should always be held by the upper edge only for insertion into the photometer.

Technology in the Laboratory

The number of medical laboratories in doctor's offices is increasing. These are called *POLs,* or physician's office laboratories. Sometimes, one laboratory assistant or technologist may be employed by several physicians and travel from laboratory to laboratory during one day or from day to day during a week. On-site testing is becoming popular within larger hospitals to speed the treatment of patients in emergency situations. Satellite laboratories can be established for intensive care units and the operating room away from the chief or central laboratory. Laboratory procedures carried out in these areas are called *point-of-care testing.*

Changes in POLs and point-of-care testing have been made possible by the development of microcomputers and microelectronics for use in automated testing equipment. At present, there are two types of technologies that are used in most automated medical laboratories. These are called continuous-flow analysis and discrete analysis. During *continuous-flow analysis,* both samples and reagents constantly flow through the equipment. They are added at specified time intervals, and samples are separated by either reagents or air bubbles.

In *discrete analysis,* patient samples are placed in individual containers, which eliminate the need for mixing of the samples. The two procedures employed in this type of analysis are centrifugal analysis and solid-phase analysis.

In discrete *centrifugal analysis,* the patient sample and reagents are brought together in a container and then centrifugal force is used to mix them during the reaction time period. The test results are obtained by reading from a spectrophotometer within the analyzer.

When *solid-phase analysis* is used, the patient sample is added to dry reagents on a slide or strip. The reagents occur in layers, which react with the sample for testing. The area where the reagents are located is called the test patch, rest area, or reagent patch. The bottom support layer on the strip may be transparent so that the instrument can read the test results. A different strip is used for each type of test and is identified by the machine through a code located on the strip. After a reaction period, the machine reads assay results, calculates, and finally displays its findings.

General Tests Performed in the Chemistry Department

There are many routine tests performed in the clinical chemistry laboratory, either manually or by automation. Some of these are the glucose or blood sugar; blood urea nitrogen (BUN); uric acid; creatine and creatinine; proteins (albumin and globulin); bilirubin and bromsulfalein (BSP); triglycerides, cholesterol, phospholipids, and fatty acids determinations; calcium, phosphorus, and magnesgium measurements; and electrolytes (chloride, sodium, potassium, and carbon dioxide).

Glucose or Blood Sugar

The oxidation of glucose provides energy for various biochemical processes. Diabetes mellitus is a disease that prevents the body from using glocuse properly. Blood glucose determinations are used for diagnosis and treatment, as well as in routine physical examinations and health screenings. When a glucose or blood sugar test is ordered, blood specimens are collected both during fasting and after eating. Tests done on blood and urine over a set period of several hours are called a glucose tolerance tests.

This test aids in diagnosing hypoglycemia as well as hyperglycemia.

Blood Urea Nitrogen (BUN), Uric Acid, Creatine, and Creatinine

The kidneys are responsible for excreting blood urea nitrogen, uric acid, creatine, and creatinine. An increase of these chemicals in urine may be an indication that the kidneys are unable to process these substances adequately. Uric acid testing is used primarily for determination of gout.

Proteins (Albumin and Globulin)

Proteins make up the support tissue of animals, protect us from disease in the form of antibodies, and are the basis for the basic functions of life. The ratio of albumin to globulin (A/G ratio) is used in the diagnosis of liver and kidney disease.

Bilirubin and Bromsulfalein (BSP)

These are tests of liver function. Biliurubin is formed when hemoglobin is broken down. Only an increase is significant.

Triglycerides, Cholesterol, Phospholipids, and Fatty Acid Determination

The body's fatty acids, or lipids, relate to fat metabolism by providing stored energy. They also form part of the structural units of cell membranes and hormones. Cholesterol and triglyceride tests are often performed if the physician suspects that the patient is suffering from artherosclerosis or has problems with fat metabolism. Cholesterol can be broken down for testing into high-density lipoprotein (HDL) cholesterol and low-density lipoprotein (LDL) cholesterol. The HDL is considered "good" because it is broken down in the liver. However, the LDL is considered "bad" because it is the type stored as fat in the tissues. Physicians often use the ratio of LDL to HDL in order to determine the patient's heart attack risk factor. The larger the ratio, the greater the risk.

Calcium, Phosphorus, and Magnesium

These minerals are important in the coagulation of blood and in the proper function of the kidneys. An increase in one results in a decrease in the other. A delicate balance must be maintained for proper functioning of body processes.

Electrolytes (Chloride, Sodium, Potassium, and Carbon Dioxide)

Chloride is important in the maintenance of osmotic pressure and is the anion present in the largest amount in the body fluids. Sodium is the cation present in the largest amount in extracellular fluid. Potassium is the largest intracellular cation. These, along with carbon dioxide, are responsible for maintaining the blood's pH. The normal range of the blood pH is 7.35 to 7.45. This range is narrow, and deviations can result in acidosis, alkalosis, or in some cases, even death.

Testing Enzymes

Enzymes are biochemical catalysts found within the body that allow it to carry out its chemical reactions at body temperature and at a pH compatible with life. They are not changed during the reaction. There are several routine tests that are performed in the chemistry lab that allow the technologist to measure these chemical reactions. They include testing for amylase, lipase, alkaline phosphatase, acid phosphatase, and transaminases.

Amylase

Amylase breaks down starches into sugars. Any abnormal results indicate that problems with the pancreas, salivary glands, or the liver may exist.

Lipase

Lipase is furnished by the pancreas and is necessary for the breakdown of fats; any elevation in lipase level is generally an indication that a disorder of the pancreas may be present.

Alkaline Phosphatase and Acid Phosphatase

Alkaline phosphatase is important in the formation of bones and is almost always elevated in bone disease. It may also cause jaundice if an obstruction is present.

The acid phosphatase level is usually elevated in cases where cancer of the prostate is present. It is particularly high if the cancer has spread to other parts of the body.

Transaminases

Transaminases are usually elevated when there is a deterioration of tissue in an organ. *Serum glutamic oxalacetic transaminase/aspartate aminotransaminase*

(SGOT/AST) is present in heart muscle, liver tissue, and other organs. Destruction of cells in these areas causes an increased release into the blood. *Serum glutamic pyruvic transaminase/alanine aminotransaminase (SGPT/ALT)* is found in liver tissue. The presence of *lactic dehydrogenase (LDH)* is used to diagnose cardiac and liver disorders, anemias, and pulmonary infarction. *Creatine phosphokinase (CPK)* is used in the diagnosis and prognosis following heart attack.

Profile Testing and Protein and Hemoglobin Electrophoresis

Combinations of general or routine tests to study the function of a specific organ are called *profiles*. When these are required, automated machines take a sample of a patient's serum and then run from 12 to 20 tests on a very small sample. A large number of tests indicates the patient's general condition and may be a combination of several profiles. Specific profiles may be ordered for liver function, kidney function, cardiac condition, carbohydrate usage, or lipid metabolism.

Electrophoresis is the process by which charged colloidal particles move through an electrical field. The particles move with different velocities because of their size, shape, and electrical charge. They are then dispersed onto a stabilizing medium by way of the electrical current so that they can be stained and studied.

Through electrophoresis, lactic dehydrogenase (LDH) can be separated into five fractions or isoenzymes. An increase in isoenzymes 1 and 2 can indicate heart trouble, while an increase in isoenzyme[3] usually indicates pulmonary infarction. Increases in fractions 4 and 5 are usually associated with liver disease.

Abnormal hemoglobins can also be detected by electrophoretic procedures. The patterns formed by the hemolyzed blood cells from a test sample can be matched against standard bands of known hemoglobin. Abnormal types of hemoglobin that may be iden-

tified are *hemoglobin S*, which results in sickle-cell anemia; *hemoglobin C*, which is responsible for a type of hemolytic anemia; and *hemoglobin F*, a type of fetal hemoglobin that persists later in life and may produce a condition known as thalassemia, an inherited abnormality causing a type of anemia.

Therapeutic Drug Monitoring by the Chemistry Department

There are many times when a physician will need to monitor the effects of the drugs he or she has prescribed for a patient. Such monitoring is usually completed by tests performed in the chemistry department. Some of the medications that require careful monitoring include digoxin, lithium, phenobarbitol, quinidine, and certain antibiotics.

Laboratories are also called on to evaluate for drug abuse, suicide attempts that may involve a drug overdose, and in cases of accidental ingestion of drugs by children. These tests are never run to be used as legal evidence; however, law enforcement agencies may perform some types of testing. The results from the clinical laboratory can given physicians indications for treatments.

Summary

In this chapter we discussed the three sections of the medical laboratory that are most responsible for identifying, testing, and analyzing most specimens brought into the lab. We identified those departments as serology, which is most responsible for studying antigen-antibody reactions in vitro, microbiology, which deals with the various methods of collecting, inoculating, streaking, incubating, and identifying different types of pathogenic microorganisms, and finally, the chemistry department, whose sole responsibility is to perform various tests and procedures that analyze different types of laboratory specimens and samples.

Review Questions

1. What is the name of a substance used in a culture medium?

2. A(n) _____ is a biochemical catalyst within the body that produces chemical changes without being changed itself.

3. What does the term *in vitro* mean?

4. What does the abbreviation *HIV* mean?

5. A(n) _____ is a protein that has developed within the body in response to a foreign substance.

6. What is the difference between *anaerobic* and *aerobic*?

7. What is the term used to describe a process that occurs when measurements or results do not agree?

8. What is the name of the test performed to determine the presence of infectious mononucleosis?

9. The study of fungi, yeast, and molds is called _____ .

10. A(n) _____ is a device used to measure light intensities in different parts of the spectrum.

23

Working in the Blood Bank

Performance Objectives

Upon completion of this chapter, you will be able to:

1. Discuss the purpose and function of the blood bank.
2. Describe the process used for screening blood donors.
3. Explain the process for properly drawing a unit of whole blood.
4. Describe the correct procedure for the processing and labeling of blood.
5. Identify the four groups used in the ABO blood grouping system and explain how the ABO blood group and Rh factor are determined.
6. Identify and describe the various components of blood.
7. Describe the correct procedure for cross-matching blood.
8. Explain why a Coombs test is performed.

Terms and Abbreviations

Agglutinins antibodies found in plasma that react with agglutinogens on the RBCs.

Agglutinogens antigens that are located on the surface of RBCs.

Autologous blood a donation of blood by an individual before surgery for his or her intended transfusion at a later time.

Components portions of the blood that have been separated from a single unit for use in different transfusions.

Cross-matching the process by which tests are performed in order to determine whether a donor's blood will be compatible with the recipient's blood during a transfusion; also called *compatibility testing.*

Cryoprecipitate the precipitate formed when plasma is frozen.

Donor someone who gives blood for use in a transfusion.

Iodophore a compound of iodine with a stabilizing agent to lessen irritation.

Plasma the liquid portion of the blood.

Recipient the person who receives blood or its components.

Red blood cells concentrated solution of blood cells used for transfusion; component of blood that has been separated from serum by centrifugation or undisturbed sedimentation.

Transfusion the replacement of whole blood or its components.

Whole blood the entire unit of blood.

Some of the larger hospitals maintain a blood bank in the medical laboratory. Others depend on local or area blood banks that serve more than one hospital. All blood banks are required by law to meet specific standards in order to ensure the delivery of a quality product and the safety of donors.

The purpose of the blood bank is to provide a location in which the proper screening, collection, testing, processing, and dissemination of blood can be completed. The blood bank functions as an integral part of the medical laboratory in order to provide patients with transfusions that may be necessary to replace blood lost through hemorrhage because of trauma or surgery, destruction of erythrocytes, or the body's inability to provide its own blood supply.

Blood Donor Screening

Any person wishing to donate blood must first be carefully screened and sign an informed consent form prior to donation. Donors are not restricted by sex or race, however, an individual can be permanently rejected for donating blood if he or she has ever been exposed to, or suffered from viral hepatitis, drug or alcohol addiction, malaria, AIDS, tuberculosis, syphilis, diseases of the heart, liver, or kidney, convulsive disorders such as epilepsy, cancer, any diseases of the blood, and diabetes mellitus. A transfusion of blood or its components, major surgery, and tattooing can also cause deferment of a donor for up to 6 months. Women who are pregnant may also be deferred for up to 6 months after delivery. People who have been recently vaccinated generally must wait for 2 to 4 weeks after receiving a vaccination or immunization, depending on the type of vaccination received. All donors generally range between the ages of 17 to 65, and most are limited to five or fewer donations per year. At least 8 weeks must elapse between donations.

Once an individual donates blood, he or she will be issued a donor card that acts as a permanent record. This card contains personal identifying information, including a social security number and the person's medical history. The date of donation and results of the screening are recorded on the card. The donor will also be assigned a number that is carefully entered in the blood bank's record system or database.

Whenever a person comes in to donate blood, he or she will be given a partial physical examination before the donation. The donor must weigh at least 110 pounds, and his or her temperature, pulse, and blood pressure must be within normal range. The hemoglobin and hematocrit are determined, and they too must be within normal limits.

Donor screenings must include questions that relate to AIDS, HIV (human immunodeficiency virus) infection, ARC (AIDS-related complex), and the high-risk behaviors associated with these conditions. Each donor is given an opportunity, in strict confidence, to indicate that the blood drawn will not be suitable for transfusion. If significant abnormalities are detected during processing, the blood bank must notify the donor.

Collection and Numbering of the Blood

Both the donor and the recipient must be protected when blood is collected for transfusion. The site selected for venipuncture must be free of lesions and made thoroughly aseptic by cleaning it with soap and 70% alcohol prior to introduction of the venipuncture needle. Finally, an iodophore is applied. An *iodophore* is a compound of iodine with a stabilizing agent to lessen irritation. A restricting band or tourniquet is placed above the collection site. Usually a sphygmomanometer is held at 40 mmHg. The needle is inserted firmly, and blood flows into a closed collecting system, consisting of a plastic bag with tubing attached.

The collecting unit contains an anticoagulant. This is usually a sterile, acidified citrate-dextrose (ACD) solution. In order to constitute a unit of blood, the proper amount must be collected. A unit should contain between 450 to 500 mL of whole blood. During collection, the anticoagulant in the plastic bag must be frequently mixed with the incoming blood to prevent formation of any clots. The donor must also watch during and after the collection process for any signs of fainting.

After the blood has been collected the needle is removed from the donor's arm with pressure and elevation applied to stop bleeding. A special tube, called a *pilot tube*, is collected after the needle is withdrawn by gently inserting the needle into a vacuum tube. This is used for donor testing. The collection tubing is heat-sealed into segments for use in cross-matching procedures (Figure 23-1).

Once the unit of blood has been properly collected, it is assigned a unique number. All test tubes, segments of tubing, and printed records are then identified by the number assigned to the unit by the blood bank. The number is in series and must therefore be carefully logged into the bank's records. Blood bank personnel must be able to locate and provide a history for any unit of blood should a question be raised later by a physician or a patient.

After collection, the blood must be placed in storage in a location with a maintained temperature of 1 to 6°C.

Processing the Blood

Each unit of blood that has been donated is tested for liver disease, different types of hepatitis, the HIV virus, and syphilis. The RPR test procedure is generally used to detect the presence of syphilis. The blood group and Rh factor are also determined. During processing, each unit of blood receives a label that must show the blood group, Rh factor, type of anticoagulant present, donor identification, date of expiration, and the name and address of the blood bank.

All units of whole blood are stored in a refrigerator. Once processing has been completed, the bags are arranged by their ABO groups, that is, into group

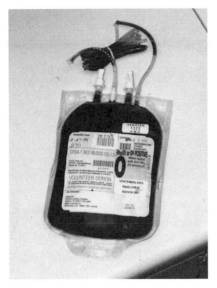 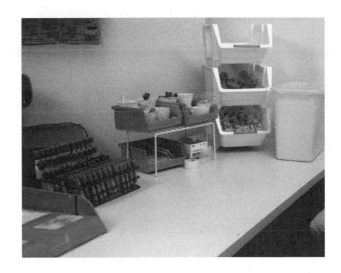

Figure 23-1
Unit of blood and rack of pilot tubes.

A, group B, group AB, and group O. These groups are also divided into Rh-positive and Rh-negative. The storage refrigerator must be maintained at a temperature of 1 to 6°C. A recording thermometer should be used to keep a continuous, permanent record of the temperature. Should the temperature exceed the accepted limit of 10°C, an alarm will sound during the day or at night.

Daily inspections are conducted on stored blood. Each unit must be inspected for clot formation; turbidity; or color changes, such as hemolysis; and findings then recorded on the daily record of inspection. Outdated blood must be discarded.

Blood units are often exchanged between banks as the need arises. Incoming blood must be added to the receiving log book or data bank. Outgoing blood is also recorded. All units must be identified as to the donor's number, the ABO type and Rh factor, and the dates of arrival and expiration.

Some people, anticipating elective surgery, may bank their own blood for future use. This blood is called *autologous blood*. If this is the case, the donation, storage, and transfusion will require the consent of both the blood bank physician and the patient's physician.

Blood Components

A unit of blood can be transfused as *whole blood*, or the blood can be separated into components so that one unit may benefit more than one person. The concentrated solution of cells, called *red blood cells*, goes to one person. The plasma can be frozen to form *fresh frozen plasma*. After freezing and thawing,

a white precipitate is found in the container. This is called *cryoprecipitate*, and contains most of the clotting factors. These blood clotting factors can be removed for use by someone with bleeding problems. *Plasma* can be given to restore blood volume or be further separated by chemical means into fractions such as gamma globulin or serum albumin. If water is removed, plasma can be dried and stored for a considerable length of time. Sterile, distilled water can then be used to restore plasma to a liquid state for transfusion.

Blood Grouping

Among the important factors in the blood are antigens and antibodies that determine blood type. An *antigen*, as we previously discussed, is a substance that reacts with its specific antibody. Antigens are named for the type of antigen-antibody reaction they may bring out. *Agglutinogens* are the antigens located on the surface of red blood cells.

Antibodies are protein substances in the plasma that react with their specific antigen. Thus, agglutinogens (antigens) will react with agglutinins (antibodies) in order to bring about agglutination. There are many different kinds of antigen-antibody reactions.

Two kinds of agglutinogens may be found on the surface of human red blood cells, called A and B. An individual may have either A or B, neither, or both. A person's blood group or type is determined by the presence or absence of these A and B antigens.

If a person has A agglutinogens on the red blood cells, then he or she will also have corresponding antibodies called anti-B agglutinins in the plasma. Per-

Table 23-1
ABO Blood Grouping System

Blood Group	Agglutinogen Red Blood Cells	Agglutinin in Serum	Cells Agglutinated
A	A	Anti-B	A, AB, O
B	B	Anti-A	A, AB, O
AB	A and B	None	A, B, AB, O
O	None	Anti-A and Anti-B	None

sons with B agglutinogens will have anti-A agglutinins. Those with both A and B agglutinogens will have no agglutinins; and those with neither A nor B agglutinogens will have both anti-A and anti-B agglutinins. Plasma could never contain antibodies against the antigens on its own red blood cells. If so, the antigen and antibody reaction would bring about the agglutination of the person's own red blood cells. Table 23-1 shows the antigens and antibodies present in the various blood groups.

Blood types are hereditary and therefore do not change during one's lifetime. The pattern of inheritance is predictable. It is possible, by determining blood types, to know whether a given person *could* be the parent of a particular child, but not that he or she *is* the parent. Research has shown that the only way to prove definite parentage is through DNA testing.

The percentage of a given blood type in various ethnic groups varies. In the United States, for example, about 47 percent have type O, while approximately 41 percent have type A, 10 percent have type B, and about 4 percent have type AB.

Understanding the Rh Factor

The Rh system is based on the presence or absence of a certain antigen on the erythrocytes. The factor was first discovered in rhesus monkeys. That is where the Rh symbol derives from. About 85 percent of the population in the United States has these antigens and will test Rh-positive. Those who lack the antigen are Rh-negative. Rh antigens are located on the surface of the RBCs as well as the A and B antigens. Thus, a person can be type A, B, AB, or O, and also be Rh-positive or Rh-negative.

The Rh factor is of little importance except in the pregnancy of Rh-negative persons, or if they receive blood transfusions. If a person who is Rh-negative receives Rh-positive blood, he or she may become sensitized to the antigen. The body is stimulated to produce specific anti-Rh antibodies. These remain in the blood. If the patient receives further transfusions of Rh-positive blood, the Rh antigen on the donor's red

blood cells and the Rh antibody in the patient's blood will react, causing the red blood cells to agglutinate, thus resulting in serious consequences or even death.

To avoid this problem, Rh determinations are done prior to transfusion with whole blood, and Rh-negative patients are given only Rh-negative blood. In that way, there can be no antigens to stimulate the production of antibodies.

A similar reaction can occur during pregnancy, when the mother is Rh-negative and the baby is Rh-positive. The inheritance of Rh types follows genetic patterns. The child of an Rh-negative mother and an Rh-positive father could be either Rh-positive or Rh-negative. If the child is Rh-positive, it is possible for the Rh antigens to cross the placental barrier during pregnancy and cause the Rh-negative mother to produce Rh antibodies. In a subsequent pregnancy with an Rh-positive fetus, an antigen-antibody reaction between the infant's RBCs and the anti-Rh antibodies in the mother's blood could cause the RBCs of the infant to break down or hemolyze, thereby releasing hemoglobin in the baby's blood. This may cause the baby to be anemic. Further damage may be caused if the disintegrating red blood cells occlude the blood vessels. If this occurs, the condition is called *erythroblastosis fetalis* or *hemolytic disease of the newborn*. It can be treated by giving the baby many small transfusions of Rh-negative blood to replace the damaged blood.

Currently, if an Rh-negative mother delivers an Rh-positive baby but has no anti-Rh antibodies, she is given anti-Rh immune globulin during the first 72 hours after delivery. These antibodies react with any fetal antigens in the mother's blood so she will not produce anti-Rh antibodies. Then, if a second pregnancy with an Rh-positive fetus occurs, there will be no Rh-positive antibodies present to cause a reaction.

Although Rh factors must be determined to provide adequate care of both mother and child, the actual numbers involved are quite small.

Cross-Matching Blood

Blood types are important in blood transfusion because if a donor's blood contains antigens and/or antibodies of a different type from that of a recipient, the RBCs will agglutinate and cause severe reaction or even death. Blood group O has no antigens. It is called the "universal donor" because theoretically the blood would not react with any cells in transfusion. In actual practice, patients are almost always transfused with their own type of blood.

The anti-A and anti-B antibodies in the serum and other factors in the blood could cause an undesirable reaction. Look at Figure 23-2. It shows the type of reactions of AB blood groups in cross-matching prior to transfusion.

When a patient needs a transfusion, the physician will write an order. The order is then placed on a transfusion request form and sent to the blood bank or requested by computer networking. A member of the blood bank will then take a sample of the patient's blood and use it to determine the ABO group and Rh factor. A unit of blood is selected that is the same group or from a compatible group. The selected donor unit is checked for compatibility with the recipient's blood by a process called *cross-matching*. Cross-matching refers to the tests performed to determine whether a donor's blood will be compatible with the recipient's blood during the transfusion process. A cross-match involves three types of testing: incubation at room temperature with a saline suspension of blood cells, high protein (albumin) incubated with cells and serum at 37°C, and an antiglobulin or Coombs test.

The Coombs Test

The Coombs, or antiglobulin, test is a nonspecific test used to detect weak or incomplete antibodies. It was first used to demonstrate weak Rh agglutinins. The indirect Coombs test detects antibodies in vitro, that is, antibodies located in the blood serum. Some-

times incomplete antibodies are not present in the routine cross-matching procedures. The indirect Coombs test can also detect the presence of incomplete antibodies that might result in incompatibility. This test is also done routinely on new obstetrical patients and then periodically on Rh-negative obstetrical patients.

The direct Coombs test is used to detect antibodies in vivo, that is, antibodies that are attached to the RBCs. In this test, the patient's RBCs are mixed with antihuman serum. The antihuman serum is usually prepared from the blood of rabbits that have been injected with human RBCs. Agglutination of the patient's RBCs is a positive test.

The direct Coombs test can also be used to determine the presence of hemolytic disease of the newborn, autoimmune hemolytic anemia, and in the investigation of hemolytic transfusion reactions.

Transfusions

Records must be kept to show routine or special testing. After the cross match has indicated compatibility, the unit of blood can then be released to the nursing unit for administration to the patient. A careful record, called a transfusion release ledger, must be kept in order to document that the cross-match was completed properly. It must include the time and date for the release of the unit, the name of the per-

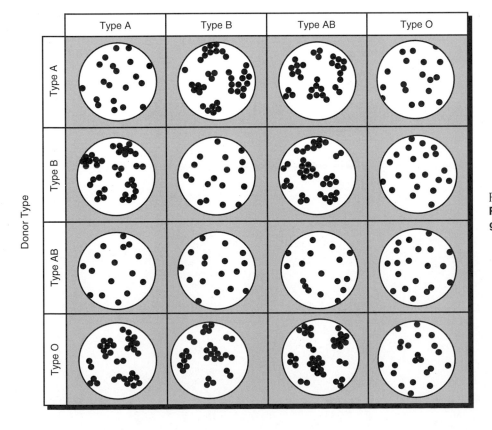

Figure 23-2
Reactions of ABO blood groups in cross-matching.

son releasing it, and the name of the person to whom it was received.

Summary

In this chapter, we discussed the purpose and function of the blood bank, that is, the department within the medical laboratory responsible for screening, collecting, numbering, processing, and testing blood that will eventually be transfused from one donor to another person. We also discussed how units of blood are typed, carefully tested for purity, and placed in the bank for future use. We talked about how blood can be divided into its components for distribution to more than one person, as well as how the process of cross-matching the blood determines its compatibility from one person to another.

Review Questions

1. A(n) _____ refers to the person who receives blood or its components.

2. What is the name of the process used to determine whether a donor's blood will be compatible with the recipient's blood?

3. The replacement of whole blood or its components, is called _____ .

4. The liquid portion of the blood is called:

    a. proteins

    b. plasma

    c. protozoa

5. A(n) _____ is someone who gives blood for use in a transfusion.

6. An entire unit of blood is referred to as _____ _____ .

7. What is the name of the compound of iodine used to lessen irritation during the collection of blood?

8. What is the name of the test procedure most often used to detect the presence of syphilis?

9. Identify the four blood groups:

    a. _____

    b. _____

    c. _____

    d. _____

10. _____ are protein substances found in the plasma that react with their specific antigen.

24

Histology and Cytology

_____
_____
_____
_____

_____

Performance Objectives

Upon completion of this chapter, you will be able to:

1. Identify the types and sources of specimens tested in the histology and cytology lab.
2. Describe the steps involved in processing tissues and cells.
3. Describe and be able to demonstrate how to mark and store slides.
4. Discuss and demonstrate the practice of safety precautions unique to the histology-cytology department of the medical laboratory.

Terms

Autopsy examination of a dead body or tissue from a dead body in order to establish the cause of death.
Biopsy pertaining to living tissue that has been removed for microscopic examination in order to aid in diagnosis.
Cytology the study of cells.
Dehydration pertaining to the removal of water.
Exfoliated cells cells that have been shed from the body, often in sheets or layers.
Frozen section process by which water content of a fresh tissue specimen is frozen to give rigidity for immediate sectioning, staining, and diagnosis; performed especially in cases where cancer may be suspected.

Fixative solution used to prevent the decomposition of tissue and to preserve it.
Histology the study of tissues.
Microtome a machine with a knife blade used for cutting tissue into very thin slices.
Mount the process of placing tissue sections on slides for staining and/or to cover with a cover slip for permanency.
Postmortem autopsy.
Staining the process of identification of tissue or cell parts by their color reaction to dyes.

In some hospitals, cytology and histology may be located together in the pathology department. In other facilities, they may be separate departments within the medical laboratory. *Cytology* is concerned with cells discarded by the body, whereas *histology* deals with tissues. Both accept tissues and cells for fixing, sectioning, staining, and mounting on slides. In most cases, it will be the technician who is most responsible for identifying normal and abnormal cell structures. However, in some smaller facilities, such as laboratories found in physician's offices, you may be required to perform some of the testing on both cells and tissues.

Specimen Collection, Recording, and Processing

Disease and infection cause changes in tissues and cells. Tissues may be removed for study after death during autopsy, as surgery is performed, or during an examination by a physician. An example of a surgical specimen is a gallbladder removed during a cholecystectomy. A *biopsy* is living tissue that has been removed from a person for microscopic examination and that can be used to aid in diagnosing a disease. Biopsies are usually obtained with a scalpel and occasionally with a needle. Other specimens that are tested in the histology or cytology lab may arrive as smears on slides, such as Pap smears, or as fluids, such as urine, amniotic fluid, nipple discharge, cerebrospinal fluid, or other body cavity fluids. Some tissues are collected into containers filled with 70% alcohol.

Keeping Accurate Records of Specimens

As tissue arrives in the laboratory, it is assigned a number and then logged into a record book by number and patient name, or is added to computer records. Copies of requisitions may also be kept and filed alphabetically by the patient's name and the case number added.

All facilities choose their own type of numbering system. The case number may include letters or numbers as part of the code used for identification. Numerals may indicate the date of collection, such as using the last two for the year and another set of two for the month. Case numbers usually change each year. In a large laboratory, numbers may change each month. However, in a smaller lab, this may not be the case. With such a system, slides can be located if the date is known.

Processing Cells and Tissues

The pathologist will study large sections of tissue or whole organs in a gross examination. He or she will then describe any conditions observed and will indicate parts that may require further study. Tissues are processed by histotechnologists and histotechnicians. Cell screening is performed by cytotechnologists. Slides are studied in order to determine the type and number of cells present, whether any are abnormal, and whether more testing may be necessary. The size, shape, general appearance, and staining qualities of cells are observed. The cell nucleus and any cellular inclusions are also examined.

The process that tissue undergoes prior to permanently mounting it onto a slide includes several steps. These include embedding, blocking, cutting or sectioning, staining, clearing, and finally, mounting. *Embedding* is a process that involves placing tissue into a medium in order to keep it intact for processing and placement on a slide for microscopic examination. The ideal size of tissue for processing is 2 cm square and 0.4 to 0.5 cm thick. Embedding includes four separate processes. The first, called *fixation*, is done with a mixture of chemicals necessary to kill the fresh tissue to prevent any decomposition by its own enzymes, and to harden it. The second process is called *dehydration*, which is the removal of water by chemical means, such as alcohol or acetone. *Clearing* is the third process involved in embed-

ding. It involves the removal of any alcohol by an agent that must also be a solvent for the paraffin in the next step of the process. The final process, called *infiltration*, allows the embedding medium to penetrate the tissue for support.

Cutting or Sectioning Tissue

The next step involved in processing tissues is called *cutting* or *sectioning*. In this process, the block of tissue is fastened to a holder on a rotary microtome. The side of the block must be parallel to the knife edge along the entire surface facing the knife in order to cut a smooth ribbon. The knife edge must be kept very sharp with no nicks, since these will show on the tissue on the slide under the microscope. As the microtome wheel is rotated, the knife will cut a ribbon of paraffin slices with tissue embedded. When the ribbon is 6 to 8 inches long, it is moved carefully with a brush to the surface of the water in a constant-temperature water bath. The best sections are then selected. A slide is slipped under the section, centered, and then separated from the ribbon. Slides may have albumin on the surface as a fixative in order to hold the tissue. They may also be blotted and placed onto a warming table for drying. Each slide must carry an identification number from the block.

Staining

The object of *staining* is to identify tissue components and cell parts by their color reaction to certain dyes. Hematoxylin and eosin are the dyes most often used for this purpose. Hematoxylin stains the nucleus a dark blue color, while eosin, which is an acid stain, colors the cytoplasm a rosy-red color. The color reaction occurs because the dye penetrated and caused a reaction, thus forming another substance with a specific color. A second dye, called a *counterstain*, may also be applied. This will add contrasting colors in order to bring out differences between elements in cells or tissues.

Slides are placed in slotted trays and moved by hand from staining dish to staining dish with washes between, as shown in Figure 24-1. In a small laboratory, only one or two slides might be stained at a time. Automatic stainers, which are run by computer, are also available for staining a large volume of slides.

Clearing and Mounting

The purpose of *clearing* is to make the microscopic preparations transparent. Clearing chemicals should be solvent in the mounting medium, which is used next.

During *mounting*, a medium is applied and a

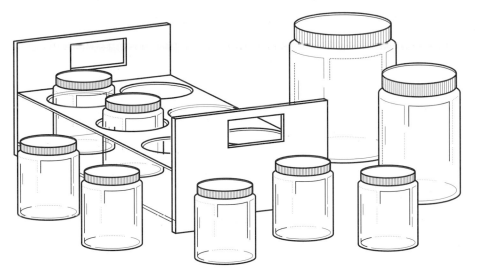

Figure 24-1
Staining jars and racks.

cover slip added. Both the mounting medium and the cover slip must be completely transparent. The mounting reagent must form a film over the tissue that is the size of the cover glass. Excess reagent is wiped away. The cover slip must be large enough to form a margin around the tissue. The slide is then allowed to dry, and the label checked for completeness.

Storing Slides

Facilities can choose their own methods for properly storing slides (Figure 24-2). They may be placed in trays, in wooden or plastic boxes, or, for long-term storage, they may be placed in metal or wooden filing cabinets. It is important to remember,

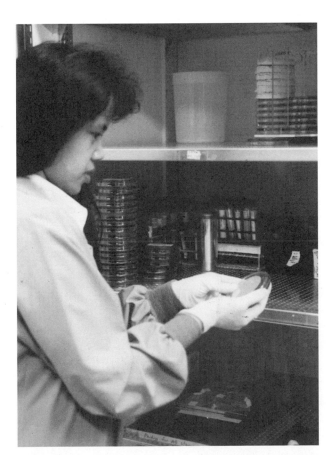

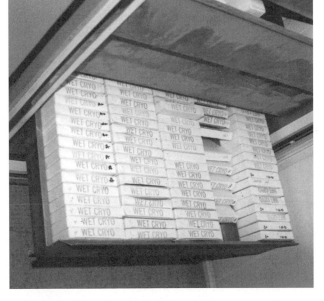

Figure 24-2
Methods of storing slides.

however, that no matter what method is employed by your facility, once a slide has been processed, it must be placed flat and in its proper numerical sequence.

Following Safety Precautions in the Histology and Cytology Lab

If you find that your responsibilities as a laboratory assistant include the testing and processing of tissues and cells in the histology or cytology laboratory, you must follow the safety precautions that are employed by all departments located within the medical laboratory. Whenever you are working with tissue or cellular specimens, the following guidelines will help you to avoid hazards and prevent accidents from occurring:

· Always put on gloves before handling body tissues and fluids.
· Make sure that all patient and tissue specimens are properly identified, and that the tissue carries the same identification number throughout the process without loss or confusion.
· Make sure that small bits of tissue are wrapped or secured while processing to prevent any potential loss of the specimen.
· Always remember to prepare ingredients carefully for reagents, dyes, and stains according to the manufacturer's directions.
· Discard solutions at the date indicated for shelflife of solutions.

· Handle all reagents carefully.
· Keep your fingers away from the knife blade whenever you are using the microtome.
· Remember to check the temperature often on water baths and the drying oven to prevent damage to tissue during processing.
· Keep the surface of the water in the tissue floating bath free of broken bits of tissue or embedding medium that could contaminate another slide.
· Never store food or drinks in the same refrigerator where tissue specimens or reagents are kept. Cross contamination can occur.
· Be certain that lids and covers are replaced on all reagents.

Summary

In this chapter, we discussed the role of histology and cytology in the medical laboratory, including the purpose and function of tissues, as well as how they are collected, recorded, and processed. We talked about the various steps involved in the testing of tissue specimens, including how they are fixed, sectioned, stained, and mounted onto a slide. We also discussed the importance of properly identifying and storing individual slides, as well as some of the general guidelines for maintaining a safe environment by practicing acceptable safety precautions.

Review Questions

1. What is the name given to the study of cells?

2. Briefly explain the process of *staining*.

3. The study of tissues is called _____ .

4. A(n) _____ is a solution used to prevent the decomposition of tissue and to preserve it.

5. _____ cells are cells that have been shed from the body, often in sheets or layers.

6. What is the name of the process by which the water content of a fresh tissue specimen is frozen in order to obtain fresh sections of it?

7. Briefly explain why it is important to keep an accurate record of a specimen entering the laboratory.

8. What does the term *embedding* mean?

9. What does the term *infiltration* mean?

10. Identify at least three safety precautions you should follow in the laboratory:

    a. _____

    b. _____

    c. _____

25

Introduction to Respiratory Therapy

Performance Objectives

Upon completion of this chapter, you will be able to:

1. Define the field of respiratory therapy.
2. Identify and discuss the various careers available in the field of respiratory therapy.
3. Discuss the educational requirements and scope of practice for a respiratory therapy practitioner and respiratory therapy assistant.
4. Identify employment opportunity and expected salary ranges available in the field of respiratory therapy.
5. Discuss the role of the respiratory therapy assistant.
6. Discuss the type of patient commonly seen by the respiratory therapy practitioner.
7. Discuss the importance of the care and maintenance of respiratory therapy equipment.

Terms and Abbreviations

AART abbreviation for the American Association for Respiratory Therapy, which is a national professional organization for respiratory therapy practitioners.

CRTT abbreviation for certified respiratory therapy technician. A CRTT has passed an NBRT credentials examination.

JCAH abbreviation for the Joint Commission for Accreditation of Hospitals. The JCAH specifies details and requirements for respiratory therapy departments in hospitals in facilities, staffing, continuing education, quality assurance, record keeping, and other areas.

JRCRTE abbreviation for the Joint Review Committee for Respiratory Therapy Education, which is the organization responsible for accrediting schools of respiratory therapy. This committee collaborates with the Committee on Allied Health Education and Accreditation of the American Medical Association in this process.

Medical Director a physician who is associated with a respiratory therapy department. This person may be a pulmonary specialist, an anesthesiologist, or other type of specialist who is interested in respiratory care. The medical director assists the department manager with implementing policies and procedures.

NBRT abbreviation for the National Board for Respiratory Therapy, which is the organization responsible for testing individuals and for providing credentials to certain practitioners in the field of respiratory therapy.

Pulmonary Function Laboratory a department within the hospital that is responsible for performing diagnostic testing for pulmonary diseases. It may be combined with the respiratory therapy department or function as a separate department.

RRT abbreviation for registered respiratory therapist. An RRT has passed the two-part NBRT credentials examination.

Technical Director the manager of the respiratory therapy department; responsible for both the clinical and the managerial functions of the department.

Respiratory therapy is a fast-paced and demanding technological and interpersonal field of study. A person considering respiratory care as a profession should be prepared for the advanced technology and sophisticated equipment used in patient care and diagnostics. Professions in respiratory therapy also require a high degree of skill development in interpersonal communications in order to provide effective patient care and education.

The respiratory therapy practitioner is an allied health specialist who works under the direction of a medical doctor or respiratory or pulmonary specialist. This person may be required to evaluate and treat patients with diseases or deficiencies of the *cardiopulmonary system* (the lungs and heart). Care provided to patients may vary from a postoperative patient requiring support until he or she recovers from anesthesia, to a premature infant showing signs of respiratory distress, or from a patient with trauma or injuries resulting from an automobile accident, to a child with pulmonary or lung complications resulting from a childhood disease such as cystic fibrosis or asthma.

As a respiratory therapy assistant, you may be required to provide assistance to patients in various states of health. Some may be outpatients who come in for education about their disease and how to administer self-care. Others may come in for diagnostic testing.

Patients may be treated intermittently, following a surgical procedure or illness, and may stay in a room on a nursing floor of a hospital. Some patients are placed in *intensive care units* (ICUs) following surgery. Other patients are critically ill or injured and require intensive care and life-support systems.

The Practice of Respiratory Care

The current practice of respiratory care encompasses all types of patients and patient care situations (Figure 25-1). It requires the therapist or assistant to have a working knowledge of the many diseases and defects that cause pulmonary problems. Therefore, in order to be successful in your career as a respiratory therapy assistant, it is important for you to become familiar with all types of diagnostic and therapeutic equipment and associated techniques. Some examples of these include the following:

- Adult and infant ventilators and patient management.
- Medical gases and administration devices.
- Humidification devices and aerosol generators and administration devices.
- Medication delivery and dosage calculation.
- Bronchopulmonary drainage.
- Airways management.
- Pulmonary rehabilitation and patient education.
- Cardiopulmonary resuscitation and all related monitoring equipment.
- Diagnostic procedures, such as arterial blood

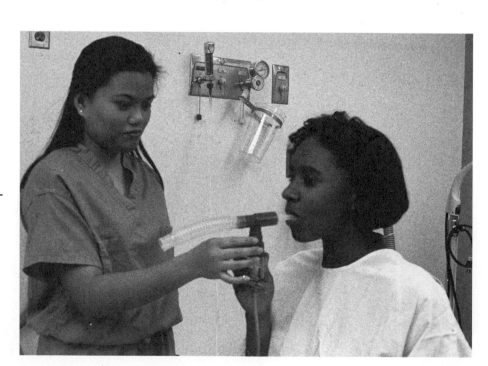

Figure 25-1
The respiratory therapy assistant.

gas, bronchoscopy, and pulmonary function techniques.

Employment and Training

Respiratory practitioners, therapists, and assistants are generally employed by hospitals in respiratory therapy departments and pulmonary function laboratories. Others may work in research, sales, and manufacturing of related equipment and for clinics and private agencies such as the American Lung Association or the American Cancer Association. A wide variety of growth and career opportunities are available, depending on the individual's interests.

Training

The field of respiratory therapy generally encompasses three levels of practitioner. These include the certified respiratory therapy technician (CRTT), the registered respiratory therapist (RRT), and the respiratory therapy assistant. The CRTT and the RRT require more advanced levels of education, and both must pass a credentials examination. The respiratory therapy assistant is not required to possess a certification or license, but must, however, be trained by a CRTT or RRT, or graduate from a formal RTA vocational training program. Both the CRTT and the RRT may work independently or under the direction of a medical doctor or specialist; however, the respiratory therapy assistant must be supervised by a licensed respiratory therapist and/or physician in the specific training or diagnostic setting.

The Respiratory Therapy Assistant

As the occupational title implies, the role of the respiratory therapy assistant is to assist the CRTT or RRT in carrying out the daily tasks related to pulmonary or respiratory care of patients. Training for the respiratory therapy assistant is generally accomplished in the vocational training classroom and usually consists of a combination of classroom study and hands-on training. In addition to learning about the various types of equipment and procedures used in the field of respiratory therapy, the assistant also receives theoretical training in basic anatomy and physiology; pharmacology, microbiology and diseases; medical terminology; patient psychology; medical ethics; administrative tasks; and personal and interpersonal techniques and adjustments to work.

As a respiratory therapy assistant, you will be required to work under the supervision of a licensed respiratory therapist and/or physician in your specific training or diagnostic setting. And many of the tasks and responsibilities you encounter may be shared with the licensed practitioner. Some of the areas in which you will receive training include working with flowmeters, general sterilization and sanitation techniques, isolation techniques, safety standards for hazardous equipment and gas cylinders, providing a safe environment for the patient and the employees, suctioning protocol for tracheostomies, mechanical ventilation assessments, medical emergency techniques, positioning and restraining patients, and procedures for keeping therapy and payment/charge records. Working under the direction of the therapist, the following is a list of tasks which you may be required to perform as part of your job responsibility:

- Escort patients to treatment rooms, or wheel equipment to patient's bedside.
- Properly answer the telephone.
- Work effectively with other employees in the department and the rest of the hospital.
- Set up, check, and maintain various types of respiratory therapy equipment.
- Administer oxygen, gases, and intermittent positive-pressure breathing (IPPB) treatments to patients.
- Practice medical ethics, be punctual and well-groomed, and avoid gossip.
- Carry out assignments skillfully and conscientiously, and provide for patient's safety.
- Clean, sterilize, store, and take inventory of equipment and supplies.
- Keep records of procedures and infection control methods.
- Follow routine respiratory therapy procedures, including oxygen therapy, aerosol therapy, IPPB, deep breathing and incentive spirometry, chest physical therapy, suctioning protocol, and mechanical ventilation assessments.
- Dissemble and clean equipment.
- Assist respiratory therapist as needed.
- Verify patient information.
- Position and explain procedures to patients.

Summary

In this chapter, we discussed the field of respiratory therapy, including the regulatory agencies responsible for setting up the standards of care in the field, as well as the different levels of education and training for the health care practitioners who work in respiratory therapy. We particularly discussed the role of the respiratory therapy assistant, outlining the various tasks and responsibilities of this person as related to working in the field of respiratory therapy.

216

Your Career in

Review Questions

1. What is the name of the organization responsible for testing individuals for certification in the field of respiratory therapy?

2. What is the name of the organization responsible for accrediting schools of respiratory therapy?

3. What does the abbreviation *CRTT* mean?

4. What does the abbreviation *RRT* mean?

5. Briefly explain the role of the Joint Commission for Accreditation of Hospitals as it relates to function of the respiratory therapy department.

6. What is the difference between the *Medical Director* and the *Technical Director* in the respiratory therapy department?

7. What do the following abbreviations mean:

   a. ICU _____

   b. CCU _____

8. List at least three functions of the respiratory therapy department:

   a. _____

   b. _____

   c. _____

9. List at least three functions of the respiratory therapy assistant:

   a. _____

   b. _____

   c. _____

10. Identify at least two places a respiratory therapy assistant may receive his or her training:

   a. _____

   b. _____

Respiratory Therapy Equipment

26

Performance Objectives

Upon completion of this chapter, you will be able to:

1. Identify the appropriate cleaning and sterilization area for a respiratory therapy department.
2. Discuss how to clean respiratory therapy equipment.
3. Define the term *sterilization.*
4. State the purpose of sterilizing respiratory therapy equipment.
5. Identify and discuss methods of sterilizing respiratory therapy equipment.
6. Explain the appropriate procedure to follow in case of an equipment failure.

Terms

Aseptic   free from disease-producing microorganisms.

Cleaning process   the use of a detergent.

Cold sterilization   the removal of all microorganisms by submerging an item into a liquid chemical agent capable of killing the microorganisms.

Disinfect   the process used to destroy all harmful or pathogenic microorganisms.

Gas sterilization   the use of ethylene oxide gas in a special cabinet in which humidity, gas concentration, temperature, and length of exposure are calculated in order to sterilize an item. The process is very effective in sterilizing heat-sensitive items.

Immersion   completely covering an item with a fluid.

Isolation   a procedure used to prevent the spread of microorgan-

isms; it protects employees and visitors from contracting disease through the use of barriers such as gowns, masks, and gloves. *Reverse isolation* is used to protect the patient from employees and visitors when he or she has weakened defenses.

Microorganism   any microscopic organisms such as bacteria, virus, or protozoa.

Pathogen   any microorganism that can cause disease.

Steam autoclave   sterilization equipment that uses hot steam under high pressure.

Sterilization   the process used to remove all living microorganisms.

M icroorganisms can multiply rapidly in a warm, wet environment. Since organisms that thrive in this type of environment may be *pathogenic*, or disease-producing, the assistant must take great care in cleaning, sterilizing, and packaging equipment. All of these processes should be monitored in the most effective manner possible.

All equipment must first be cleaned. Then, following a rinse, the equipment may be sterilized in any one of several ways.

Sterilization

Sterilization is defined as removal of all living microorganisms. Respiratory therapy equipment is exposed to patients' exhaled air that contains respiratory pathogens and organisms that grow in the mouth. Often equipment is filled with fluid and heated.

There is more than one method of sterilizing respiratory therapy equipment. The one chosen will depend greatly on the needs of the respiratory therapy

217

department, its capabilities, and procedures. It may be a single method or a combination of two or more methods. The three most common methods include cold sterilization, ethylene oxide gas sterilization, and steam autoclaving.

Cold Sterilization

Cold sterilization involves immersing items in liquid chemicals in order to kill all existing microorganisms. *Gluteraldehyde* in a 2% aqueous solution is generally the most common liquid chemical sterilizing agent used in the respiratory therapy department. For a sterilizing agent to be most effective, exact concentrations and contact times must be used. To avoid recontamination, great care should also be taken with rinsing, drying, and packaging.

If an agent is used for a shorter time or in a more diluted concentration, it is considered a disinfectant. A *disinfectant* is an agent that destroys all harmful or disease-producing microorganisms. It is used after the removal of all organic materials from the items to be disinfected or sterilized. The items are then submerged in the liquid chemical for a set time period. The items are then removed, rinsed, dried, and packaged.

Agents used in cold sterilization are very irritable to the skin. Therefore, anyone using them should always wear gloves and follow the manufacturer's recommendations for length of contact for sterilization and disinfection should be followed exactly.

Ethylene Oxide Gas Sterilization

A second commonly used sterilization method for respiratory therapy equipment is the use of ethylene oxide. Ethylene oxide gas is widely used for sterilizing all heat-sensitive items. This is very important in respiratory therapy because of the great use of plastic materials in the manufacture of equipment. Sterilization takes place in a special cabinet in which the temperature (49 to 60°C), humidity (50%), length of exposure (time), and concentration of ethylene oxide gas is controlled. Sterilization should be performed strictly according to the manufacturer's instructions, since ethylene oxide residue is toxic to human tissues.

Steam Autoclave

Steam sterilization is not widely used for respiratory therapy equipment. Since much of the equipment is made of plastic, it cannot withstand high temperatures (121°C). The steam autoclave is a special chamber in which all the air can be exhausted. Then the air is gradually replaced by steam at a high pressure. The sterilizing time is usually short and the process is very effective. But because most rubber and plastics products are distorted by the heat, the steam autoclave is usually not used for most respiratory therapy equipment. Monitoring strips innoculated with bacteria are run in both gas sterilizers and steam autoclaves in order to check the effectiveness of the sterilizing process.

Respiratory therapy uses liquid reservoirs to deliver medication; aerosol; or warm, humidified air to patients. Because of the warm temperature and liquid, these reservoirs may favor the growth of bacteria, such as the gram-negative rods *Pseudomonas*.

To prevent the growth and spread of organisms in respiratory therapy equipment, the assistant should follow specific guidelines, including

1. Carefully handling patient equipment only after washing the hands thoroughly.
2. After equipment is used, rinsing it free of any unused medication before storing it in the patient's room.
3. When refilling any larger reservoir, all the unused fluid should be discarded before refilling with fresh fluid.
4. Using an ongoing program for monitoring equipment, so that it can be checked for growth of microorganisms.
5. Checking all respiratory therapy equipment on a regular basis, especially high-risk equipment such as nebulizers and life-support equipment, and replacing it on an established time schedule.

Equipment repair is generally assigned to a specific person within the department. Everyone setting up or placing equipment in use, however, is responsible for checking it to see that it functions adequately before it is used on a patient. Any broken or malfunctioning equipment should be distinctly marked as to the problem encountered and then directed to the repair department. All electrical equipment is safety-tested by the repair department for electrical leakage, But with each use, the cord and plug should be examined for loosening and wear.

Even with adequate repair and testing procedures, equipment failure will sometimes occur. In the event that a failure does occur, the patient should be cared for first. In other words, if the life-support equipment fails, such as the ventilator, the patient's uninterrupted mechanical ventilation with a resuscitation bag or another ventilator should be ensured before troubleshooting the equipment failure.

If the patient is receiving oxygen, the oxygen delivery device should be adequately replaced before trying to troubleshoot the broken equipment.

Remember, always provide uninterrupted support for the patient before doing anything else. After that, the equipment should be repaired or removed from use and marked as to the problem encountered.

Because respiratory therapy is a highly technological field, equipment maintenance is an important aspect of the work, and it is a responsibility shared by all members of the respiratory therapy department. Equipment maintenance is divided into two separate categories: cleaning and sterilization and equipment checkout and repair.

Cleaning and Sterilization

First, you will need to understand the layout of the cleaning and sterilization and equipment storage areas of the respiratory therapy department. There should be a distinct separation between the "dirty" area, where used equipment is received, sorted, and cleaned, and the "clean" area, where the sterilized equipment is packaged and stored. Widespread use of disposable equipment has decreased the amount

of processing in these areas, but many items are still cleaned and sterilized in the respiratory therapy department.

In most hospitals, respiratory therapy equipment is received at a door or window used only for the return of used equipment. All disposables are discarded into their smallest parts, and these parts are then submerged in a detergent solution and cleaned in order to ensure the removal of all organic material.

Summary

In this chapter, we discussed how respiratory therapy equiment is maintained, particularly as it relates to removal of microorganisms by sterilization. In our discussion, we talked about various types of sterilization methods, including cold sterilization, gas sterilization, and autoclaving.

Review Questions

1. What does the term *aseptic* mean?

2. A(n) _____ is any microorganism that can cause disease.

3. _____ _____ involves the use of ethylene oxide gas as part of its process in sterilizing items.

4. Sterilization of items using hot steam under high pressure is called _____.

5. What is the name of the procedure used to prevent the spread of microorganisms by protecting both the employees and the visitors from contracting the disease?

6. _____ _____ is the process of immersing items in liquid chemicals in order to kill all existing microorganisms.

7. What are the two categories that all respiratory therapy equipment maintenance must fall under?

   a. _____

   b. _____

Administration of Medical Gases, Humidity, and Aerosol Therapy

Performance Objectives

Upon completion of this chapter, you will be able to:

1. Describe the regulations regarding manufacture, transport, testing, and storage of medical gas cylinders.

2. Discuss cylinder usage, with regard to the identification, handling, transport, sizes, safety systems and use in patient areas.

3. Explain the operation of pressure-regulating devices and flow-regulating devices.

4. Discuss and demonstrate how to calculate use time for an E cylinder and an H cylinder.

5. Discuss oxygen as a drug and how it is manufactured, and explain how oxygen toxicity and retrolental fibroplasia occur.

6. Describe two types of bulk oxygen systems.

7. Identify, describe, and explain the most commonly used oxygen delivery devices.

8. Explain oxygen analysis and identify and discuss two types of oxygen analyzers.

9. Explain when to use humidity therapy.

10. Describe the relationship between absolute humidity, temperature, potential humidity, and relative humidity.

11. Define humidity deficit.

12. Identify and describe commonly used humidification devices.

13. List the indications for aerosol therapy, and briefly discuss the hazards of using aerosol therapy.

14. Describe the following types of aerosol generators: jet nebulizer, ultrasonic nebulizer, and hydrosphere nebulizer.

15. Discuss the following aerosol delivery devices: enclosure, mask, face tent, and Briggs T.

16. Discuss the delivery of oxygen with aerosols.

Terms and Abbreviations

Absolute humidity   the actual amount or weight of water contained in a given volume of gas.
Aerosol   particles suspended in a gas; in respiratory therapy, refers to liquid particles suspended in air or in an oxygen mixture.
Color code   a scheme that uses colors to identify cylinder contents. For example, oxygen is shown as green or white (international).
Flowmeter   a device that measures and meters the flow of gases from a 50-psi source.

220

Humidifier a device used to add water vapor to a dry gas for delivery to a patient.

Hydrostatic testing testing a cylinder by submerging it in water and increasing pressure to 3000 psi. This measures the elastic expansion of the cylinder to determine if it should remain in use.

Nebulizer a device used to generate an aerosol that either is bland (water or saline) or contains a medication.

Oxygen analyzer a device used to measure oxygen concentration.

Oxygen toxicity a lung disorder caused by breathing high concentrations of oxygen.

Potential humidity the maximum amount of water vapor that can be contained in a volume of gas at a given temperature.

Pressure regulator a device used to reduce cylinder pressure (2200 psi) to working pressure (50 psi).

psig pounds-per-square-inch gauge; used to measure pressure.

Relative humidity the ratio of absolute humidity to potential humidity times 100, expressed as percent.

Retrolental fibroplasia varying degrees of blindness in infants, presumably caused by a high PaO_2.

Safety connection systems the pin index (for D and E cylinders), and American Standard (for large cylinders). These systems prevent the use of the wrong gas with a piece of equipment designed for another gas.

As a respiratory therapy assistant, your responsibilities include becoming familiar with the various types of materials, equipment, and procedures used in the respiratory therapy department. You should make every effort to observe both the respiratory therapist and the physician as they use certain equipment and machinery, administer medical gases, and even perform diagnostic tests and surgical procedures on patients. Whether or not you actually participate in any of these procedures is strictly a matter of policy and specific rules, as set forth by the hospital, clinic, or other diagnostic setting in which you are employed.

Administration of Medical Gases

Use of Cylinders

One of the most important tasks of a respiratory therapist is to administer medical gases. This includes the administration of oxygen, compressed air, and some gas mixtures such as helium and oxygen and carbon dioxide and oxygen. Cylinder gases are also used in the pulmonary laboratory as *calibration gases* for various types of equipment, such as blood gas analyzers. It is necessary to transport and connect cylinder oxygen systems such as those used in most major hospitals. Therefore, it is important for a respiratory therapy assistant to know about all aspects of these devices.

The Department of Transportation (DOT) is the government agency that regulates the manufacture, testing, transportation, and marking of medical gas cylinders in the United States. These cylinders are manufactured from a special seamless steel called chromemolybdenum steel.

A method called *hydrostatic testing* is used to test cylinders for wall thickness and strength by measuring elastic expansion. This is accomplished by first submerging the cylinder into water, and then pressurizing it to about 3000 psi (for a cylinder normally filled to 2200 psi). After the pressure is relieved, the amount of elastic expansion is measured. If it exceeds the DOT requirements, the cylinder cannot be used.

Government Regulations and Cylinders

The regulations for storage of cylinders and for maintenance of bulk oxygen systems are established by the *National Fire Prevention Association (NFPA)*. Some of the regulations for storage of cylinders are:

· Separating storage areas for flammable gases and those such as oxygen that support combustion.
· Providing storage areas that are located on an outside wall and have at least a 1-hour fire resistance rating.
· Providing storage areas that cannot be used for anything except cylinder storage.
· Providing for storage areas that separate full and empty cylinders and that have retainers to keep cylinders from falling over.

Color-Coding System

To help determine the contents of medical gas cylinders, the government established a color-code system that has been accepted throughout the world. Chemicals are coded as follows:

· Oxygen—green or white.
· Air—yellow or black.
· Helium/oxygen—brown and green.
· Carbon dioxide/oxygen—gray and green.

· Nitrous oxide—blue.
· Cyclopropane—orange.
· Helium—brown.

Although using a color coding system is a good way to make sure that the appropriate gas cylinder is used, it is not always a foolproof system. Therefore, before using a cylinder for gas, even though it has been identified by color, the respiratory therapy assistant should always make sure that the label has been checked. You must read the label to determine the true contents of the cylinder.

Size and Safety

Commonly used medical gas cylinders generally come in three sizes: small, medium, and large. Although all three cylinders are filled with 2200 psi, each contains a different amount of cubic footage, thereby making its capacity to hold gas, different. Small cylinders, which contain approximately 22 ft^3, hold about 622 L of oxygen. Larger, or G cylinders, contain about 187 ft^3, or 5260 L of oxygen. Large, or H, cylinders contain about 244 ft^3 or 6900 L of oxygen.

Cylinder valves employ two types of safety systems. The first, a valve relief system, is used to vent excess pressure to the atmosphere. The other, known as a safety connection system, prevents the connection of the wrong equipment to the cylinder.

Types of Valve Relief and Safety Connection Systems

There are different types of valve relief and safety systems used in gas cylinders. The two types of valve relief systems are called a *frangible disc* and a *fusible plug*. The frangible disc is a metal disc usually made of copper that bursts when exposed to a pressure of 3000 psi. The fusible plug is a safety relief device that melts at a temperature of above 150°F.

The two types of safety connection systems found on most cylinder valves are the *American Standard Compressed Gas Cylinder Outlet and Inlet Connection System* and the *Pin Index Safety System*. The American Standard Compressed Gas Cylinder Outlet and Inlet Connection System is a threaded connection system used with equipment operating at pressures in excess of 20 psi. It is generally used with large cylinders (G and H) in order to prevent accidental connection of administering equipment to the wrong gas cylinder. The Pin Index Safety System is always used on D and E cylinders or the small cylinders. Specific pin hole placements on the cylinder valve have corresponding pins on the yoke of the reg-

ulator. These are also used to prevent accidental connection of equipment to the wrong cylinder.

Steps for Properly Using a Cylinder in a Patient's Room

No matter which cylinder is used to administer medical gases, there are basic steps that the respiratory therapy assistant must take prior to administering the gas. These include the following:

1. Always make sure that the cylinder is taken from the storage area with the cylinder cap in place. It should be moved and secured on a cylinder cart.
2. While outside the patient's room, always make sure you remove the cylinder cap first, and then *crack* the cylinder valve. Cracking the valve means you must open it slightly and then quickly, in order to blow out any debris in the valve opening.
3. The regulator, which is a pressure-reducing device, is then applied, and the cylinder is secured, or placed in a ring stand or cart in order to keep it in an upright position in the patient's room or other area of use. This is an important safety consideration.
4. The final step is to connect the administration device to the cylinder regulator.

Cylinder Pressure Regulator

The cylinder pressure regulator, or pressure-regulating device, is used to decrease the cylinder pressure to a working pressure of 50 psi. A *single-stage regulator*, the type most commonly used in the respiratory therapy department, works in the following way (Figure 27-1):

1. Gas enters the regulator through the nozzle and into the upper chamber of the regulator.
2. When the gas pressure in the upper chamber reaches 50 psi, the diaphragm is moved down; this closes off the nozzle so that no more gas is able to flow into the regulator.
3. Therefore, the gas leaving the regulator is stabilized at 50 psi.

Flow-Regulating Devices

In order to function properly, some respiratory therapy equipment may require the use of *flow-regulating devices*. The two most commonly used flow-regulating devices, or flowmeters, are the *Bourdon flowmeter* and the *Thorpe tube flowmeter* (Figure 27-2). Bourdon flowmeters are often used for patient transportation, since they can be used in any position. These devices measure pressure but read flow.

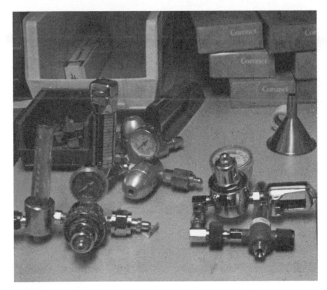

Figure 27-1
Pressure regulator.

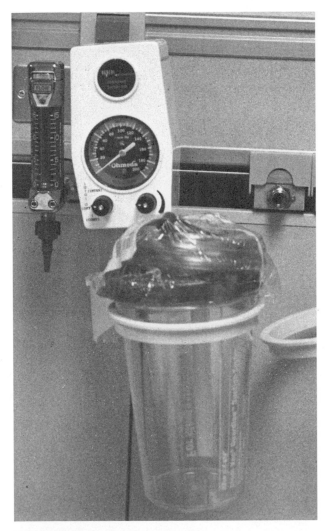

Figure 27-2
Thorpe tube flowmeter.

Because of this, any restriction to outflow causes an increase in back pressure and in the gauge reading. Therefore, this type of device may read inaccurately high when used with equipment attached to the outflow device.

There are two types of Thorpe tube flowmeters most often used by the members of the respiratory therapy department. The first, called the *nonpressure compensated flowmeter*, is rarely seen in the clinical setting today, since they are no longer being manufactured. Although some are still available in research and laboratory areas, this type of flowmeter is hardly ever used with patients because of its tendency to indicate a lower flow rate than is actually being delivered when it is used in conjunction with equipment attached to the outflow device.

A pressure-compensated Thorpe tube flowmeter uses calibration in its operation. The opening is adjusted, or calibrated, to 50 psi, rather than to atmospheric pressure. The valve that turns the flow on is located between the gas outlet and the indicator float. For the flowmeter to show an inaccurate flow, the back pressure would have to exceed wall-line pressure. Wall-line pressure refers to the pressure in the piped-in oxygen system in the hospital.

Calculating Use Time

In order to understand how long a cylinder can be used before it should be changed, you must first be able to calculate the *use time* for the remaining cylinder contents at the current rate of use. This can easily be done by using a factor for each cylinder size.

For an E cylinder, the factor is 0.28 L leaving the cylinder for each psi drop in pressure. For an H cylinder, the factor is 3.14 L leaving the cylinder for each psi drop in pressure.

An H cylinder contains 1500 psi on the gauge. Keeping that figure in mind, how long will it last if it is being used at the rate of 10 L/min? In order to solve that question, let's look at the following equation:

$$\frac{1,500 \times 3.14}{10} = \frac{471 \text{ min}}{60} = 7.85 \text{ h}$$

An E cylinder shows 2000 psi on the gauge. It is being used at a flow rate of 3 L/min. How long will it last?

$$\frac{2,000 \times .8}{3} = \frac{186 \text{ min}}{60} = 3.1 \text{ h}$$

The cylinder will be changed at a pressure of 500 psig since below that pressure the pressure gauge may not be accurate. Therefore, before you can begin your calculation, you must first subtract the 500 from the psi reading:

$$\frac{1,000 \times 3.14}{10} = \frac{314 \min}{60} = 5.23 \, h$$

$$\frac{1,500 \times .28}{3} = \frac{140 \min}{60} = 2.33 \, h$$

Administration of Oxygen

Oxygen is a drug that must be measured and delivered carefully and monitored often. As with other drugs, when properly administered, oxygen can help people live through disastrous illnesses. But it can also cause dramatic and devastating side effects. A high-inspired oxygen tension, for example, can cause lung disease similar to the adult respiratory distress syndrome (ARDS). It can also damage the alveoli and the capillary membranes in the lungs, as well as cause *interstitial edema*, or excessive fluid in the tissues. In the late stages, excessive administration of oxygen, can also cause scarring of the lung itself.

Oxygen administration in infants may result in both lung disease and in disorders of the eye. This problem occurs most often in premature infants. When the immature arterial system of the infant's eye is exposed to higher than normal PaO_2 for a prolonged period of time, retinal vasoconstriction may occur. This can cause varying degrees of blindness, thus resulting in a condition called *retrolental fibroplasia*, or retinopathy of prematurity.

Oxygen is manufactured by a complex commercial process called *fractional distillation* that takes advantage of differences in the boiling points of oxygen and nitrogen. Other gases contained in air have lower boiling points than oxygen and will evaporate and leave pure oxygen behind.

Oxygen Systems in the Hospital

Bulk oxygen systems are used in hospitals in order to provide them with large supplies of oxygen. This oxygen, which is ready for use with a flowmeter, is piped into individual hospital rooms at 50 psi. This method of "piping in" the oxygen is accomplished by yoking together many large cylinders or by using a liquid oxygen reservoir piping system.

There are five delivery devices commonly used by hospitals for administrering oxygen to patients. These include the cannula, the simple oxygen mask, the nonrebreathing mask with reservoir bag, the partial rebreathing mask, and the Venturi mask (Figure 27-3).

An oxygen cannula, sometimes called nasal prongs, has one prong that fits into each naris on a plastic tube. The tube, which fits around the ears, is easily acceptable for use by the patient, because it is comfortable and well tolerated. It also allows the patient the ability to eat, talk, and go on about his or her regular routine without any disruption from the influx of oxygen. A cannula provides the patient with an oxygen concentration of between 22% and 50%, at flow rates of between 0.5 and 6 to 8 L/min. The amount of oxygen actually received by the patient using the cannula will depend upon the rate and depth of ventilation because of the air drawn in when the patient breathes.

The simple oxygen mask allows for the delivery of approximately 35% to 55% oxygen at flow rates of 6 to 10 L/min. The final concentration depends on the amount of air drawn in by the patient. A major drawback of the mask is that it is sometimes very uncomfortable to the patient, thereby causing great frustration and interruption of the flow of oxygen during routine tasks, such as eating and talking.

A nonrebreathing mask with a reservoir bag is generally used to deliver high oxygen concentrations. It requires a fairly tight-fitting mask, and oxygen therapy must be interrupted for such tasks as suctioning or eating. As much as 70% to 90% oxygen can be delivered with a tight-fitting mask.

The partial rebreathing mask consists of a face mask to which a reservoir bag has been added. Oxygen is directed into the reservoir. When the patient inhales, oxygen from the reservoir is used, and atmospheric air can then enter the mask by way of the exhalation ports. At expiration, about one-third of the exhaled air enters the bag and is inhaled in the next breath. A 60% concentration of oxygen can be delivered by using a partial rebreathing mask.

The final method used for administering oxygen to the patient is through a device called a Venturi, or air entrainment, mask. The major advantage of this device is that it is able to deliver an exact oxygen concentration at a high enough flow rate so that the patient will not drawn in room air. These masks can deliver 24%, 28%, 31%, 35%, 40%, and 50% oxygen. This type of mask also guarantees that the patient will never receive more than the ordered concentration. A Venturi mask uses a jet principle, that is, oxygen is delivered through a nipple with a restricted orifice, or opening. When the oxygen goes through the opening, the pressure on the sides of the gas flow is decreased, and thus room air is entrained, or drawn in. The Venturi mask is designed so that an exact oxygen concentration results.

Since in the respiratory therapy setting oxygen is considered a drug that must be continuously monitored, the process of *oxygen analysis* is used, It is an

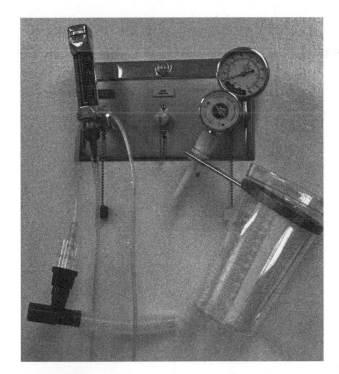

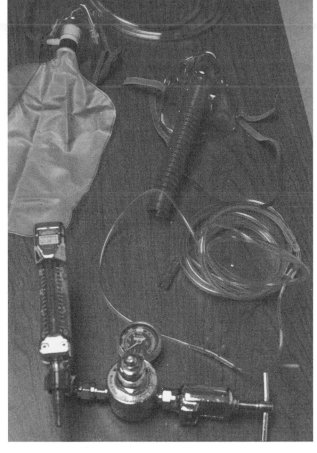

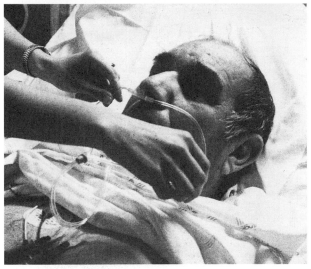

Figure 27-3
Oxygen delivery devices.

important part of respiratory therapy. There are three basic types of oxygen analyzers, the two most common types, the physical analyzers and the electrical analyzers, and the least used electrochemical analyzers.

A physical analyzer uses the *Pauling principle*. One type is called the Beckman D-2. In this analyzer, a glass dumbell filled with nitrogen is suspended on a quartz fiber in a magnetic field. Since one characteristic of oxygen is its ability to alter a magnetic field, when the oxygen enters, the dumbbell rotates, thus reflecting a light onto a scale.

The electrical analyzer uses the principle of *thermal conductivity*. It has a Wheatstone bridge that compares the resistance to current flow through a reference wire and a simple wire that is cooled when exposed to oxygen and conducts more current. One example of an electrical analyzer is the MIRA.

Electrochemical analyzers, which are the least used by most respiratory therapy departments, include two types: the *galvanic fuel cell* and the *polarographic analyzer*. Both of these operate similarly. Oxygen enters the electrode of the analyzers, and through a chemical reaction, electrons are released.

Humidity and Aerosol Therapy

When you are required to deliver medical gases that are *anhydrous*, that is, contain no water, they must be humidified before they can be delivered to the patient. This process is generally accomplished in one of two ways: either with a humidifier, which adds water vapor to the gas, or with a nebulizer, which generates an aerosol. Any time medical gases are administered, they should, with very few exceptions, be humidified in the same manner.

Humidity

Humidity is defined as the amount of moisture in the air or the water vapor content of the air. *Absolute humidity* refers to the actual amount or weight of water contained in a given volume of gas. It is usually expressed as milligrams of water per liter of gas.

Relative humidity (RH) refers to the ratio of absolute humidity to potential humidity times 100. This is expressed as a percentage. *Potential humidity* is the maximum amount of water vapor that can be contained in a gas at a given temperature.

The amount of water that can be contained in a gas, its saturation, depends upon the temperature of the gas. At higher temperatures, gas can hold more water vapor, and at lower temperatures, gas can hold less water vapor.

Since relative humidity can be calculated by using the actual weight of water vapor in milligrams per liter (mg/L) or the partial pressure of water vapor in mm Hg, you must first learn the formula for calculating it. That formula is RH = Absolute humidity divided by potential humidity multiplied by 100. Remember, the same measurement must be used for both absolute humidity and potential humidity to perform the calculations.

Types of Humidifiers

There are two basic types of humidifiers commonly used in hospitals. They are the bubble humidifier and the cascade-type humidifier (Figure 27-4).

The bubble humidifier may be a disposable type or a permanent piece of respiratory therapy equipment. In this type of humidifier, oxygen passes under the water, usually through a diffuser that breaks the gas into very small bubbles. It picks up water as it passes to the surface and out of the humidifier. Some examples of this type of humidifier include the Ohio, Puritan, Bubble/Jet (permanent), McGaw, and Inspiron (disposables). Some of these can be heated to increase their humidity output.

Cascade-type humidifiers are heated and used routinely as the humidifiers on ventilator system cir-

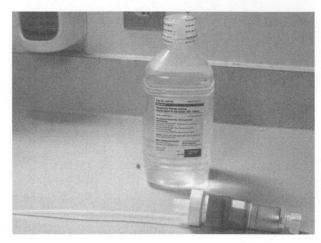

Figure 27-4
Bubble humidifier and Cascade-type humidifier.

cuits. The ventilator outflow is forced under the water. Because of a special grid in the humidifier, there is more of a mixing or cascade effect between the gas and the water. This agitation, along with the heat, increases the humidity output to 100% relative humidity. Examples of cascade-type humidifiers include the Bennett Cascade and Bourns, both of which are nondisposable.

Aerosols

An *aerosol* is a suspension of particles in a gas. Therapeutic aerosols are suspensions of water, normal saline, or medications in a gas such as oxygen, compressed air, or an oxygen-air mixture. Aerosol therapy is used when there is a need to add water to the respiratory tract and when assistance is needed in the delivery of oxygen.

When aerosol therapy is delivered to the patient, there are some hazards that you must be aware of. These include the possibility of overhydration, swelling of mucous membranes, bronchospasm, and transport of microorganisms, which may ultimately cause contamination of the equipment.

Nebulizers

As we have previously discussed, aerosol therapy is generated through a piece of equipment called a *nebulizer*. There are three basic types of aerosol nebulizers: jet nebulizers, ultrasonic nebulizers, and hydrosphere nubulizers.

Jet nebulizers operate using the *Bernoulli principle,* which states briefly that as the velocity of a gas stream increases, the pressure perpendicular to the gas stream decreases. Oxygen is forced through the inlet tube. The pressure at the top of the siphon tube is decreased so that fluid is drawn up through the tube and into the gas stream. The liquid is then broken down into smaller particles by impacting the baffle and then is finally carried out of the nebulizer.

The *ultrasonic nebulizer* uses high-frequency sound waves in order to produce an aerosol. Energy is applied to a ceramic disc that changes one type of energy to another through vibration. Thus, the liquid is broken into small particles.

In the *hydrosphere nebulizer*, a thin film of liquid is spread over a hollow glass sphere. The nebulizer has a small orifice that is placed in the midportion of the sphere, and a baffle placed just in front of it. The gas is able to escape through the orifice and eventually breaks the film of liquid, producing an aerosol.

Summary

In this chapter, we discussed how medical gases are administered, including how they must be regulated by law. We also talked in depth about gas cylinders, including the various types of cylinders currently in use by most respiratory therapy departments, the steps for properly using them in patient's rooms, and the different types of regulators and devices made for administration of medical gases to patients. Additionally, we talked about the administration of oxygen in patient's rooms, and its administration by way of humidifiers, aerosol therapy, and nebulizers.

Review Questions

1. The actual amount or weight of water contained in a given volume of gas is called:

   a. absolute humidity

   b. relative humidity

   c. potential humidity

2. The maximum amount of water vapor that can be contained in a volume of gas at a given temperature is called:

   a. absolute humidity

   b. relative humidity

   c. potential humidity

3. A(n) _____ is a device that is used to measure and meter the flow of gases from a 50-psi source.

4. A(n) _____ is a device used to generate an aerosol that either is bland or contains a medication.

5. A lung disorder caused by breathing high concentrations of oxygen is called:

   a. pneumonia

   b. atalectasis

   c. oxygen toxicity

6. What is the name of the instrument used to measure oxygen concentration?

7. What is the name of the disease seen in infants, which often causes varying degrees of blindness, presumably because of a high PaO_2 concentration?

8. What is the name of the device used to add water vapor to a dry gas for the delivery of a patient?

9. Briefly explain how a color-coding system is used in delivering respiratory therapy.

10. What is the purpose of a safety connection system?

28

Intermittent Pulmonary Therapy

Performance Objectives

Upon completion of this chapter, you will be able to:

1. Define intermittent positive-pressure breathing (IPPB), and discuss why it is used.
2. Identify the hazards of using IPPB.
3. Describe the delivery of IPPB treatments and how the patient should be educated in their use.
4. Discuss the mechanical devices used to deliver IPPB treatments, including the Bird Mark-7, the Bennett PR-2, and the Bennett AP-5.
5. Define incentive spirometry and identify the indications for its use.
6. Discuss how incentive spirometry is delivered to the patient.
7. Identify mechanical devices used to deliver incentive spirometry.
8. Define chest physical therapy (CPT) and list the indications for its use.
9. Discuss the hazards of CPT.
10. Identify postural drainage positions.
11. Discuss mechanical and manual percussion.
12. Identify and discuss the techniques of vibration, segmental resistance, tussive squeeze, breathing exercises, pursed lip breathing, graded exercise and breathing control, and assisted breathing during CPT.

Terms and Abbreviations

Apnea   the absence of respiration.
CPT   abbreviation for chest physical therapy; pertains to the use of positioning and clapping and vibrating the chest in order to remove secretions.
Gastric insufflation   the distention of the stomach with air.
Hemoptysis   the coughing up of frank (bright red) blood from the lungs.
Incentive spirometry   process of using a mechanical device to encourage and coach a patient to take slow, deep breaths.
IPPB   abbreviation for intermittent positive-pressure breathing; pertains to the delivery of a series of positive pressure (above

atmospheric pressure) inhalations, which inflates the lungs and thereby allows passive exhalation.
Patient application or adjunct   the delivery device used for IPPB, such as a mouthpiece or a mask.
Percussion   the clapping of the chest wall in order to set up a vibration necessary to help remove mucus from the airways.
Pneumothorax   the condition in which air is in the pleural space, causing a collapsed lung.
Postural drainage   positioning a patient so that gravity can assist in the drainage of secretions.

Intermittent positive-pressure breathing, or IPPB, is a method used to assist the patient in his or her breathing. It is a process that involves delivering a series of positive-pressure inhalations to the patient through a device that has been connected to a mask, a mouthpiece, or an endotracheal adapter. This inflates the lungs, thereby allowing passive exhalation to the atmosphere when pressure is released.

IPPB can be used for a number of purposes, such as hyperinflation of the lungs, decreasing the workload of a patient's breathing, and delivery of aerosolized medications. No matter what reason for delivery of this type of treatment, as a health care professional, you should always remember that any effective therapy is dependent on both your skill as a respiratory therapy assistant and how well your patient has been taught the procedure. If the patient is relaxed and knowledgeable about how the therapy works, IPPB can be very beneficial.

Any time a new patient is to receive IPPB treatments, it is important to first thoroughly explain the procedure. Following the explanation, the patient can be oriented to the equipment. If at all possible, try to assist the patient into a comfortable sitting position, either in bed, on the side of the bed, or in a chair.

Procedure for Delivering IPPB Treatments

IPPB treatments involve a process which, when delivered properly, provides for slow, deep breaths with a pause before exhaling. The procedure, as well as the results, should always be monitored for patient effectiveness and tolerance. For maximum benefit, it is important to "coach" the patient on every part of the maneuver.

Prior to delivering the treatment to the patient, it is important that you spend a few minutes explaining how the IPPB machine works. Patients who have an understanding of how the machine works generally reap greater benefits from the treatment.

The correct procedure for using the IPPB machine is as follows:

1. Place the mouthpiece in your mouth, on top of your tongue.
2. Sip on the mouthpiece in order to start the flow of air from the machine; then relax.
3. Apply a nose clip or pinch the nose closed, if necessary.
4. Seal your mouth tightly around the mouthpiece.
5. Allow the machine to fill the lungs with air. It will stop by itself when the lungs are filled.
6. When the machine stops, try to hold your breath for a couple of seconds. This allows the medication to adhere to your lungs so that it will not be exhaled. Then exhale very slowly.
7. Begin the process again.

Mechanical Devices Used to Deliver IPPB Treatments

Depending on the physician's order, there are several different types of mechanical devices that can be used to deliver IPPB treatments. The most commonly used devices include the *Bird Mark-7*, the *Bennet PR-2*, and the *Bennett AP-5* (Figure 28-1).

The Bird Mark-7 is generally used for IPPB treatments in which an emergency has occurred; however, it may also be used to support a patient's breathing for a longer period of time. In this machine, the pressure that builds in the patient-respirator system and the flow rate of the machine interact to determine the amount of tidal volume the patient will receive. The air mixture allows the respiratory therapy practitioner to choose a mixture of oxygen and air. If the machine is powered by compressed air, it will only deliver compressed air. In an emergency situation, the expiratory time for apnea, that is, absence of breathing, allows you to set a rate for a patient who is not breathing.

The two types of Bennet IPPB machines, the Bennett PR-2 and the Bennett AP-5, are also devices that can be used to deliver IPPB treatments. The PR-2, when equipped with a humidifier, may be used at times for continuous ventilatory support.

The Bennett AP-5 is one of the most commonly used IPPB devices. It is powered by electricity, rather than by gas. It makes home therapy easier and does not require the use of cylinder gas.

Incentive Spirometry

Incentive spirometry is a method of using coaching, encouragement, and/or a mechanical device (incentive) in order to get the patient to take slow, deep breaths with no assistance, such as from an IPPB, and to cough. Many devices are used to help patients accomplish these tasks, or goals. Some are disposable items, while others are nondisposable. The *Marion Spirocare*, an electronic device that converts flow to a volume measure, is most commonly used for incentive spirometry. The Spirocare has lights that reflect various volumes. When the patient reaches his or her goal set, a clown lights up at the top of the machine and stays lit for 1 second. This is the time in which

230

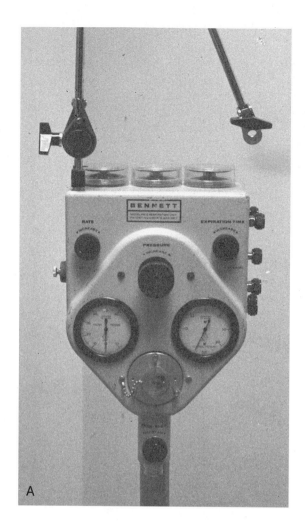

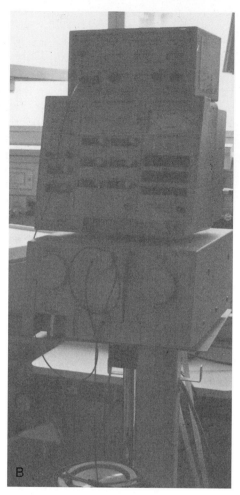

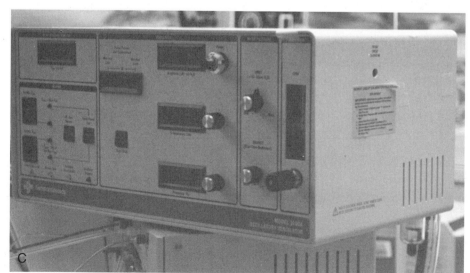

Figure 28-1
Bird Mark-7 (A), Bennett AP-2 (B), Bennett AP-5 (C).

you should be encouraging the patient to hold his or her breath.

Disposable spirometry devices are usually plastic and include items such as a Ping-Pong ball held suspended in a tube or a small bellows that can be filled with air.

Incentive spirometry has one main purpose: to get the patient to take slow, deep breaths and hold each breath at the top of inspiration. Doing this allows inflation of all areas of the lungs and improved distribution of air in the lungs. It also gets the patient to cough, thereby removing any mucus in the airways.

Incentive spirometry is most often used following surgery. After surgery, patients attempting deep breathing may experience pain from the surgical site. Therefore, the effectiveness of incentive breathing will require coaching on your part, as well as effort on the patient's part.

Procedure for Teaching Incentive Spirometry

In order for the patient to receive the maximum benefit, incentive spirometry must be taught properly. The procedure includes:

1. Prior to surgery, introduce the patient to the equipment and the proper method for performing the procedure.
2. Have the patient completely exhale.
3. Inform the patient to take slow, deep breaths through the incentive device.
4. Following maximum inhalation, tell the patient that he or she should hold the breath for one to three seconds.
5. Tell the patient to exhale slowly and completely.
6. Advance the patient's goal to a higher volume as he or she is able.

As with IPPB treatments, for incentive spirometry to be most beneficial, it is important that you not only teach this maneuver, but also that you continue to encourage and coach the patient throughout the procedure.

Chest Physical Therapy

The purpose of chest physical therapy, or CPT, is to both remove excess mucus from the airways and to assist the patient with coughing, thereby improving ventilation. It involves positioning the patient for secretion drainage. *Postural drainage* and the use of adjunct procedures such as *percussion* and breathing exercises, both help move the secretions out of the lungs and airways at a faster rate and strengthen the respiratory muscles.

CPT must be modified for some patients. A patient who has suffered a head injury or a stroke, for example, should not be positioned with the head down because it may increase *intercranial pressure*. CPT should never be administered just prior to eating and should be delayed for at least 1 hour following a meal. This is necessary in order to avoid regurgitation of the patient's stomach contents. Patients with traumatic injuries, broken limbs, and traction, as well as other types of patients, may not be able to tolerate standard positions because of the pain and fatigue they suffer. During the administration of CPT, a patient should always be monitored very carefully for any changes in his or her heart rate, respiratory effort and difficulty, anxiety, and color.

Supplementary Techniques for CPT

There are several different types of ancillary or supplementary techniques that are sometimes used in conjunction with CPT. These include percussion, vibration, segmental resistance, tussive squeeze, breathing exercises, pursed lip breathing, graded exercise and breathing control, and assisted breathing during CPT. The most frequently used technique during CPT is percussion. It can be done either manually with cupped hands, or with a mechanical device. When done properly, percussion causes a vibration of the chest wall in order to dislodge and help move mucus out of the airways so that it can be coughed out.

Summary

In this chapter, we discussed some of the most commonly used techniques involved in administering pulmonary therapy, determining that IPPB, or intermittent positive-pressure breathing, is by far the most frequently used mechanical method because of its ability to improve the patient's breathing ability. We also talked about some of the mechanical devices used to deliver IPPB treatments, including the three most commonly used, the Bird Mark-7, the Bennett PR-2, and the Bennett AP-5. Another method we discussed was the use of incentive spirometry, which is generally used to encourage the patient to take deep, slow breaths, and cough. This method is most often used after a patient has had surgery in order to prevent any potential for pneumonia. Finally, we talked about the use of chest physical therapy, including the use of postural drainage, percussion, and breathing exercises, all of which are used to help move secretions out of the lungs and airways at a faster rate, thus strengthening the respiratory muscles.

Review Questions

1. Define the following abbreviations and terms:

   a. Apnea

   b. CPT

   c. IPPB

   d. Percussion

   e. Incentive spirometry

2. What is the name of the condition in which air is in the pleural space and causes a collapsed lung?

3. What is the name of the process of positioning a patient so that gravity can assist in the drainage of secretions?

4. What does the term *hemoptysis* mean?

5. List at least three devices that can be used to deliver IPPB treatments:

   a. _____

   b. _____

   c. _____

29

Pulmonary and Respiratory Disorders

Performance Objectives

Upon completion of this chapter, you will be able to:

1. Identify and define the types of pulmonary and respiratory disorders and abnormalities in adults, children, and neonates.
2. Describe airway obstruction.
3. Describe pulmonary restriction.
4. Identify the features of the following respiratory disorders: asthma, chronic bronchitis, and emphysema, adult respiratory distress syndrome, pneumonia, tuberculosis, pleural disease, occupational lung disease, pulmonary edema, and congestive heart failure.
5. Identify the features of the following neuromuscular diseases as they relate to respiratory distress: drug overdose, Guillain-Barré syndrome, and other neuromuscular diseases.
6. Describe the pulmonary complications of surgery and trauma.
7. Discuss the etiology, pathophysiology, functional abnormalities, clinical features, diagnostic testing, and treatment of the following childhood and neonate respiratory diseases: idiopathic respiratory disease syndrome (IRDS), bronchopulmonary dysplasia (BPD), meconium aspiration, congenital heart abnormalities, asthma, croup and epiglottitis, and cystic fibrosis.

Terms and Abbreviations

Asphyxia   suffocation; nonbreathing state, without enough oxygen to live.

Aspiration   breathing a substance other than air into the airways and lungs.

Complication   a second disease that develops in a patient who is already ill. Although the second disease is not specifically related to the original disease, it may modify or affect its outcome.

Congenital   existing at birth; resulting from abnormal development before birth.

Diagnosis   the identification of a disease based on history, physical findings, laboratory findings, and other relevant information.

Dysplasia   impaired or abnormal function or development of various tissues.

Etiology   the cause of a disease.

Exacerbation   the increase in the severity of a disease or any of its symptoms.

Genetic   hereditary; transmitted from parent to offspring; inherited.

Gestation   period of carrying the young in the uterus from conception to birth.

Hypercapnia   an increase in the amount of carbon dioxide in the blood.

Hypercarbia   an increase in carbon dioxide.

Hyperreactivity   greater than normal response to stimulus.

Hypersecretion   excessive secretion.

Inflammation   tissue reaction in injury, infection, or irritation; characterized by redness, pain, heat, and swelling.

Obstruction   narrowing of airways causing a decrease in exhaled flow rates, measured by spirometry.

Pathogenic   structural and functional changes caused by disease.

Pilocarpine iontophoresis   a stimulation of sweat production.

Chloride content of sweat has been determined to aid in the diagnosis of cystic fibrosis.

Prognosis   the predicted course or outcome of a disease.

Relapse   the recurrence of a disease after apparent recovery.

Remission   the period during which the symptoms of a chronic disease subside.

Restriction   a decrease in lung volumes, such as vital capacity, as measured by spirometry.

Sequela   a condition following and resulting from a disease (e.g., heart valve damage following rheumatic fever).

Sign   objective evidence of disease or dysfunction (fever, increased heart rate, and others).

Symptom   the indication of disease as perceived by the patient (pain, shortness of breath, and others).

Syndrome   a combination of symptoms, always occurring in a complex.

The respiratory system has two basic functions: moving air in and out of the lungs, known as ventilation, and allowing gas exchange at the alveolar-capillary interface. Any disturbance in either of these two functions presents a significant abnormality in the patient's pulmonary function. Any pulmonary or respiratory disease or complication can alter functions in different ways.

Some pulmonary diseases, such as *asthma, chronic bronchitis,* and *emphysema,* can cause *obstruction* of the airways. With this type of abnormality, air flow in and out of the lungs is impaired, as well as drainage of pulmonary secretions. Because the airways normally become narrowed during exhalation, the airway obstruction caused by these diseases may become worse during the exhalation phase of breathing.

Some pulmonary diseases, such as *pneumonia, ARDS (adult respiratory distress syndrome), occupational lung diseases,* and *pleural disease,* affect the volume of the lungs. These are known as *restrictive diseases.* They make the expansion of the lungs more difficult than normal. They may also cause a decrease in the measured lung volumes such as the vital capacity and functional residual capacity.

Diseases than cause *pulmonary complications* can also affect the pulmonary function in different ways. Patients who suffer from some *neuromuscular diseases,* for example, may have normal lungs but lack the function of the muscles to move air in and out of the lungs. Patients who have had *surgery* or suffered *trauma* from an accident may not be able to take a deep breath because of pain.

Respiratory Disorders Seen in Adults

As a member of the respiratory therapy team, you may encounter patients suffering from some type of respiratory or neuromuscular disorder or complication that would require the delivery of some type of respiratory therapy treatment. The most frequently seen disorders, which generally affect patients not requiring the confinement of care in an intensive care

or critical care unit, include asthma, chronic bronchitis, emphysema, pneumonia, tuberculosis, pleural disease, occupational lung diseases, congestive heart failure, and in some cases, pulmonary edema, Guillain-Barré syndrome, and some neuromuscular diseases and pulmonary complications following surgery or trauma.

Asthma

Asthma is a disease characterized by intermittent obstruction of the airways with episodic dyspnea caused by hyperactive airways, and almost always accompanied by wheezing. Changes that may occur in the airways as a result of asthma include muscle contraction, vasoconstriction, hypersecretion of mucus, and inflammation of the tissue. Changes that may occur in the ventilatory function include a marked obstruction to air flow during exhalation, and in some cases, mild hypoxemia.

There are two forms of asthma. The first type, called *extrinsic asthma,* is an allergic form of asthma that is almost always linked with a family history of allergy. Patients usually respond well to specific antigens that produce antibodies, particularly when inhaled. Extrinsic asthma usually occurs in childhood and up through the age of 20.

The second type of asthma is called *intrinsic asthma.* It usually occurs later in life, in individuals with no family history of allergy. Respiratory tract infections may play a key role in this type of asthma.

In rare instances, some patients may suffer from a condition known as *status asthmaticus.* This is a severe clinical form of asthma that does not respond to usual types of therapy for reversal. It is considered a medical emergency and may require continuous monitoring in the intensive care unit.

Chronic Bronchitis

Chronic bronchitis is a disease characterized by chronic cough and excessive sputum production that is not the result of other specific causes, and that has occurred for more than 3 months each year, for two or more successive years. The cause is not completely understood; however, there does seem to be a link to chronic irritation.

Chronic irritation seen in this disease may be due to any one or a number of predisposing factors, including, but not limited to, heavy, long-term cigarette smoking; exposure to industrial irritants; and chronic upper respiratory tract infections, causing sinus drainage. Pathologic changes generally include hypertrophy of the bronchial mucous glands and goblet cells, a decreased ciliary activity, and a hypersecretion of mucus production. Changes to the patient's ventilatory function include an obstruction to air flow, hyperinflation, increased residual volume, and variable hypoxemia and hypercarbia.

Treatment for chronic bronchitis almost always includes some type of bronchial hygiene and decreased exposure to irritants and cessation in smoking.

Emphysema

Emphysema is defined as a destruction of the respiratory portion of the lung, distal, or farthest away from the center, to the terminal bronchiole. There are two types of emphysema. The first, called *centrilobular emphysema*, occurs most often in the upper portion of the lungs, causing an enlargement and destruction of respiratory bronchioles. It is generally associated with chronic bronchitis and cigarette smoking. The second type of emphysema, called *panlobular emphysema*, involves the entire area below the terminal bronchioles. In this condition, the alveoli and alveolar ducts are usually destroyed.

Emphysema is believed to develop with long-term bronchiolar obstruction from inflammation, mucosal edema, infection, secretions, and air entrapment. With these chronic changes, more lung tissue is destroyed.

Although administration of bronchial hygiene and decreased exposure to irritants may slow down the emphysema, there is no real treatment that will reverse the destruction that has already taken place. All treatment is generally supportive and is the same as that for chronic bronchitis.

Adult Respiratory Distress Syndrome

Adult respiratory distress syndrome (ARDS) is an injury to the lung that can be caused by a variety of disorders, including shock, trauma, aspiration, inhalation of noxious gases, blood transfusions, cardiopulmonary bypass, and pancreatitis. Pathological changes that may occur include an increased permeability of the capillary walls in the lungs, an increased

permeability of the alveolar walls, and formation of fibrous tissue. There may also be severe hypoxemia (lack of blood oxygen), that may or may not respond well to usual methods of oxygen administration.

Treatment for adult respiratory distress syndrome usually includes adequate oxygenation; ventilatory support; PEEP (positive end-expiratory pressure) in order to increase functional residual capacity toward normal and to restore the openness to collapsed alveoli and small airways; fluid management; and in some cases, corticosteroid medications.

Pneumonia

Pneumonia is an acute infection of the lung tissue that may be caused by bacteria, viruses, or mycoplasmas (bacterialike organisms that cause pneumonia). In this disorder, there is a marked decrease in the compliance and vital capacity. Hypoxemia and dehydration also occur. Treatment for pneumonia usually involves administration of the appropriate antibiotic therapy, oxygen, ventilation support if needed, and rehydration.

Tuberculosis

Tuberculosis is an infectious pulmonary disease transmitted by airborne droplets expelled when a person with tuberculosis coughs or sneezes. The organism that causes tuberculosis is called *Mycobacterium tuberculosis*. Diagnosis of tuberculosis is usually done with a skin test, chest X-ray, and, finally, a positive sputum culture for *Mycobacterium tuberculosis*.

Treatment for tuberculosis is usually given for 18 to 24 months after the onset of the disease. Effective chemotherapy rapidly decreases infectiousness. First-line drugs are also used for the treatment of tuberculosis. They include INH (Isoniazid), ethambutol, rifampin, and streptomycin. Most patients are treated with at least two drugs for the period of treatment. Proper patient education is necessary in order to ensure compliance with the appropriate drug therapy.

Pleural Disease

Pleural disease occurs as fluid, pus, blood, or air in the potential space between the parietal pleura (which covers the chest wall) and the visceral pleura (which covers the lungs). The four most common pleural diseases include *empyema*, in which there is frank pus in the pleural space; *pleural effusion*, in which there is fluid in the pleural space; *hemothorax*, in which there is blood in the pleural space; and *pneumothorax*, in which air is trapped in the pleural space.

Treatment for pleural disease includes drainage of the pleural space by a procedure called *thoracentesis*, in which a surgical puncture of the chest wall is made, a chest tube is inserted in order to remove the fluid, and any underlying conditions causing the pleural disease are treated.

Occupational Lung Diseases

Occupational lung diseases are caused by exposure to occupational and industrial hazards and pollutants. Some of the more common of these include *asbestosis*, caused from inhaling asbestos; *pneumoconiosis*, caused from inhaling dust particles; and *silicosis*, caused by inhaling quartz (silica) dust.

People in many occupations are exposed to these types of hazards. Workplace standards are based on maximum allowable concentrations. These diseases cause pulmonary restriction. The best treatment for them is *prevention*.

Congestive Heart Failure and Pulmonary Edema

Congestive heart failure and pulmonary edema have several possible causes, but the most common cause is *cardiac disease*. Pulmonary edema is an excessive accumulation of fluid that has built up in the alveoli and bronchioles. Failure of the left ventricle of the heart causes an increase in the capillary hydrostatic pressure in the lungs. This results in the fluid moving from the capillaries into the alveolar spaces.

Changes in ventilatory function seen in these two disorders include decreased lung compliance and vital capacity, thereby causing an increase in the work of breathing. There may also be moderate to severe hypoxemia.

Drug Overdose

In drug overdose, the main problem with ventilatory function is depression of the central nervous system and, as a result, decreased ventilation. Treatment depends on the drug involved, but it always includes protection of the airways from aspiration of stomach contents, and ventilatory support of the patient until central nervous system function can return to normal.

Guillain-Barré Syndrome

Guillain-Barré syndrome is an acute *ascending polyneuritis*, or acute inflammation of the nerves. It usually begins shortly after a mild viral illness such as an upper respiratory infection, and it is believed to be the body's immune system's own attack on the peripheral nerves. The patient may experience a range of symptoms from muscular weakness to complete paralysis. Although the patient may experience no loss of function or a decrease in vital capacity, there may be complete paralysis of the muscles of respiration.

Treatment of Guillain-Barré syndrome generally includes continuous monitoring for loss of ventilatory function and, when necessary, ventilatory support until the paralysis subsides.

Guillain-Barré syndrome most commonly reverses, and the patient recovers over a period of time. However, this generally depends upon the severity of the episode.

Pulmonary Complications of Surgery and Trauma

In some instances, pulmonary complications may occur following surgery or trauma. Many complications resulting from surgery can generally be prevented by maintaining an appropriate recovery period from anesthesia. Patients may need ventilatory support until they become alert and awake following extensive surgery and anesthesia.

Some of the complications that may occur following surgery or trauma include adult respiratory distress syndrome, and postoperative pulmonary complications such as *atelectasis* (partial collapse of lung tissue) usually due to inadequate expansion of the lung and poor cough because of pain. This may also occur with chest trauma caused by broken ribs and similar problems.

Respiratory Disorders in Children and Neonates

Many respiratory therapy assistants choose to work with neonates (newborn infants, some born prematurely), and small children with various respiratory and pulmonary disorders. This can be a particular challenge that tests not only your technical skills, but also your interpersonal communication skills.

A small child cannot always understand what is happening and may not be able or willing to cooperate fully with his or her care. You must work with both the child and the parents who are, at best, apprehensive and anxious about their child's illness. Special understanding, kindness, and support must be given in these circumstances, whether the patient is an infant or a child who is very ill and requires specialized care.

As with adults, the disturbances in pulmonary function are either in the infant's or child's ability to move air in and out of the lungs (ventilation), or in the gas exchange at the alveolar-capillary interface, or both.

Some of the more common disorders in which such disturbances may occur in infants or children, include *neonatal respiratory distress syndrome, bronchopulmonary dysplasia, meconium aspiration, congenital heart defects, asthma, croup, acute epiglottis,* and *cystic fibrosis.*

Neonatal Respiratory Distress Syndrome

Neonatal respiratory distress syndrome is sometimes called *hyaline membrane disease* or *idiopathic respiratory distress syndrome.* It is considered the most pressing respiratory problem in neonates, and it most commonly occurs in infants of less than 35 weeks of gestation who weigh between 1 and 1.5 kilograms.

The syndrome most often occurs in premature infants, infants of diabetic mothers, and in infants who experience asphyxia *in utero* (inside the uterus). These infants may have any number of respiratory complications, including, but not limited to, decreased lung compliance, increased work of breathing, alveolar instability and collapse, increased fluid in the lungs, decreased alveolar ventilation with increased minute ventilation, and decreased lung volumes. All of these factors may result in *hypoxemia* and *hypercarbia.*

The disease progresses fairly rapidly after birth and usually stabilizes in about 3 days. Then the infant may begin to improve. The support these infants need varies with the severity of the disease. Some infants may require only oxygen administration, usually delivered by a "halo" (oxyhood). Others may require a continuous positive airway pressure with nasal prongs or the insertion of an endotracheal tube, and humidified oxygen-enriched gas. Still others may require continuous ventilatory support with PEEP, or oxygen administration, endotracheal intubation, suctioning, and bronchial hygiene.

Whatever support may be required, with each improvement, the infant's support is decreased appropriately until weaning from the support is completely achieved.

Bronchopulmonary Dysplasia

Bronchopulmonary dysplasia is a chronic pulmonary disease that is a complication of contemporary therapy for sick neonates. It was first thought to be caused by prolonged exposure to high oxygen concentrations, however, now it is believed to be a result of high oxygen administration, positive pressure of ventilatory support, and prematurity of the infant's lungs.

Infants with this disease usually have severe neonatal respiratory distress syndrome and experience a prolonged disease course and a gradual recovery. Treatment is generally supportive and includes oxygen, diuretics, and digitalis.

Because the lungs have grown and developed to such a small degree at this age, the child suffering from bronchopulmonary dysplasia may eventually outgrow his or her chronic respiratory problems.

Meconium Aspiration

Meconium is the contents of the colon of a fetus *in utero.* If intrauterine stress or asphyxia occurs, the meconium may be released into the amniotic fluid, and the infant may breathe it in. It is a thick, sticky material that may block the airways, and may cause pneumonia in an infant after birth.

Treatment for meconium aspiration involves prevention of aspiration. When an infant is born with meconium staining, the mouth, pharynx, and airways should be suctioned prior to stimulating the infant to breathe. Positive-pressure breathing should follow good bronchial hygiene.

Congenital Heart Defects

There are many congenital heart defects that an infant may be born with. Some of them may cause hypoxemia in the infant, and some may not. Some of the more commonly seen congenital heart defects include *patent ductus arteriosus, coarctation of the aorta, ventricular septal defect, atrial septal defect, tetralogy of Fallot, aortic stenosis, pulmonary stenosis,* and *tricuspid atresia.*

Patent Ductus Arteriosus

The ductus is a normal passageway between the pulmonary artery and the aorta. It usually closes after birth. When it does not close, the heart must work harder, because some blood goes back to the lungs from the aorta instead of to the body. Treatment is accomplished by surgically closing the ductus.

Coarctation of the Aorta

In this disorder, there is a narrowing of the aorta where it leaves the heart. Treatment of the narrowed section of the aorta involves excising, and the aorta is then sewn back together. This defect can cause heart failure if not corrected.

Ventricular Septal Defect and Atrial Septal Defect

In ventricular septal defect (VSD), a hole exists between the right and left ventricles. The heart has to pump harder because part of the oxygenated blood from the left ventricle is pumped back into the right ventricle and back through the lungs. In atrial septal defect (ASD), a hole exists between the two atria that may cause the same problem as VSD. Treatment for these two defects require open heart surgery for correction. This is usually deferred until childhood.

Tetralogy of Fallot

Tetralogy of Fallot is a combination of four defects: VSD, pulmonary valve stenosis (narrowing), right ventricular enlargement, and unoxygenated blood passing into the aorta. This defect causes hypoxemia. Total correction of the defect is deferred until late childhood, when a temporary opening is made between the aorta and the pulmonary artery.

Aortic Stenosis and Pulmonary Stenosis

In aortic stenosis, there is a narrowing of the aortic valve. A surgical opening of the valve is necessary when left ventricular pressures rise.

Pulmonary stenosis exists when there is a narrowing of the pulmonary valve. Surgical intervention is also required by making an opening of the valve. This must be done when right ventricular pressure increases.

Tricuspid Artesia

Tricuspid artesia is caused by an absence of the opening between the right atria and ventricle. Blood flows through an ASD and unoxygenated blood is pumped to the body. This defect causes hypoxemia. The disorder cannot be completely corrected, but blood can be diverted into the pulmonary artery so that more blood is oxygenated by the lungs.

Asthma, Croup, Acute Epiglottitis, and Cystic Fibrosis

Asthma

Asthma in children is very similar to asthma in adults. It is a disease characterized by intermittent obstruction of airways with episodic dyspnea, and almost always accompanied by wheezing. It is a disorder that may be caused either from an allergy (extrinsic asthma), or may occur later in life, as a result of an infection (intrinsic asthma).

Croup

Croup is a disease of infants and young children that causes inflammation from the larynx to the bronchi. About 85% of croup is caused by a *Parainfluenza virus*. It usually is seen in children 3 months to 3 years old. Bacterial croup, usually caused by an organism called *Hemophilus influenzae*, is generally seen in children 2 to 12 years of age. Bacterial croup, which is about 15% of all croup, is more severe.

Croup is generally a result of the laryngeal airway being to small. It may also be caused by an increased vascularity occurring in the mucous membranes lining the epiglottis and the vocal cords.

Treatment for croup usually includes the use of aerosolized epinephrine, humidity, antibiotics for bacterial croup, and in severe cases, intubation.

Acute Epiglottitis

Acute epiglottitis is a life-threatening pediatric emergency. It must be recognized and treated immediately. Fifty percent of patients require an artificial airway during peak symptoms. The condition is usually caused by *Hemophilus influenzae*. The rapid onset of symptoms lasts less than 24 hours. The child has fever, may be apprehensive, prefers to sit up, drools, and refuses to swallow, and the voice is muffled rather than hoarse. The epiglottis is enlarged and red. The child should not be forced to lie down, and any examination that might provoke the child should only be done with adequate provision for intubation or tracheostomy.

Cystic Fibrosis

Cystic fibrosis is a genetic disorder that involves the *exocrine glands*. It causes chronic pulmonary disease, pancreatic deficiency, and high electrolyte concentration in the sweat. Patients with severe pulmonary disease have thick, sticky secretions that cause *obstruction of the small airways*. The mucus is a growth medium for bacteria such as *Pseudomonas*. This *chronic bacterial infection* causes more mucus production and obstruction and less ability to evacuate the mucus from the lungs. This disease may progress to respiratory failure with other problems, such as hypoxemia, hypercapnia, and right heart failure.

Some patients with cystic fibrosis have a less severe pulmonary disease. With good bronchial hygiene, including home respiratory care, excercise, and diet control, they are able to live with their disease for many years.

Summary

In this chapter, we focused on some of the most frequently seen respiratory disorders. We determined that some of these disorders, such as asthma, chronic bronchitis, and emphysema can cause obstruction of the airways. We also talked about other diseases, such as pneumonia, adult respiratory distress syn-

drome, occupational lung diseases, and pleural diseases that affect the volume of the lungs. We determined that some pulmonary diseases can also be a result of other disorders, and thus may cause complications in different body systems, such as the neuromuscular system. In addition to discussing many of the disorders seen in adults, we also talked about some of the more commonly seen respiratory diseases in children and neonates, including neonatal respiratory distress syndrome, bronchopulmonary dysplasia, meconium aspiration, congenital heart defects of the newborn, and asthma, croup, acute epiglottis, and cystic fibrosis.

Review Questions

1. What is a medical term used to describe suffocation?

2. Briefly explain the difference between *hypercarbia* and *hypercapnia*.

3. _____ describes the structural and functional changes caused by a disease.

4. A(n) _____ is a combination of symptoms, always occurring in a complex.

5. Briefly explain the difference between a *sign* and a *symptom*.

6. What does the term *remission* mean?

7. Define *diagnosis*.

8. Define *gestation*.

9. Define the difference between *hyperactivity* and *hypersecretion*.

10. What does the term *etiology* mean?

30

Airways, Suctioning, and Ventilation

Performance Objectives

Upon completion of this chapter, you will be able to:

1. Explain the need for using an artificial airway.
2. Identify the various types of artificial airways available for patient use.
3. Discuss the indications for using an oral airway versus a nasal airway.
4. Discuss endotracheal intubation, its hazards, indications, and complications, and identify the necessary equipment.
5. Discuss the differences between nasotracheal and oral endotracheal intubation.
6. Explain the process, indications, hazards, complications, and equipment necessary for tracheostomy.
7. Describe the care of a tracheostomy site.
8. Describe the role of the respiratory therapy assistant in the process of intubation and tracheotomy.
9. Discuss a rational approach to use with a patient with an artificial airway.
10. Identify equipment used for suctioning an airway.
11. Explain the procedure for suctioning through an endotracheal and tracheostomy tube.
12. Describe the procedure for nasotracheal suctioning with no artificial airway in place.
13. Explain the procedure for suctioning a patient on ventilatory support.
14. Discuss the hazards of suctioning.
15. Identify precautions that should be observed when suctioning a patient.
16. Define continuous mechanical ventilation and identify the indications for its use on an adult patient.
17. Discuss the special care required for a patient receiving continuous ventilatory support.
18. Explain the general functions of a ventilator suitable for use in an ICU.
19. Describe the Bennett MA-1, the Bourns Bear 1, and the Bird Mark 14 ventilators, and identify other adult ventilators currently in common use.

Terms and Abbreviations

Alarm any device that alerts the therapist or assistant to a deviation from normal operation of the patient-ventilator system.
Arrythmias abnormalities of the heart rate and rhythm.
Artificial airway a device used to maintain an open, functional breathing passage; also used as a passage to remove excess mucus from the airways.
Assist-control mode of continuous ventilation in which the patient is allowed to cycle the ventilator into inspiration.

Barotrauma   injury or injuries to the lung, mainly related to the pressure exerted during continuous mechanical ventilation.

Bevel   the slanted or patient end of an endotracheal tube.

Bradycardia   pertaining to an abnormal slowing of the heart rate.

Compliance   distensibility of the lungs; volume change per unit of pressure change, usually measured in liters per centimeter of water (cm H_2O).

Cuff   the inflatable balloon located just above the patient end of a tracheal tube that is used to provide a seal or no-leak fit between the the tube and the patient's trachea.

Electrically powered   a ventilator that is operated mainly by electrical power.

Endotracheal intubation   placement of a proper-sized plastic or silicone tube through the mouth or nose into the pharynx and through the vocal cords; used to provide a patent (open) airway for continuous ventilation, suctioning, and other uses.

Expiratory phase   the phase of the respiratory cycle during which there is no volume delivery to the patient.

15-mm adapter   a device that allows the tracheal tube to attach to a continuous ventilator circuit or other airway device.

Flange   the neck piece surrounding the tracheostomy tube, which helps to maintain the correct placement of the tube and allows for movement of the neck.

Flow rate   the speed at which the volume of air from the ventilator is delivered to the patient; measured in liters per minute.

Guedel airway (oropharyngeal airway)   a hard rubber or plastic device placed into the mouth over the tongue.

Hyperinflation   deep inspiration; the breath is delivered by a ventilator or taken spontaneously by the patient.

Hypoxemia   the decrease in the amount of oxygen in the arterial blood.

Hypoxia   the decrease in the amount of oxygen in the alveoli.

I:E ratio   the ratio of inspiratory time to expiratory time; normally, inspiration should be shorter than expiration.

IMV/SIMV   method of continuous ventilation or weaning in which the ventilator delivers a certain number of mandatory breaths per minute, and the patient breathes spontaneously between ventilator breaths.

Inflation tube   a thin tube that is attached to the tracheal tube, used to fill the cuff with air so that a no-leak fit between the tube and the trachea is established.

Inner cannula   a separate tube that fits inside the standard tracheostomy tube and allows for removal of the inside tube for cleaning.

Inspiratory phase   that phase of the respiratory cycle during which a volume of air is delivered to the patient.

Laryngoscope   an instrument used to visualize the glottis and vocal cords of a patient so that an endotracheal tube can be properly placed.

Machine/proximal end   the end of the tube with a 15-mm adapter; the portion that attaches to an oxygen-administering device or a continuous ventilator.

Manometer   the gauge device on the face of a ventilator that measures system or proximal airway pressure, usually measured in cmH_2O or mm Hg.

Minute volume   a measure of the amount (volume) of air inhaled and exhaled by a patient in a one-minute period, usually measured as exhaled volume.

Nasal trumpet (nasopharyngeal airway)   a soft, rubber airway that is inserted through the naris into the nasopharynx.

Nasotracheal intubation   placement of a special tube through the nose.

Obturator   a device that fits inside the tracheostomy tube in order to allow for atraumatic insertion of the tube into the opening of the skin.

Oral endotracheal intubation   placement of a special tube through the mouth.

Oxygen concentration   control that allows the therapist or assistant to deliver a precise amount of oxygen to the patient, usually measured in percent oxygen, from 21 to 100%.

Patient-distal end   the end of the tracheal tube that is inserted into the patient; the bevel end of an endotracheal tube.

Peak pressure   the highest pressure reached on the manometer of a ventilator during the inspiratory phase of a respiratory cycle or during the delivery of a volume of gas to a patient.

PEEP   abbreviation for positive end-expiratory pressure; positive pressure exerted on the airway during the expiratory phase of the respiratory cycle used to normalize the functional residual capacity and gas exchange.

Pilot balloon   a small balloon on the end of the inflation tube that indicates the amount of inflation of the tube cuff.

Pneumatically powered   a ventilator that is operated mainly by a high-pressure gas source.

Pneumothorax   abnormal accumulation of air in the pleural space.

Pressure-cycling   cycling mechanism of a ventilator that switches from inspiration to expiration when a preset volume of gas has been delivered from it.

Pressure-regulating valve   a mechanism on the pilot balloon or inflation tube that allows air to escape if pressure in the tube cuff builds.

Radiopaque   impenetrable by X-ray or other forms of radiation.

Respiratory rate   the number of breaths or cycles per minute delivered by the ventilator, or taken by the patient.

Sensitivity   amount of negative inspiratory force the patient must exert to cycle a ventilator into the inspiratory phase.

Sigh   a deep inspiration; the breath is delivered by a ventilator or delivered spontaneously by the patient.

Stenosis   abnormal narrowing or stricture (of the trachea). Tracheal stenosis may be caused by damage from a tracheal tube.

Sterile   being free from all living microorganisms.

Stylet   a metal guide wire used to give rigidity to an endotracheal tube so that it can be moved more easily through the airway.

Subcutaneous emphysema   abnormal accumulation of air in the instertitial space (under the skin) which is caused by a tear in the trachea or lung.

Suction catheter   a plastic or rubber tube that is used in the suctioning procedure.

Suctioning   procedure for removing secretions or assisting the patient in the removal of secretions when an artificial airway is in place, the cough reflex is decreased, or the patient has lung disease.

Time-cycling cycling mechanism of a ventilator that switches from inspiration to expiration when a preset time interval has elapsed.
Tracheotomy the surgical opening into the trachea for the purpose of placing a tube to provide a patent airway.
Tracheostomy the opening present in the trachea following the surgical procedure of tracheotomy.

Vacuum pressure below atmospheric pressure.
Volume-cycling cycling mechanism of a ventilator that switches from inspiration to expiration when a preset volume of gas has been delivered from it.
Xylocaine a local anesthetic agent that is sometimes used when suctioning through the nose.

If you find yourself working in a hospital setting, you will soon discover that many of your patients may require airway or breathing assistance. These patients' situations may vary from one whose tongue is occluding his airway, to one who is unable to breathe on her own and requires ventilatory support. Although your job description may or may not preclude you from being able to insert certain types of airway tubes, you must still become familiar with how they are inserted, as well as their care, limitations, and possible complications.

Types of Airways

The five most commonly used airways include the *S-shaped* or *Guedel* (oropharyngeal) airway (which is considered the most complex of the five), the *nasal trumpet*, the *oral endotracheal* (nasopharyngeal) *tube*, the *nasotracheal tube*, and the *tracheostomy tube* (Figure 30-1).

The S-shaped or Guedel airway is a hard plastic or rubber device that is placed into the patient's mouth, between the teeth and over the tongue. When placed appropriately, this type of airway maintains

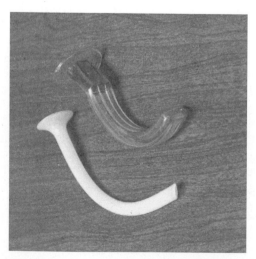

Figure 30-1
Types of airways.

the tongue position, keeping it from falling back and closing off the airway. It also allows for suctioning and removal in the oropharynx. Generally speaking, the Guedel airway is almost always used for patients who are semialert or comatose, since many of these patients require assistance with removal of secretions and maintenance of the tongue position.

A similar type of airway is the nasal trumpet, which is placed through the naris, or opening of the nose, into the nasopharynx. This airway is made of soft, pliable rubber and is therefore best used for patients requiring assistance in removing secretions by suctioning through the nose. It is also used on patients who may require suctioning because of a hyperactive gag reflex, or for initial treatment of a facial trauma.

Intubation

Endotracheal intubation is the process of placing a semirigid tube through the patient's mouth or nose, into the trachea, and between the vocal cords. Although it is a procedure which is usually done by a physician, with the assistance of a respiratory therapist or nurse, it is important that you have a general understanding of technique involved in intubation, since you may be required to assist either the physician or the therapist during the procedure.

Endotracheal intubation is performed by first placing the patient in a supine position, with the physician or therapist standing at the head of the bed. The laryngoscope blade is then placed into the patient's mouth, and the oropharynx is lifted in order to expose the glottis. The tube is then inserted into the right side of the mouth. It is then advanced through the vocal cords into the trachea and placed so that the cuff is below the vocal cords. Finally, the cuff is inflated, and the tube secured in place (Figure 30-2).

An oral endotracheal tube is inserted through the mouth with direct visualization of the airways. A nasotracheal tube is inserted through the nose in a slightly different manner. It is usually inserted without the use of a laryngoscope, with the physician following along the airway and listening for airway sounds.

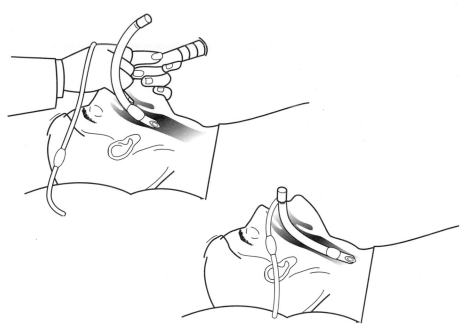

Figure 30-2
Oral endotracheal intubation.

Purpose of Intubation

Patients may require either nasotracheal or oral intubation when they are in need of maintaining an open airway, require protection from aspiration of the airway, are connected to long-term ventilatory support, or are in need of effective suctioning and removal of secretions. However, if intubation is used as a therapy, it is important that you understand that such a procedure does not come without its risks or complications. Endotracheal intubation, for example, may result in a misplacement of the tube into the esophagus or right mainstem bronchus. It may also cause fractures of the teeth, or even a mispositioning of the tube, causing a complete obstruction of the airway.

There may also be long-term complications, such as damage to the vocal cords, airway edema, tracheal stenosis, or even obstruction of the tube with secretions.

Damage to the airways can be prevented by careful placement of the tube and by minimizing tube and patient movement following tube placement. Obstruction and misplacement of the tube can also be prevented by using a good suctioning technique. Also, tube placement should be checked immediately after intubation with a chest x-ray. Following this, the physician or therapist should listen often with a stethoscope for bilateral equal aeration.

As a respiratory therapy assistant, in order for you to be able to properly care for the intubated patient, you must become thoroughly familiar with the functional parts of an endotracheal tube. Figure 30-3 is a diagram of a conventional tube with all the functional parts labeled.

Tracheotomy

Tracheotomy is the surgical procedure for making an opening into the trachea. The procedure should be done in an operating room with the patient orally intubated if at all possible. In some cases, however, it

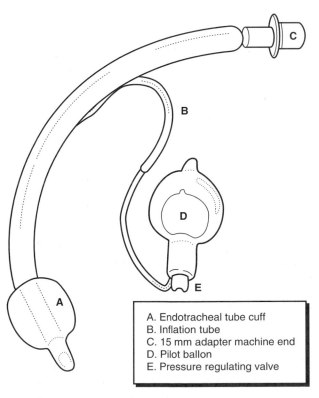

A. Endotracheal tube cuff
B. Inflation tube
C. 15 mm adapter machine end
D. Pilot ballon
E. Pressure regulating valve

Figure 30-3
Parts of an endotracheal tube.

may be done in the intensive care unit. In either case, it is always done under sterile conditions.

Using local anesthesia, an incision is made in the skin of the lower neck above the sternum (A), the trachea is exposed and incised between the second and third tracheal cartilages (B), and a tracheostomy tube is inserted (C), and is anchored (D). The incision is dressed and covered with a gauze pad between the tube and the skin.

The placement of the tube is checked with a chest x-ray and by listening often for bilateral equal air movement with a stethoscope.

Although the respiratory therapy assistant should never be responsible for performing the tracheotomy, the task of maintaining and cleaning the tracheostomy site is shared by all members of the respiratory therapy team. The site must be cleaned and have a dressing applied often in a sterile manner. It is usually done every 8 to 24 hours following the surgery.

Indications for Tracheostomy

When a patient is unable to breathe independently for a very long period of time, a tracheostomy tube may be placed in order to prevent long-term airway damage of an endotracheal tube. Often, airway secretions cannot be effectively evacuated through an endotracheal tube. In those cases, a tracheostomy tube may be placed for more effective airway clearance.

In addition to many of the same complications that endotracheal intubation causes, tracheostomy may also cause bleeding, subcutaneous emphysema, pneumothorax, cardiac arrest, and infections.

Artificial airways are uncomfortable at best, and the patient's inability to communicate is extremely frustrating. Remember, that even though the patient may not be able to communicate, he or she can still hear, understand, and feel, and therefore should be treated gently and with dignity. Every procedure initiated should be thoroughly explained prior to beginning in order to alleviate fear and anxiety as much as possible. Developing a bond of humanity and trust between yourself and the patient is as important as the technical aspects of giving care.

Airway Care and Suctioning

Patients suffering from lung diseases and those that may require artificial airways and ventilatory support often have abnormally increased mucus production or an abnormally decreased ability to cough.

In either of these circumstances, a patient may need your assistance in order to remove secretions. Suctioning, either through an artificial airway or through the nose or mouth, is the procedure we use in order to help remove excess secretions from the patient's airways.

Suctioning Equipment

Suctioning is a very exact procedure and involves both an exact technique and the use of the appropriate equipment. Using the wrong equipment or not following the exact procedure may cause the patient both undue discomfort, and in some cases, even harm. Before beginning the procedure, you must first make sure you have secured all of the proper equipment (Figure 30-4). This includes the following:

· Sterile, disposable suction kit containing a sized, sterile catheter and one or two sterile gloves; all of the items are for single-patient use.
· Connecting tubing.
· Disposable suction vial.
· Vacuum source and bottle; either piped wall outlet or electrically generated pump.
· Manometer.
· Oxygen source.
· Resuscitation bag.
· Water-soluble lubricant.

The suction catheter is a very important and integral part of the equipment necessary for the suctioning procedure (Figure 30-5). Many different types of catheters are commonly used today. A basic suction catheter is a sized plastic tube that is very flexible. It should have a small hole on one side close to the end of the catheter and a small hole in the tip of the catheter in order to prevent adherence and damage to the tracheal mucosa. The most commonly used sizes are 1.5 and 8 French, which are most commonly used for infants and small children, and a 10 and 14 French, used most commonly for adults and larger children.

A suction catheter should be as large as possible in order to accommodate thick secretions. But it should not be more than one-half to two-thirds the size of the internal diameter of the tube or airway through which the suctioning will be done.

Performing the Suctioning Procedure

Suctioning should not become a routine procedure. It should be approached as a complex task which, at best, is uncomfortable for the patient, and in some cases, can be very hazardous.

Patients with artificial airways should be suctioned only when necessary. Generally this is when secretions can be heard or seen at the tube, when breath sounds on auscultation indicate the need for

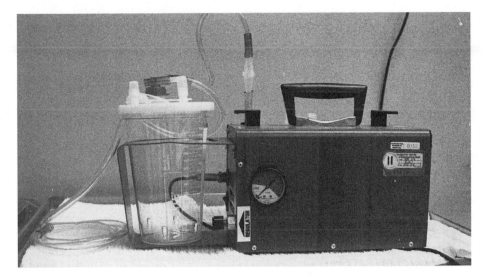

Figure 30-4
Suctioning equipment.

suctioning, or when a change in the ventilator parameters indicates the need for suctioning. A patient without an artificial airway is usually suctioned either when he or she is unconscious or comatose or when he or she is unable to cough out secretions with proper coaching, encouragement, and assistance.

As with any patient care procedure, you should never attempt to undertake the task until you have received proper instruction and training in it. Prior to beginning it, you must always make sure that you have thoroughly washed your hands.

Once you have gathered all of the appropriate equipment, washed your hands, and thoroughly ex-

plained the procedure to the patient, you are ready to begin. To complete the task of suctioning, you should follow the guidelines listed below:

1. Assemble all equipment, and make sure that the suction is on and adjusted properly.
2. Hyperinflate the patient with several breaths of 100% oxygen.
3. Open the catheter and glove.
4. Glove one hand.
5. Connect the catheter to the connecting tube without contaminating the catheter or glove.
6. With the suction machine off, gently insert the catheter until resistance is met.
7. Apply suction, while removing the catheter, with a rotating motion for no more than 10 to 15 seconds.
8. Remove the catheter without contaminating it.
9. Hyperinflate the patient with several breaths of 100% oxygen.
10. Repeat the above steps.
11. Dispose of the catheter and glove when finished.
12. Wash your hands.

The suction catheter can be used for suctioning as long as it has not touched any surface outside the airway. Remember, suctioning must be as sterile as possible in order to prevent the introduction of pathogens into the patient's airway.

When a patient is being supported by a ventilator, the suctioning procedure is the same as the guidelines listed above. However, it is usually better to have two people present when suctioning. While the first person suctions, the second person sighs the patient with 100% oxygen and removes and replaces the ventilator adapter onto the tube quickly, and

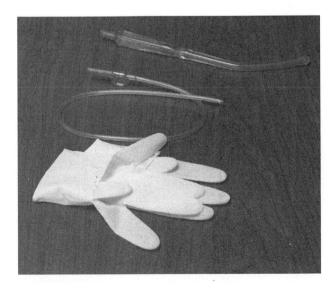

Figure 30-5
Suction catheter.

sighs the patient with 100% oxygen again. This process may be repeated if necessary.

It is important to remember that a patient who is dependent upon ventilatory support should never be disconnected from it longer than a few seconds. The second person can quickly reconnect the patient to the ventilator.

Suctioning through a Nasal Passage

Suctioning a patient through the nasal passage without the use of an artificial airway, as is the case of a patient with either an endotracheal or tracheostomy tube, is a more difficult and complex procedure. Patients who require nasal suctioning should be on a cardiac monitor in order to allow the visualization of any arrythmias that may occur more often with this type of suctioning. Prior to beginning the procedure, it is important to make sure you take enough time to position the patient properly at a 30° to 45° angle, with the head elevated. After that, the first part of the procedure is the same as for other suctioning, with three very important exceptions:

1. Even more care should be taken to explain the procedure to the patient; how it will feel, what he or she needs to do to help, and coughing during the procedure.
2. The catheter may be lubricated with sterile water-soluble lubricant or xylocaine jelly.
3. Oxygenation should continue throughout the procedure with the patient instructed to breathe 100% oxygen in deep breaths through the mouth.

Once the catheter has been inserted into the opening of the nose, it should be slowly and gently advanced until it is in the trachea. This is done by listening for air flow or by having the patient cough while inserting the catheter. This is a difficult, time-consuming maneuver, and should never be undertaken without first having received proper instruction.

Once the catheter is in the trachea, suctioning proceeds normally, every 10 to 15 seconds, with oxygen being administerd continuously to the patient's airways.

Hazards of Suctioning

Whenever you are required to undertake the task of suctioning a patient, whether it be through an artificial airway or while the patient is on ventilator support, you must be aware of some of the more common hazards that can accompany this procedure. These hazards may include, but are not limited to, hypoxia, cardiac arrhythmias, trauma to the nasal mu-

cosa and the tracheal mucosa, catheter size being too large, resulting in atelectasis or the lung to collapse partially or completely, and in rare cases, cardiac arrest.

Problems can be avoided when suctioning is not treated as a routine procedure. Therefore, you must remember that great care should always be taken when choosing an appropriately sized catheter and in hyperinflating and oxygenating the patient. Also, make sure you carefully observe the cardiac monitor. The catheter should be inserted very gently into the airway in order to avoid trauma to the membranes and unnecessary stimulation of nerve endings.

And finally, always remember that being suctioned is uncomfortable and can be painful and hazardous. It is similar to forced breath-holding and can make a patient feel as though he or she is suffocating. So try to suction as carefully and gently as possible. Always communicate the procedure to the patient in a gentle, comfortable, and reassuring manner.

Mechanical Ventilation

While providing ventilatory care and support is considered one of the major areas of responsibility of the respiratory therapist and is generally most often seen in the intensive care unit, as a respiratory therapy assistant and member of the health care delivery team, it is important for you to have a clear understanding of the purpose, care, and maintenance of continuous mechanical ventilation.

Since adults, children, and infants may all suffer from different types of respiratory difficulties, you should understand that the goal of all mechanical ventilation is the same: to support life until patients are able to breathe well enough on their own. The physician, respiratory therapist, nurse, as well as yourself must all work very closely in order to make a patient's ventilator course as smooth as possible.

Continuous mechanical ventilation can be defined as the support of a patient's breathing with a mechanical device. This process may be necessary in a variety of clinical situations, such as chronic obstructive pulmonary disease, chronic bronchitis, drug overdose, cervical and head injuries, heart failure, trauma to the chest wall or abdomen, major surgery and anesthesia, adult and infant respiratory distress syndrome, and certain neuromuscular diseases such as Guillain-Barré syndrome and myasthenia gravis.

In any of these diseases or disorders, patients who are unable to breathe effectively may have respiratory or ventilatory failure. If that occurs, continuous mechanical ventilation may become necessary.

Continuous mechanical ventilation is a procedure that can be hazardous for the patient. An artificial airway is necessary for continuous ventilation. As we have already mentioned, there may be several hazards associated with artificial airways. In addition to those discussed, there may be other complications of continuous mechanical ventilation. Some of these may include, but are not limited to, equipment failure, infection, and decreased cardiac output and blood pressure.

Patients receiving continuous ventilatory support will require much care and support in addition to the nursing and respiratory care needed for the primary disease or disorder. These patients are unable to communicate effectively their pain, fears, and frustrations. It is very difficult for adults and children to cope with feeling helpless and dependent and not knowing what is happening to them.

Whenever you are required to work with a patient on continuous ventilatory support, be supportive, try to calm fears, and explain each procedure to them. A little caring means a lot.

There are many different types of ventilators used in most intensive care units. The type of ventilator chosen is based upon its ability to provide certain controls or paremeters (measures) of ventilatory support. Most of the ventilators used today include sophisticated controls, monitors, and alarms that assist the patient. It is the physician who is responsible for ordering the continuous mechanical ventilation, and the respiratory therapist who is responsible for setting up the appropriate ventilator.

Types of Ventilators

For adults, there are three ventilators used most commonly for patients requiring continuous ventilatory support. These are the *Bennett MA-1* (Figure 30-6), the *Bourns Bear I*, and the *Bird Mark 14*.

Bennett MA-1 Ventilator

The Bennett MA-1 is probably still the most commonly used ventilator in hospitals and clinics today. It is an electrically powered, volume-cycled ventilator that can be an assistor, controller, or assistor-controller. It has a system of warning lights that allows the therapist to know when the patient is assisting the ventilator, when the high-pressure limits have been exceeded and the volume delivery to the patient has stopped, and when the inspiratory-expiratory ratio is less than 1 or the inspiratory time is longer than expiratory time. It also lets the therapist know when a sigh breath is delivered and when an oxygen concentration that is greater than 21% is in use.

Bourns Bear I

The Bourns Bear I is a newer, more sophisticated ventilator than the MA-1. It has many built-in capabilities. On the MA-1, extra pieces of equipment, such as alarm systems, are required. The Bear I is also electronically operated and volume-cycled, and is capable of assisting and controlling the patients' ventilation. It has a much more comprehensive alarm system than the MA-1.

Bird Mark 14

The Bird Mark 14 is a pneumatically powered pressure-cycled ventilator. It can, with additional equipment and therapist experience, be used in much the same manner in an intensive care unit as the MA-1 and the Bear I. Exceptions to this are situations in which the patient has low lung compliance and high resistance.

In order to use the Mark 14 in the intensive care unit, several pieces of equipment must be added to it. Therefore, its usefulness as a patient support system may not be as great as that of the MA-1 and the Bear I.

Infant and Child Ventilators

Ventilators that are used for infants and small children are time-cycled, not volume-cycled. In an infant ventilator system, exhaled tidal volumes cannot be measured as with adults, because the volumes are so small. Therefore, monitoring an infant or a small child on a ventilator requires close patient observation and close attention to all other parameters that can be monitored. Some of these include arterial blood gases, chest movement, peak pressure, respiratory and cardiate rate and rhythm, and blood pressure.

Because complications in infants and small children that receive continuous ventilatory support occur so rapidly and can be life-threatening, these patients must be monitored very closely. Oxygen concentration must be checked at least every 2 hours, and tube placement and breath sounds must be checked often since an exhaled volume measurement cannot be seen.

A ventilator suitable for providing continuous mechanical ventilation for an infant or small child should provide accurate control of oxygen concentration and respiratory rate, peak pressure, manometer, continuous flow with a controlled flow rate, humidification, and appropriate alarms and monitors. Such ventilators include the *Baby Bird Ventilator*, the *Bourns BP 200*, and the *Healthdyne Ventilator* (Figure 30-7).

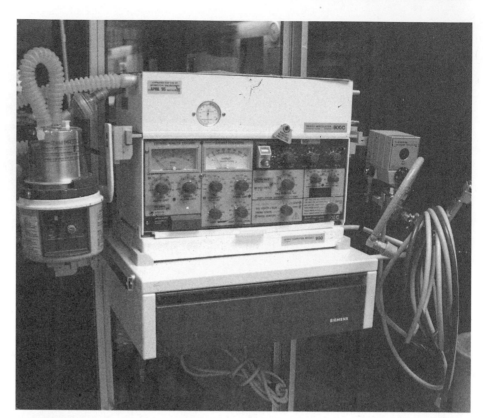

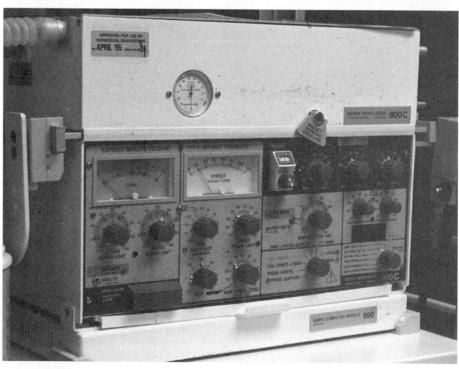

Figure 30-6
Bennett MA-1 ventilator.

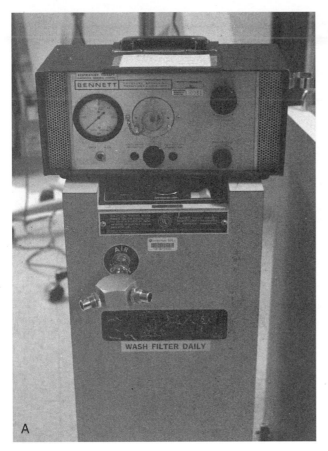

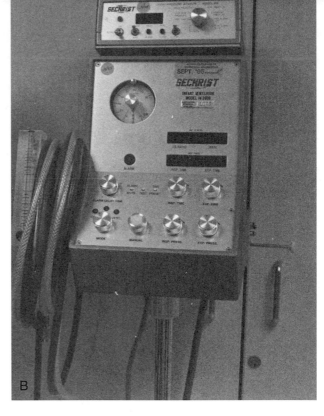

Figure 30-7
Baby Bird (A) and Sechrist (B) infant ventilators.

Baby Bird Ventilator

The Baby Bird ventilator is a pneumatically powered, time-cycled, constant-flow ventilator for infants and babies under 20 pounds. It incorporates a high-pressure reed valve alarm and relief, a low-source gas pressure alarm, and an inspiratory time limit alarm.

Bourns BP 200 Ventilator

The Bourns BP 200 is a pneumatically powered, electrically controlled, time-cycled, continuous-flow infant ventilator. To be safely used, this ventilator needs an added low-pressure audible alarm system.

Healthdyne Ventilator

The Healthdyne ventilator is a pneumatically operated, electronically controlled infant ventilator that can also be used effectively with larger babies and small children. A major advantage of the Healthydyne ventilator over the Baby Bird and the BP 200 is that is incorporated both an audible and a visual alarm system.

As you observe adult and infant ventilators in use, you will note that most of them all operate very similarly. All are continuous-flow systems, and all have some mechanism for timed closure of an exhalation valve. This allows pressure to build to a certain point in the system and then to deliver a volume of gas to the patient's lungs

Summary

In this chapter, we spent a great deal of time discussing the purpose and function of assisting the pulmonary patient with artificial airways, suctioning, and mechanical ventilation. We discussed various types of artificial airways available for patient use, as well as what the indications were for using them. We also talked about the differences between endotracheal and nasotracheal intubation, as well as the process, indications, hazards, complications, and equipment used for a tracheostomy. We described what suctioning was, including some of the hazards and the precautions that must be followed when suctioning. Finally, we talked about mechanical ventilation, noting some of the special care required for patients receiving continuous ventilatory support.

Review Questions

1. Define the following:

   a. barotrauma _____

   b. bradycardia _____

   c. hypoxemia _____

   d. hypoxia _____

   e. pneumothorax _____

   f. subcutaneous emphysema _____

2. Describe the difference between a *tracheostomy* and a *tracheotomy*.

3. Briefly explain how endotracheal intubation is performed.

4. Briefly explain the difference between an *oropharyngeal airway* and a *nasopharyngeal airway*.

5. What does the abbreviation *PEEP* mean?

31

Cardiopulmonary Resuscitation

Performance Objectives

Upon completion of this chapter, you will be able to:

1. Describe the procedure for establishing unresponsiveness.
2. Describe the procedure for opening the airway of an unconscious victim.
3. Describe the procedure for rescue breathing.
4. Identify and describe the steps for artificial circulation (external chest compressions).
5. List some of the problems that may occur during cardiopulmonary resuscitation.
6. Explain when to begin and when to end cardiopulmonary resuscitation.
7. Describe the procedure for cardiopulmonary resuscitation on infants and children.
8. Describe the universal distress signal for choking.
9. Describe how to obtain certification in cardiopulmonary resuscitation from the American Heart Association or the American Red Cross.

Terms and Abbreviations

ACLS abbreviation for advanced cardiac life support; the use of adjunct equipment and procedures in addition to cardiopulmonary resuscitation (drugs, defibrillation, and others).

AHA abbreviation for the American Heart Association; an organization that provides many services, including cardiopulmonary resuscitation training.

ARC abbreviation for the American Red Cross; an organization that provides many services, including cardiopulmonary resuscitation training.

Artificial circulation providing external cardiac compression for the victim of a cardiac arrest.

Artificial ventilation breathing for the victim of arrest with mouth-to-mouth resuscitation or a resuscitation device.

BLS abbreviation for basic life support; externally supporting the circulation and respiration of a victim of respiratory or cardiac arrest using cardiopulmonary resuscitation.

CPR abbreviation for cardiopulmonary resuscitation; a procedure for maintaining blood flow and oxygenation to the body when a victim is not breathing and has no effective heartbeat.

ECC abbreviation for emergency cardiac care.

EMS abbreviation for emergency medical services; a system in a community for emergency care, including on-site care, transportation, and extended care.

Gastric distention filling of the stomach with air during artificial ventilation.

Obstructed airway an airway blocked either by an anatomical structure or by a foreign body such as a food particle.

Ventricular fibrillation condition in which the ventricles of the heart vibrate in an asynochronous fashion, in which no more effective blood flow to the body can occur; leads to complete cardiac standstill if not treated. CPR must be instituted and electric shock (defibrillation) delivered to the heart to convert to an effective heartbeat.

Author's Disclaimer Regarding Cardiopulmonary Resuscitation

The information being presented in this chapter was written and designed to be presented as an introduction to cardiopulmonary resuscitation. If you do participate in any of the activities and procedures covered in this chapter, in order to receive the most up-to-date and current information regarding CPR, the author recommends that you contact your local American Heart Association or American Red Cross.

Cardiopulmonary resuscitation, or CPR, is an important skill for everyone working in the hospital or clinical setting. It is particularly important for individuals, who work as members of the respiratory therapy team. The Joint Commission for Accreditation of Hospitals suggests that all hospital personnel, especially those with patient care responsibilities, should be certified in CPR.

Both the American Heart Association and the American Red Cross provide CPR courses for people in all walks of life. To become certified, you must pass either the AHA or ARC basic life support course.

CPR certification must be renewed yearly. The skills that you will be required to learn can only be learned properly through the use of mannequins and through performance practice with a qualified instructor.

Adult One-Person CPR

Adult one-person CPR should only be used when there is one rescuer involved. To provide one-person CPR, it is recommended that you follow the guidelines listed below:

1. *Shake and shout!* If you encounter someone who appears to be unconscious, gently shake his or her shoulders and ask, "Are you okay?" This is to establish unresponsiveness, and to make sure that the person is not just sleeping.
2. *Call out for help!* Maybe someone will hear and come to assist you.
3. *Position the victim.* Gently move the victim onto his or her back, being careful to support the head and neck.
4. *Start CPR!*
5. *Open the airway.* It is recommended that the head tilt–chin lift maneuver be used.
6. *Check for breathing.* Sometimes all that is needed is for the airway to be opened, and the victim will begin breathing spontaneously on his or her own. You must look, listen, and feel. Look for chest movement, listen for air movement, and feel for breathing by placing your cheek next to the victim's nose.
7. *Begin rescue breathing.* If there is no breathing, maintain the airway position, pinch the nose, and give four quick breaths using the mouth-to-mouth method.
8. *Check for a pulse.* Using the tips of your fingers, check the victim's carotid artery, located on the neck, for a pulse.

9. *Activate the emergency medical services system.* Designate a specific person to call the ambulance. If you are still alone, perform CPR for 1 minute, and then call for help.
10. *Begin chest compressions.* If your victim does not have a pulse, begin chest compressions at a ratio of 15 : 2 (15 compressions to 2 breaths). Be certain that your hand placement is correct according to AHA and ARC Standards.

Adult Two-Person CPR

The procedure for performing adult two-person CPR is exactly the same as for one-person CPR until chest compression is begun. With two-person CPR, the ratio of compressions to rescue breathing is 5 : 1, or 5 compressions to 1 breath.

Adult (Obstructed Airway)

If the rescuer is unable to ventilate the victim, that is, make the victim's chest rise, he or she should follow the guidelines listed below:

1. *Reposition the head and open the airway.* Try to ventilate the victim again. If unsuccessful,
2. *Activate the EMS.*
3. *Apply four back blows in rapid succession.*
4. *Apply four manual thrusts.*
5. *Apply the finger sweep to remove any debris.*
6. *Reposition the head.* Attempt to ventilate again. If successful, continue CPR. If unsuccessful, repeat the whole sequence.

CPR for Infants and Children

The basic procedure for performing CPR is the same for an infant or child as it is for an adult, with the following differences:

1. Rescue breathing may be done mouth to mouth and nose in an infant or small child.
2. The breathing rate is faster, once every 3 seconds, or 20 times per minute for infants. It is once every 4 seconds, or 15 times per minute for children.
3. An infant's pulse should be checked at the brachial artery, located on the inside of the upper arm, rather than at the carotid artery, as for adults.
4. The hand position is two fingers at mid-sternum, rather than two hands, as for adults.
5. The compression rate is faster for infants.

A Final Note on Performing CPR

To learn how to administer CPR properly, you must practice the techniques involved thoroughly on mannequins in order to build your skill development and speed. CPR is an urgent procedure and must be implemented with speed and skill.

As a member of the health care delivery team, you are urged to enroll in a CPR course with your in-hospital instructor or contact your local American Heart Association or American Red Cross in order to find out when the next CPR course will be taught, or when one can be provided to your class.

Summary

In this chapter, we dealt specifically with cardiopulmonary resuscitation, or CPR, noting that it was extremely important for all health care providers to check with their local American Red Cross or American Heart Association to make sure they receive the latest and most up-to-date information on the implementation of CPR. We briefly talked about the procedures involved in administering adult one-person and two-person CPR, assisting an adult with an obstructed airway, and administering CPR to an infant or a child.

Review Questions

1. Define the following abbreviations:

   a. ACLS _____
   b. AHA _____
   c. CPR _____
   d. EMS _____
   e. BLS _____
   f. ARC _____

2. Briefly explain what an *obstructed airway* is.

3. Briefly explain what *ventricular fibrillation* is.

4. What is the ratio for performing one-person CPR on an adult? On a child?

5. What is the ratio for performing two-person CPR on an adult? On a child?

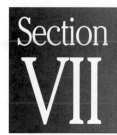

Section

VII

Administrative Skills in Cardiovascular Technology: Concepts and Applications

32

Administrative Management and Office Maintenance

Performance Objectives

Upon completion of this chapter, you will be able to:

1. Discuss factors that influence the effectiveness of an administrative medical office environment.
2. Describe the purpose of maintaining all areas within a health care facility or medical office.
3. Explain why it is important to maintain an equipment maintenance program.
4. Discuss the purpose and function of a supply and inventory ordering system.
5. Identify responsibilities of the cardiovascular worker as they relate to drugs and their storage in a department or health care facility.
6. Discuss the purpose and function of a department office procedure manual.

Terms and Abbreviations

EPA abbreviation for the Environmental Protection Agency, a government agency responsible for outlining the correct procedures and products required by all health care facilities, to help them avoid accidents and hazardous conditions to both patients and medical staff personnel.

Inventory a list of all supplies and equipment on hand in an individual department or health care facility, usually updated either on a monthly or annual basis.

Office procedure manual a written guide kept in an individual department, a private medical office, or a health care facility, which provides information related to all office procedures and routines.

PDR abbreviation for *Physician's Desk Reference*, a guide to all pharmaceutical drugs.

Preventative maintenance in health care, pertains to a maintenance contract that can be purchased for specific equipment, in which a service person comes to the department or facility on a regular basis to check the equipment and, if necessary, make minor adjustments, and repairs.

Whether you are employed in an individual department within a health care facility or by a private medical doctor, you should understand that care for the physicial environment in which you work is the responsibility of all members of the staff. A facility that is adequately lit and maintains a temperature that is comfortable and pleasant to all members of the staff and the patients, is a much healthier and more enjoyable place to work.

As you progress through your career in cardiovascular technology, you may be given the opportunity to manage a department or even a private practice. If you can show your supervisor that you possess both the leadership qualities required of a supervisor, as well as the committment to not just perform your job, but just as important, increase the productivity of both your work and your employer, you may find yourself in a very exciting and rewarding management position.

Physical Maintenance of the Health Care Environment

Maintenance of both a healthy and a comfortable environment is a task often delegated to the administrative medical worker; however, in most individual departments within a hospital or clinic, it also becomes the responsibility of all members of the health care team. As a member of this team, it is important for you to become sensitive not only to the basic housekeeping duties of the facility, but to other factors that influence both the staff and the patients in their quest to feel comfortable in the facility.

When dealing with the physical maintenance of a health care facility, there are four areas that you must be concerned with. These include *lighting*, *sound*, *temperature*, and *flooring*.

All health care facilities require excellent lighting in order to accomplish the daily tasks required of the facility. The best lighting is generally uniform, and in the case of most medical facilities uses fluorescent lights. If you are working for a private physician, you may want to maintain the reception area by using separate lamps strategically placed throughout the area. If you are using separate lamps, you must also remember to place them at reading level, where the light will not shine into the eyes of the reader or other patients waiting to see the doctor.

In planning for an effective maintenance program for your department or office, you will also need to be concerned with ensuring the privacy of all patients coming into the facility. This means maintaning a facility in which there is adequate soundproofing of walls in order to prevent confidences between patients and medical staff from being overheard. If you find that talking and conversations can be heard through the walls or between treatment or examination rooms, you will need to be sensitive to it, and let your supervisor or the doctor know as soon as possible.

One area in which patients seem to be most concerned is the proper maintenance of the facility's temperature. For most facilities, 70°F seems to be the optimum temperature for the patient reception area. If your facility or department treats a number of senior citizens, you may want to recommend that the office be kept at a temperature that is a little higher. It is also important to maintain the correct flow of air throughout the facility. Air should be kept circulating, either by an air conditioning system or by open win-

dows. You must, however, be careful not to allow drafts to enter the facility, as many patients are very intolerant of them and may become quite uncomfortable.

The last area that you must be concerned with in dealing with the physical maintenance of your facility has to do with the adequacy of your facility's flooring. In most cases, carpeting is used to cover the floor in a reception room and office area. In treatment and examination rooms, however, washable flooring is often used for hygienic purposes. When working in areas that are not covered by carpeting, it is important to make sure that these areas are not covered by a slippery wax coating that could ultimately cause both patients and staff members to slip and fall. Additionally, it is never a good idea to use rugs in the treatment or exam rooms, especially if they are not tacked down, since they can be easily moved, creating the possibility of patients or members of your staff tripping or falling.

Cleaning and Maintenance

As a professional health care provider, your duties will not require you to be responsible for the heavy-duty cleaning of your facility; however, you may be responsible for performing basic cleaning tasks that involve the maintenance and "top cleaning" of such areas of your department or facility as the reception and administrative areas, the clinical areas, such as the lab, examination, and treatment rooms, the restrooms, and storage areas. These tasks may include such things as picking up toys and magazines in the reception area and performing minor housekeeping duties that keep the reception area clean, tidy, pleasant, and free from odors.

If your job also includes basic maintenance and cleaning of other administrative and clinical areas, you will need to consult with your supervisor as to what is required. You may be responsible for the reception desk, the telephone, various business machines, and record storage areas. If this is indeed the case, you should make sure that steps are taken to keep desks neat and items are not moved out of their original place. All records should be kept out of sight of patients in order to assure complete privacy. Remember, an organized and well-maintained office gives both your patients and your coworkers the immediate impression that you are in control and that your facility runs in an efficient and effective manner.

Maintaining the Clinical Areas

Maintaining the clinical areas of a department or a private health care facility generally involves the basic cleaning and organization of treatment and examination rooms, the laboratory, restrooms, and storage areas. There is nothing more upsetting and devastating to a patient who may already be anxious than being ushered into a treatment or examination room that is completely disorganized or dirty. This means taking responsibility for seeing to the appropriate cleaning and removal of specimens of prior patients before new ones enter the room, providing areas which are spotless and free of clutter, such as soiled linen, towels, and tissues, and making sure that all examining tables have clean, fresh paper or linen on them before the patient enters the room.

One of the best and perhaps easiest ways to ensure the proper maintainence of your facility is to perform periodic checks of the facility's physical appearance and cleanliness. These periodic services generally include replacing light bulbs, cleaning out refrigerators, reorganizing cabinets and drawers, and watering plants. Most health care facilities have a specific plan for assigning such infrequent and basic tasks. Your responsibility will be to make sure that you are clear on what is assigned to *you,* and follow through when such duties are assigned.

Maintenance and Care of Equipment

If you are working in an individual department of a health care facility or are employed by a small private medical office, chances are you may be responsibile for maintaining the service agreements for equipment used by your facility. These agreements are usually kept in individual files, along with instructions for their proper maintenance, operating instructions, and invoices for repairs that might be necessary.

Another aspect of maintaining and caring for equipment is controlling supplies used in the facility. Most facilities have a variety of supplies that need to be counted, or inventoried, on a monthly or annual basis. Inventories are listings of all equipment and supplies found in the facility. They contain valuable information that may be needed for preparing income taxes, and other information that might be necessary for providing specific details regarding equipment that has been stolen or damaged.

The time an inventory is taken will depend upon the needs of your individual facility. In most cases, all capital purchases, such as furniture, medical equipment and instruments, laboratory equipment, office machines, and large decor items, such as wall paintings, are inventoried on an annual basis. Other smaller, less costly items, such as syringes and thermometers, may be inventoried more frequently.

All inventory systems generally include a method of ordering supplies. If you are responsible for completing the inventory, chances are that you will also be responsible for ordering supplies. Most of these supplies are itemized into three categories: *office supplies*, which include stationery, accounting supplies, desk items, and appointment materials; *medical supplies*, which often include such disposable items as gowns, drapes, towels, lubricants, tongue blades, syringes and needles, bandages, and in some cases, medications; and *general supplies*, which usually consist of such items as soap and towels for the restrooms, tissues, cleaning supplies, and coffee for the employees.

It is important to keep separate forms for each individual category of supplies. Each form should provide you with information and space for diminishing supplies, so that you will know when it is time to reorder. Oftentimes, salespeople, or "detail" men or women will come by your department or office, which will make your ordering a great deal easier. Mail-order houses are also available that will allow your facility to provide your orders over the telephone.

Maintenance and Storage of Drugs and Medications

Depending upon your position and employer, in some instances, you may be responsible for the proper maintenance and storage of drugs and medications used in your facility. This is often the case in situations in which the cardiovascular worker is employed by a clinic or a private medical office. If you are responsible for maintaining the storage of drugs and medications, you should start by keeping an accurate inventory of what is on hand, making sure that all drugs are accounted for and that supplies do not run out. This may mean that you may also be in charge of contacting a pharmacy or drug salesperson to plan an order.

Some smaller medical offices keep a low inventory of drugs and medications and generally rely on free samples provided to them by drug companies. Other offices, such as those not as accessible to the drug supplier, may keep larger inventories. Drug and medication supplies in hospitals are often kept in a locked drug cart or storage area within the nursing station.

In many cases, different drug companies may provide your facility with their own ordering system. Their salespeople, who are often referred to as "pharmaceutical representatives" or "detail representatives," can be given access to the drug storage area and stock the drugs themselves. If your department or facility does not allow this practice, you may be responsible for restocking and checking the expiration dates in order to make sure that your facility is not giving out expired medications. If a patient has a drug reaction and notices that the drug has expired, there may be a great potential for a lawsuit.

Depending upon your job duties and responsibilities, you may also be responsible for organizing the drug storage area. All drugs can be organized by their name in an alphabetical system. They can also be organized according to the system listed in the *PDR*, or *Physician's Desk Reference*, as to their classifications. Categories in the *PDR* include such areas as analgesics, antiemetics, cardiogenics, and antibiotics.

No matter where you work, accidents do happen, and the proper storage and usage of drugs and medications in the health care facility, is no exception. If, for example, during storage a drug's label is accidently removed, the drug in its package should be immediately discarded. Most can either be poured down a drain or flushed down the toilet. They should never be left in the trash where unauthorized people can easily take them. Of course, when drugs are discarded, you must always keep a careful record as to their disposition.

Maintaining the Office Procedure Manual

All health care facilities, individual departments, and private medical offices keep procedural manuals that provide important information regarding everything from office tasks to in-depth instructions for performing various clinical treatments and procedures. An office manual must be kept up to date, and doing so is often the responsibility of the office or department manager. In addition to providing information regard-

ing how specific procedures are performed, manuals often contain job descriptions to help guide each staff member in performing his or her specific tasks. A well-designed manual makes clear to all employees what exactly is expected of them. It is also a valuable document for training new employees and can provide assistance to a substitute employee.

Updating of all office and procedure manuals, including job descriptions, is mandatory in our rapidly changing health care environments. If you are responsible for maintaining these manuals, you should ask each staff member to assist you by updating his or her assignment listings. Remember that suggestions from the entire staff can be used to create the most current manual possible.

Summary

In this chapter, we discussed the factors that most effectively influenced the efficiency of the administrative medical office environment, noting that maintenance of the facility is the key to efficiency of a smooth-running facility. We also talked about how such maintenance is performed, including how to maintain the physical and hygienic appearance of the facility, how to maintain a running inventory and ordering system for supplies and equipment, and how to store and order drugs and medications properly. Finally, we discussed the importance of the office procedure manual, noting that such manuals must be kept updated as to job descriptions, employee tasks, and instructions pertaining to specific procedures and treatments, on a regular, ongoing basis.

Review Questions

1. What branch of the federal government is responsible for outlining the correct procedures and products required by all health care facilities, in order to help them avoid accidents?

2. What does the abbreviation *PDR* mean?

3. Briefly explain the concept of *preventative maintenance*.

4. A(n) _____ is a list of all supplies and equipment on hand in an individual department or health

care facility, and which is usually updated either on a monthly or annual basis.

5. Briefly explain the maintainence and storage of drugs and medications in a department or private medical office.

6. What is the purpose of an *office procedure manual?*

7. Who is generally responsible for maintaining the office procedure manual?

33

Administrative Management and Communications

Performance Objectives

Upon completion of this chapter, you will be able to:

1. Discuss how to receive and direct patients, their family members, and visitors.
2. Explain how to communicate effectively using the telephone, a pager, and an intercom system.
3. Describe and be able to demonstrate how to record telephone messages.
4. Explain how to receive mail and process outgoing mail in the health care setting.
5. Discuss the purpose of making duplicate copies in the health care setting.
6. Briefly explain how to prepare monthly statements.

Terms and Abbreviations

Beeper also referred to as a personal pocket pager; an electronic device that is carried by a person and can be activated by a radio signal in order to produce a "beep" or buzzing sound.
Fax (facsimile) a machine designed to transmit information or a document over telephone lines to a terminal.
Intercom also referred to as an intercommunication system, which is used to send and receive messages, using a loudspeaker and a microphone at each location.
Paging a process by which a loudspeaker system is used to summon a person by name, number, or beeper to a telephone.

Screening mail the process of separating mail into specific categories.
Screening telephone calls the process used to identify a telephone caller before permitting him or her to speak to the person who called, and then referring or handling the call in the correct manner.
Statements requests for payment for services performed or rendered.
Transfer the process of switching a caller to another telephone number in a facility.

The patient's first contact with a health care facility almost always occurs in the reception area. The receptionist, whether he or she works in a private doctor's office, the business office of a large medical facility, or a single department within a hospital, must be prompt, friendly, tactful, and knowledgeable in dealing with people. In general, most people will be cooperative, keep their appointments, and pay their bills as obligated. In general, all patients prefer to have a relaxed and friendly relationship with the people they encounter in the health care facility, and

such a relationship starts with the very first person they encounter.

Receiving and Dealing with Patients, Family Members, and Visitors

Health care workers who are assigned to work in the administrative or reception area of a clinic or private medical office, are generally responsible for reviewing the appointment sheet either at the beginning of each new day, or prior to that day (Figure 33-1). This is important because this person must be aware of which patients are expected into the office. If you are uncertain as to who is expected into your facility, and in some cases, how their name is pronounced, you may want to consult with your coworkers. In fact, you may even want to write down a phonetic pronounciation in order to help you to better address the patient.

If you are the first person who is responsible for making contact with the patient, you may want to follow the guidelines listed below:

· If possible, always call the person by his or her last name, for example, "Mrs. Green," or "Mr. Jones."
· If a person who is not scheduled suddenly appears at your facility, you must still appear gracious and find out why the patient has arrived;

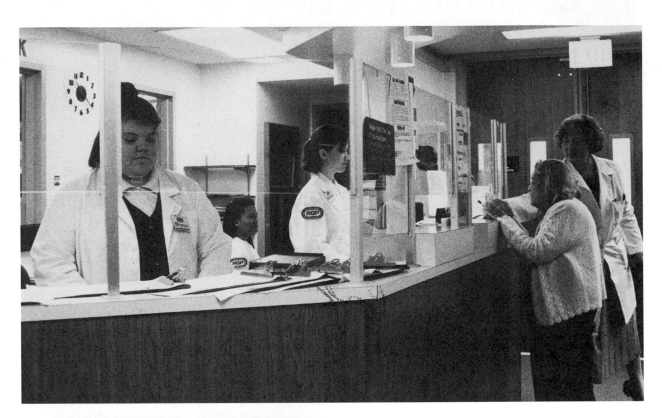

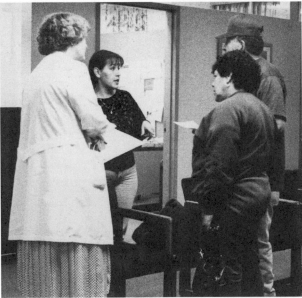

Figure 33-1
Receiving family members and patients.

for example, you might say "Good afternoon, Mr. Jones. How may I help you?"

· If a person makes a request without giving you his or her name, you should pleasantly inquire as to the person's name; for example, "May I have your name please?"

· Never call the patient by his or her first name unless you are certain this familiarity is acceptable; older patients may expect to be addressed as "Mr." or "Mrs." by members of the office or department who are younger than they are.

· It is generally acceptable to call children and teenagers by their first names.

· Whenever possible, you should always wear a name tag, since this is a considerate gesture and allows new patients to learn your name quickly.

· If there must be a delay in an appointment, explain the reason to the patient as soon as possible, and estimate the length of time that may be involved.

In addition to following the guidelines listed above, you should try to get into the practice of never allowing a patient to feel hurried. On the other hand, neither can you allow anyone to consume long periods of time in needless conversation. It is important for you to learn to read behavior and to be able to work with patients so that each individual patient looks forward to a visit in your office or department.

Dealing with Family Members and Visitors in the Hospital

If you are required to work in the administrative or reception area of your individual department, you may be required to provide information and assistance to family members and visitors of patients in the hospital. Try to make everyone you encounter feel that you are there to serve. Many relatives and friends are already worried about the illness of their loved ones. They may seem angry or upset. Your job is to be as courteous and polite as possible. Some family members may ask you questions or made demands that are not within your scope of practice to respond too. Listen to them politely. Some demands may be valid, while some may not be. Always refer medical inquiries to the patient's doctor, and try not to become involved in any private family matters or disputes.

Whenever you are dealing with family members and visitors of patients in the hospital, it is also very important to remember to respect the confidentiality of all information that may be relayed to you by the patient's family friends. All patient information is confidential. If a member of the patient's family or his or her friends persist on asking you questions pertaining to the patient, inform the person that the physician will discuss the patient's condition and progress with those entitled to know.

Communication Systems Used in the Health Care Environment

Telephone Techniques

The telephone is an essential communication tool that is used in all health care settings. It, along with personal paging systems and remote mobile telephones, are the most rapid means of communication. All members of the health care delivery team are responsibile for learning how to properly answer, transfer, and respond to telephone calls, as well as accurately record and relay messages to the appropriate person.

The most common type of telephone used in most health care facilities and physician's offices is the multibutton or multiline telephone (Figure 33-2). This type of telephone allows calls to come in and go out at the same time. A lighted button generally indicates that a line is in use.

When a call comes in on the multibutton system, the telephone will ring, and the line will be indicated by a lighted button. When this occurs, you should depress the button, lift the receiver, and answer the call.

When answering the telephone, always identify the name of the health care facility or deparment, followed by your own name. For example, if you are working in the ECG Department, you may say, "ECG Department, Mrs. Jones speaking."

If you are required to place an outgoing call, always plan what you want to say prior to placing the call. Think about what questions you are going to ask and what points you want to cover with the caller. Al-

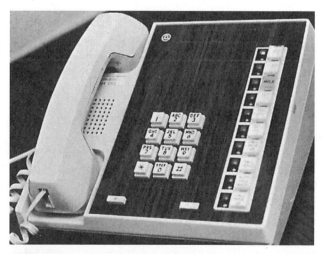

Figure 33-2
The multiline telephone system. (Reprinted with permission from LaFleur, M. W. and Starr, W. K. *Health Unit Coordinating*, 2nd ed. Philadelphia: W. B. Saunders, 1986, p 44.)

ways have a pen or pencil and paper close by, in case you want to make some notes. Also, you may need to decide the time at which the person you are calling is most likely to be available. All of your calls, of course, should be made during business hours, and you should never use the business or department's telephone to make personal calls.

If you are using a multibutton or multiline telephone system, and you wish to place a call, punch an unlighted button, pick up the receiver, and punch in the number. Identify yourself and your department and the name of the health care facility as soon as you reach the desired number. Give the reason for your call. If you must ask any questions, always make sure that they are asked in a tactful manner, yet to the point. At the end of the call, make sure that you take time to express thanks for the call recipient's time and response to any questions. You should end the conversation with a simple "good-bye." Replace the telephone receiver quietly, and remember, that the caller is the person who should end the call.

Holding and Transferring Telephone Calls

The "hold" button is used to close off one call from all the other lines. To place a call on hold, simply pick up the receiver and ask the caller if he or she would please hold. If the person cannot hold, offer to call back. When the caller agrees to hold, depress the key two to three seconds and then release it. A flashing light generally indicates that the line is on hold.

It is important to return to the caller often with a progress report, such as "I'm still looking for your report," or "Dr. Smith will be with you as soon as possible." Get the caller's attention when you return to the line by saying, "Thank you for holding." If you do not use a hold button, remember that the caller can hear everything you say.

If at all possible, try to help the caller. If you cannot, offer to transfer the call to someone who can. Tell the caller why you must transfer and to whom he or she should speak. In most cases, your facility will have a specific procedure for you to follow in order to transfer calls. If not, you can generally assist the caller by dialing the new number or by going through the facility's switchboard operator.

Telephone Etiquette

Whenever you are required to speak on the telephone, you should remember that the listener is the person who immediately forms an impression of you and your entire facility. A good telephone personality imparts friendliness, concern, sincerity, and helpfulness. The caller should be made to feel that the call is important to you.

Your telephone call will be much more effective if you also remember to use short, simple, business-like descriptive words, such as "yes" and "of course," instead of "OK" or "sure." You should also try to avoid the use of abbreviations or lengthy terms that the caller may not understand. Never use slang. Always try to be brief if the situation requires an explanation, and remember to use "please" and "thank you" during your conversation. When speaking on the telephone, use a normal conversational tone, and if at all possible, use the person's name during your discussion. Also, try to remember to speak directly into the mouthpiece so that your words will be clear and distinct.

Oftentimes, if you are answering your department's telephone or if you are working in the reception area of the private medical office, you may be required to take a message. If this is indeed the case, always make sure you have a message pad and pen or pencil closely at hand. Make notes as you receive information, and if you are not certain that you understand, ask to have the information repeated. If names are unusual, verify the spelling, and always be sure that the telephone number and dates are correct. You may even want to repeat the entire message back to the caller in order to ensure the accuracy.

Information on a telephone message should always include the date and time of the call, as well as the name and telephone number of the caller. In some cases, it may also be necessary to record the caller's address. And above all, always make sure you record an accurate message and any action that the caller may require. The message recording is generally completed by making sure that the person who recorded it also initials it at the bottom of the message form.

Screening Telephone Calls

Screening telephone calls deals with first identifying the caller before permitting him or her to speak to the person called. While this is a common practice in many health care facilities and private doctor's offices, many callers often find it irritating. If screening is practiced where you work, never say, "who's calling please?" Instead, answering the caller with "may I tell him or her who's calling, please?" tends to be less disturbing to the caller. Screening also involves handling the call correctly by relaying it to the person or to someone else, or obtaining information for calling back. Acceptable phrases such as "she's not at her desk," or "he's out of the office for a few minutes," are often used during the screening process.

Paging Systems

Large medical centers and health care facilities often have a telephone switchboard, referred to as a PBX board, that employs an operator responsible for controlling the flow of telephone communications throughout the facility. Paging of physicians, directors of departments, and emergency personnel is generally done through this system. *Paging* deals with the use of a loudspeaker system to summon a person by his or her name or number to the telephone.

At night, or during holidays, many hospitals and private physician's offices also use a telephone answering service. In these cases, the telephone operator takes information from the caller and notifies the doctor, who in turn returns the patient's call.

Most physicians and other hospital personnel often carry a small beeper. A *beeper* or small pocket pager, is an electronic device that can be easily activated by a radio signal in order to produce a "beep" or buzzing sound. Each person has an individual call

number that can be activated by the PBX operator or the telephone answering service, and the individual carrying the pager can then be alerted to telephone the hospital or office.

Intercom Systems

An *intercom* system is a type of communication system that allows both patients and your coworkers or other staff members to communicate with one another throughout different areas within a health care facility (Figure 33-3). For each location at which the intercom is used, there must also be a loudspeaker and a microphone. These systems can be used either in a doctor's office to communicate between examining rooms or between examining rooms and offices,

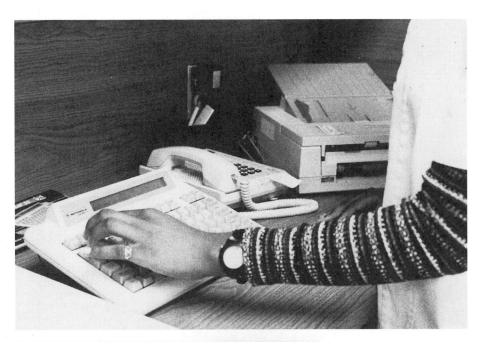

Figure 33-3
The intercom system.

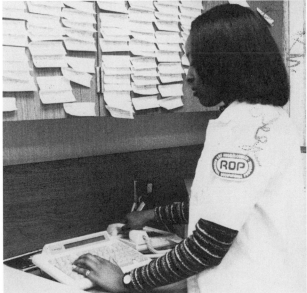

or, as they are most often used, in the hospital setting. In the hospital, the intercom is generally located at the nurse's station, and is almost always accompanied by a patient's call light system. The panel connects to a signal cord that has been attached to a wall panel near the head of the bed in the patients' rooms. The end of the cord has a button that the patient can use in order to flash a light on the panel. Once the signal has been activated by the patient from his or her room, the health unit coordinator or the person in charge of running the nurse's station should immediately respond to the signal by turning it off and answering the patient's request.

Intercoms, like telephones, are also considered to be a "first line" of communication between the patient and the health care professional; therefore, it is important that whenever you are responding to the patient via the intercom system, you should address the patient by his or her name. Once you have answered the patient's signal, it is just as important to provide the assistance as requested, or relay the message to the appropriate person. Also, don't forget to cancel the call at the nurses' station once you have completed your communication.

Communicating by Fax Machines

A type of communication system that has recently become valuable within the health care setting because of its ability to send documents from place to place via the telephone, is the fax machine. A *fax*,

or *facsimile machine*, is designed to copy a document placed in it and then transmit the information over telephone lines to a waiting terminal (Figure 33-4). A major advantage of the fax machine is that all types of records can be easily transmitted to physicians or to medical records rooms from any location.

Processing Written Communications Within the Health Care Environment

If you are ever involved in the day-to-day administrative tasks of your department or your individual health care facility, you will soon discover that being part of the health information management team also includes the processing of mail and other types of written communication. Such tasks always require that you use great speed, accuracy, and efficiency in your work. Processing mail involves both incoming and outgoing mail. No matter what department or facility you are working in, you must also remember that all correspondence from your facility or department must be grammatically correct and neat in appearance. All incoming mail must be conveyed to the addressee and dealt with in order of priority.

Processing Outgoing Mail

It is always important to establish some type of central collection point for processing all outgoing mail. All correspondence should be deposited there

Figure 33-4
The fax machine.

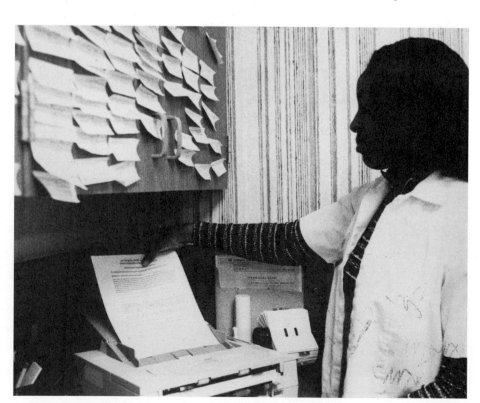

so that it can be easily picked up by a postal worker for delivery to a post office.

Most of the mail that you will be processing includes correspondence that generally falls under one of five categories. These include informational correspondence, referrals, reminders, account due statements, and interoffice mail. *Informational* correspondence is generally used to request or provide information to a patient regarding his or her care or treatment. *Referrals* are often used between one health care professional and another in order to request the second professional to examine an individual patient. A *reminder* is a type of correspondence that can be used either to inform the patient that it is time for a periodic examination or provide the time and date of the patient's next scheduled appointment. *Account due* statements are "friendly" reminders to a patient that his or her account is past due. *Interoffice mail* is a type of office memorandum and usually includes all memos and correspondence between members of your depeartment or your individual health care facility.

Most health care facilities require that all mail first be presorted into specific categories before the mail can be sent out. These categories generally include local mail, out-of-town mail, and metered mail. Bulk mail is also sorted according to zip codes. First-class and third-class mail is often separated before it is processed and mailed.

Postage Meters

Some health care facilities with a large volume of daily mail, often choose to use postage meters to help save time and facilitate the processing of their mail. When a postage meter is used, payment for postage is made in advance to the post office, and the machine is set. The postage meter imprints postage on envelopes, and then records the amount used on a meter. The date on the imprinter must be changed daily. All mail that is metered is generally stacked separately, with all addresses facing in the same direction, and five or more pieces, according to U.S. Postal regulations, must be bundled together.

Types of Mail

The U.S. Postal Service offers health care facilities many different types of mail services. If you know that you will be required to process mail as part of your responsibilities, you should become familiar with the various classifications of mail and how to use the services offered by the postal service.

There are nine types of services offered by the postal service. These include mail that is classified into first-, second-, third-, and fourth-class, special delivery mail, certified and registered mail, express mail, and mailgrams. *First-class mail* consists of letters, business reply mail, bills, and statements of accounts. *Second-class mail* includes all newspapers and published periodicals. *Third-class mail* includes all books, catalogs, and printed materials weighing less than 1 pound. *Fourth-class mail* is made up of printed matter and packages weighing more than 1 pound. *Special delivery mail*, which can be delivered 7 days a week, including holidays and weekends, may be purchased for all classes of mail for which the doctor or facility wishes to ensure a rapid delivery from the post office.

Mail that is sent either certified or registered means that the sender wishes to go one step further to ensure the prompt and exact delivery of the mail. *Certified mail* offers the sender proof of both mailing and reception. The sender receives a receipt, and the receiving post office keeps a record of the delivery on a receipt signed by the addressee. *Registered mail* goes a little farther by assigning a registration number to each item being mailed. The item's value must be specified, and the sender receives a receipt, while the receiver or addressee is required to sign upon the delivery.

The post office's fastest service is called *express mail*. Special labels are provided for each item being sent by express mail, and the item is required to be received by the post office before a specified time (usually before 5:00 p.m.) at the express window for delivery by 3:00 p.m. the following day.

A *mailgram* is a combination of a night telegram service and a postal service, and is not often used, except in situations where the facility must notify the addressee during an "off hour" of regular mail service delivery.

Processing Incoming Mail

If you are working for a private physician, you will find that in most cases, doctors require their administrative staff person to screen their mail and separate those items that require immediate attention. Any mail marked *personal* or *confidential* is usually given to the physician unopened, unless he or she has predesignated another member of the staff to open such mail. Other mail must be sorted, opened, and directed to the appropriate person for action.

Opening, Removing, and Dating Mail

When mail is first received, it must be placed on the desk in a specific order for easy recognition and for opening. The order for opening is (1) telegrams,

(2) special delivery letters, (3) regular mail, (4) advertisements, and (5) magazines, newspapers, and other periodicals. If there are only a few letters, they may be opened with a hand letter opener. If there are many, you may want to use an electronic letter-opening machine. To use most electronic letter-opening machines, you must first turn the envelopes upside down lightly to get the top edges even, and then run them through the machine for opening.

To remove mail from an envelope, you must first place the opened edge to the right. Remove the letter, unfold it, and carefully fasten any enclosures to it. If the enclosures mentioned in the letter are missing, you must write the word "NO" beside the enclosure notation in the margin of the letter. If a letter is opened by mistake, it should be resealed with tape, and marked "Opened by Mistake," and initialed.

All mail that is to be opened must be checked to ensure that the name and return address of the sender are provided in the letter. If not, the envelope should be attached to the back of the letter and not discarded. Other reasons to save an envelope include incorrectly addressed envelopes, return address in the letter appears different from that on the envelope, no signature is found in the letter, the letter date appears different from the date stamped on the envelope by the postal service, an enclosure mentioned has not been included in the envelope, and a letter containing a bid, an offer, or acceptance of a contract. It is always important to keep the envelope, since it could be needed as legal evidence should the need arise.

In addition to properly removing and categorizing mail, some health care facilities also require that all incoming mail be dated as to when it was received. If this is the case, a rubber stamp or dating machine generally provides dating. If your facility does require this procedure, information included usually consists of the date, time, and other departmental information. If you are using a dating method, you must also remember never to allow the stamped date to cover any other information.

Processing Incoming Payments

In some cases, you may find that payments for services rendered by your department or facility may arrive as part of your daily incoming mail. If this is the case, remember that all payments received should be handled immediately. Cash payments should be counted as soon as you receive them, and then recorded, so that the prompt credit is given. Checks should be endorsed immediately, using a "For Deposit Only" stamp, and then credited to the patient's account, and held for your routine deposits.

Office Machines Used in the Health Care Environment

In addition to computers and fax machines, there are two types of office machines that are frequently used in the health care environment. These are the office duplicating or copying machine, and the office calculator. In many health care facilities, a fax machine may be used to duplicate documents going to distant points. However, when copies are needed locally, you may be required to use a photocopier for duplicating specific patient data or other types of office or departmental communications. A *photocopier* or *copying machine* is a device that makes a photographic reproduction of printed material. Copiers may have other capabilities, such as printing on both sides of a sheet of paper, sorting pages, printing overhead transparencies, and printing on various sizes and types of paper stock.

When more than one person or department is required to share patient data, you may be able to provide such information more rapidly and accurately. All health care workers should be familiar with the machines so that they can troubleshoot minor disruptions in a service.

Some health care facilities, generally those that choose to perform their own billing and insurance services, often use an electronic calculator to process numbers. *Calculators* perform the basic functions of mathematics, that is, addition, subtraction, multiplication, and division. Some calculators also have the ability to provide the user with a spreadsheet that may be needed for accounting services. If you are the person required to perform any of the billing services in your facility, it would be in your best interests to learn how to use the calculator from the operations manual provided by your employer. However, you must also remember that all health information must be accurate. This means, that even if you do use the calculator to perform your mathematical equations, you must still check all your work. If your calcultor has paper tape for recording, you can easily check the calculations comparing them with the printed hard copy found on the paper tape.

Summary

In this chapter, we discussed the importance of knowing that the patient's very first contact with any health care facility, department, or private physician's office, is in the reception area or over the telephone. We also talked about how it is the responsibility of any person working in the administrative or clerical department to be prompt, friendly, tactful, and knowledgeable in dealing with people, noting, that besides dealing with the public personally or by telephone, this person must also be able to communicate by intercom or paging, and must be able to record messages for others properly and accurately.

In addition to talking about the telephone as a means of communication, we also discussed how the written word is a form of communication used by all health care facilities. This type of communication involves receiving and screening incoming mail, processing outgoing mail, recognizing types of mail and postal services, and imprinting with postage meters. Finally, we talked about different types of machines that can also be used in the health care facility, noting that such machines generally included a fax machine, photocopiers, and calculators.

Review Questions

1. Briefly explain the following communication systems used in a health care facility:

   a. beeper _____

   b. intercom _____

   c. paging _____

   d. fax _____

   e. telephone _____

2. Briefly explain the process of screening mail.

3. Briefly explain the process of screening telephone calls.

4. Briefly explain the process involved in holding and transferring telephone calls.

5. Define the following types of mail:

   a. first-, second-, third-, and fourth-class mail

   b. special delivery mail

   c. certified mail and registered mail

34

Billing and Banking Procedures

Performance Objectives

Upon completion of this chapter, you will be able to:

1. Discuss the purpose of banking procedures used in the health care environment.
2. Describe and be able to demonstrate, basic bookkeeping and billing principles and procedures used in the health care environment.
3. Identify the basic duties of the health care provider responsible for billing and banking procedures in the health care facility.

Terms and Abbreviations

A/C   abbreviation for *accounts payable*, that is, amounts owed to a creditor for regular business operating expenses.

A/R   abbreviation for *accounts receivable*, claims which arise from services rendered.

Assignment of benefits   an agreement by which a patient agrees to assign all insurance benefits over to another party, usually a medical care provider.

ATM   abbreviation for *automated teller machine*, a machine installed on the outside of a bank or other facility, allowing for deposits and withdrawals 24 hours a day.

Bank statement   a periodic list of transactions of a checking or savings account.

Bill   a statement of fees owed by a patient for services rendered.

Bookkeeping   the analysis and recording of business transactions that are necessary to report the financial condition of a business at a later date.

Check   an order for a bank to pay against an existing checking account.

Checking account   account against which checks can be written, often with no interest being paid.

CPT-4 Codes   abbreviation for current *Physician's' Procedural Terminology*, which is a listing of medical procedures and treatments.

Credit   a bookkeeping entry that shows payment from a patient, and that is entered on the right-hand side of an account.

Cycle billing   a billing procedure in which itemized statements are sent to patients according to an alphabetical breakdown.

Daily record   a record of daily business transactions; also called a *daybook* or a *day sheet*.

Debit   a bookkeeping entry for charges to a patient, which is entered on the left-hand side of an account; also referred to as a *liability*.

Deposit slip   a form used to itemize deposits made to a bank.

Disbursement   the chronological listing of monthly and yearly business expenses.

Double-entry system   a type of bookkeeping method that involves the maintenance of equality of both debits and credits.

DRGs   abbreviation for *diagnosis-related groups*, a classification coding system in which patients are grouped according to their diagnosis.

Endorsement   the process of signing one's name or the name of a business on the back of a check, indicating that all rights in the check are transferred to another party.

General ledger   a record containing all financial statement accounts.

HCPCS   abbreviation for *Health Care Financing Administration Common Procedures Coding System*, which is a coding system used primarily for Medicare insurance billing.

HMO   abbreviation for *health maintenance organization*, a health organization that offers prepaid medical services, generally with its major emphasis being on disease prevention.

ICD-9-CM Codes   abbreviation for *International Classification of Diseases, 9th Edition, Clinical Modification*, which is a coding system for classifying diseases and diagnoses.

Maker   the person who signs a check, ordering the bank to pay funds from an account; also known as the *payor*.

Medicaid   a government health insurance program that covers the indigent and people unable to pay for other insurance; also referred to as *MediCal* in California.

Medicare   a government health insurance program that provides coverage for people over the age of 65, and others with specific disabilities.

Medi-Medi   a patient receiving insurance coverage from both Medicare and Medicaid.

Payee   the person or institution named on a check who will receive the amount shown on the check; also known as the *bearer*.

Pegboard system   a type of bookkeeping system used in most health care facilities, which uses a lightweight board with pegs and forms layered one on top of the other.

Petty cash   a small amount of cash kept in a health care facility, which should only be available for small office expenses.

Postdated check   a check that has been dated for some time in the future, and which is not considered to be valid until the date noted on the check.

Professional courtesy   a discount or no-charge policy extended to certain people by a health care facility or a physician.

Provider   the person or institution who provides medical care.

Release of information   the process of a patient signing a form that allows information pertaining to him or her to be given out to an insurance company, attorney, or another third party; also known as an *authorization form* or *consent form*.

Service charge   a charge authorized by a banking institution, used for the purpose of maintaining accounts and processing transactions.

Single-entry system   a type of simple bookkeeping system that uses a daily record, checkbook, and an accounts receivable ledger.

Skip   a patient who has an outstanding bill, and who disappears, leaving no forwarding address.

Superbill   a comprehensive list of examinations, procedures, and treatments, and the corresponding fee listing, which a patient receives for services rendered.

Third party check   a check that has been made out to a patient from an unknown party.

Withholding   deductions made by an employer from an employee's paycheck.

Worker's compensation   a type of insurance program that provides both income and health care insurance coverage, and which has been established by law in each state to ensure employees against occupational diseases or job-related injuries or death.

I f you find yourself employed by a health care facility or a clinical department that deals with a number of patients, and you discover that part of your job description also includes billing, banking, and insurance processing, you will soon realize that being involved in these aspects of health care is one of the most challenging and in some cases most difficult tasks that may be required of your position.

In the health care industry, we often say that the person who takes care of the billing and banking is worth his or her weight in gold, because it is this person who is most responsible for ensuring the monetary livelihood of all the members of the health care team. This includes the doctor, the clinical and administrative staff, and yes, even yourself! It is the billing and banking person whose sole task generally evolves around seeing to it that bills and statements are sent out to patients, owed monies are paid out to the appropriate people and organizations, and employees are paid for their services.

Principles of Bookkeeping in the Health Care Environment

It is impossible for any business, including the business of delivering health care, to function effectively and efficiently without well-kept financial records. To be able to meet such a goal requires a person who is not only professional but also one who is capable of paying attention to details, well organized, and possesses the ability to maintain consistency throughout the completion of his or her workload.

If you are required to perform bookkeeping tasks in your facility, you must realize that to do so requires a well-established routine. You must also realize that there are certain guidelines, or principles, which are used in bookkeeping, and if you follow these rules, you should be able to perform your responsibilities in an orderly and efficient manner. The key principles of bookkeeping include:

- Always record all charges and receipts into the daily record immediately upon receiving them.
- Always endorse all checks as soon as they are collected.
- Make sure you prepare receipts in duplicate for all currency received.
- Be sure you pay all facility bills before they are due, and remember to record the date the bill was paid and the check number on the paid bill receipt.
- Post all charges and receipts to the general ledger on a daily basis.
- Deposit all monies received on a daily basis.
- Always check to make sure that the amount you have deposited into the bank, plus the money you have on hand in petty cash, equals the amount you have recorded in your daily ledger.

- Only use your petty cash fund for small expenses. Pay all other expenses by check, so that you will have an immediate record of the expenditure.
- Make all bookkeeping entries in ink, and always check your arithmetic to make sure you are keeping columns of figures straight and carrying decimals out correctly; *never* rely completely on a calculator!
- Never erase an error. If you find you have made an error, draw a straight line through the incorrect figure and then rewrite the correct figure above it.

Bookkeeping Systems

There are four basic types of bookkeeping systems employed by most health care facilities. These include *computerized* bookkeeping systems that utilize either a batch type of service or a telephone-linked service that is shared by others; a *single-entry* system, which is considered the easiest to use; a *double-entry* system, which involves the concept that assets minus liabilities always equals net worth; and the *pegboard* system, the most popular of all the systems, because of the ease at which bookkeeping procedures can be completed.

Accounts Receivable and Accounts Payable

All health care facilities must be concerned with accounts receivable and accounts payable. *Accounts receivable*, commonly abbreviated *A/R*, are monies or claims that arise as a result of services rendered. *Accounts payable*, or *A/P*, deal with monies or amounts owed to creditors for regular business operating expenses. When you are dealing with accounts receivable and accounts payable, you must also be concerned with the *accounts receivable control*, which is a summary performed on a daily basis of what remains unpaid on all the health care facility's accounts. An important point that you should remember too is that accounts receivable are an important and integral part of both the pegboard and the double-entry systems of bookkeeping; however, when you are using the single-entry system, accounts receivable are always given separate consideration.

Whatever is spent by your facility must also be recorded on a daily basis. These amounts are generally itemized on a form called a *disbursement record*. This record usually has columns for the date, name of supplier or vendor, amount of the charge, amount of the check and check number, deposits, and bank balance. In most cases, there are also columns for putting in a category for every business expense,

such as rent, taxes and licenses, dues and meetings, medical supplies and equipment, office expenses, utilities, travel, and employee payroll.

Petty Cash

If you work in a smaller private health care facility, such as a doctor's office or a clinic, there's a very good possibility that the facility will have a petty cash fund set aside for small office expenses, such as parking, postage fees, and less frequently used office supplies. Money should never be taken out of this fund for major expenses.

If you are using a petty cash fund, you will probably use some type of *petty cash voucher* system, which will help you to control your expenditures. The voucher provides space to record the expenditure date, the amount paid, the purpose, and the name of the person to whom the payment has been made. All vouchers should also be numbered.

If you are required to handle petty cash, chances are that your supervisor or employer will request that you become bonded by an insurance company. This guarantees payment of a specified amount to an employer in the event of financial loss caused by an employee.

Payroll and Employee Deductions

Payroll procedures, like bookkeeping methods, can be handled in a variety of ways, depending upon the type and size of health care facility in which you are employed. Some institutions may be set up for a bank to be responsible for handling all payroll, while others may hire an accountant to process the employee's payroll. Larger institutions, such as hospitals and multispecialty clinics, frequently have their payroll processed entirely by computer. This is the method of choice for many facilities, because the computer not only issues the payroll checks, but can also automatically calculate deductions for each employee.

If you are responsible for processing payroll, you will need to have a basic understanding of income tax laws and employment regulations. This means taking the time to learn about federal taxes, such as FICA; disability and unemployment insurance deductions; state tax deductions; and how to calculate an employee's gross salary into a net payroll check.

All payroll checks must include specific information regarding the employer's identification number, withholding allowance, FICA taxes, income tax deductions, unemployment compensation disability deductions, and unemployment taxes.

Employer's Identification Number and Employee's Withholding Allowance Certificate

An *employer identification number* is used for federal tax purposes. Form SS-4 from the Internal Revenue Service is used to receive this number. The employees use their Social Security number as their individual identification number. If an employee has no Social Security number, he or she must apply for a number immediately.

Upon employment, each new person hired by your facility must complete an *Employee's Withholding Allowance Certificate*, also known as a *Form W-4*. This form provides the employer with the number of exemptions claimed by the employee. Employees should be asked by December 1 of each year whether or not there has been a change in the number of exemptions since the last form filed the previous year.

FICA and Income Tax Deductions

The *Federal Insurance Contributions Act*, also known as Social Security, has three programs financed from one payroll tax in which employers and employees contribute at a rate as specified by the law. *Old Age Survivors Insurance (OASI)* provides senior citizens and their surviving dependents with retirement benefits, while *Medicare* provides them with hospitalization insurance. The *Disability Insurance Program (SDI)* provides workers who become disabled during their working years with insurance benefits.

Under federal law, all employers are required to withhold from their employee's salaries an advance payment on income taxes. This money is remitted periodically to a regional Internal Revenue Service office.

Unemployment Compensation Disability and Unemployment Taxes

Unemployment compensation disability deductions, which is a type of insurance policy that provides for temporary cash benefits for employees suffering a wage loss because of a non-work-related injury or illness, are mandatory in some states. At the present time, these states include California, Hawaii, New Jersey, New York, Puerto Rico, and Rhode Island. About 1 percent of an employee's gross salary goes to unemployment compensation disability by way of a monthly deduction.

Under the *Federal Unemployment Tax Act (FUTA)*, most employers pay a federal tax that is used to pay for administrative costs of state employment programs. Employers may also be required to pay for a state unemployment tax program.

Preparing Tax Reports

Health care professionals who are responsible for processing employee's payroll are often involved in preparing the employer's tax reports. All health care facilities are required to prepare and file these reports, which are commonly referred to as an *Employer's Federal Tax Return*, on a regular quarterly basis. The report must include the total number of employees, along with their names and Social Security number, the total wages paid, the amount of withholding tax paid, the amount of wages subject to FICA and the amount of FICA taxes that have been paid, the total periodic tax deposits, and the amount, if any, of underdeposited taxes that are due.

In addition to preparing the employer's tax report, you may also be required to prepare the employee annual reports. According to federal law, these reports, commonly referred to as *Form W-2, Employee's Wage and Tax Statement*, must be provided to the employee no later than January 31. The form must show the employer's identification number, the employee's Social Security number, the amount of total wages and other compensation, and the total income tax and social security tax paid in by the employee for the year preceding January 31.

Billing and Collecting Procedures in the Health Care Environment

An important aspect of all health facilities deals with the proper billing and collection of fees for services rendered. Larger institutions, such as hospitals, often have specially trained people and departments whose sole responsibility involves the billing and collection of patient fees. Smaller facilities, such as private physician's offices and urgent care centers, frequently designate a member of the administrative staff to be responsibile for billing and banking procedures. If you find yourself in the position of having to bill or collect payments from your patients, it is important that you become knowledgeable in just how such a task is completed.

The effective use of interpersonal skills and tactfulness are essential in dealing with issues involved in billing and collection. This involves being businesslike in your dealings with patients, particularly in cases in which patients may be having difficulties in paying for their health care services.

Internal and External Billing Practices

Most health care facilities generally use either one of two ways of billing patients. The first method involves having the billing procedures handled within the health care facility for which the patient has been seen or treated. This is called *internal billing*. Internal billing can be very simple, as in the case of billing in a small private doctor's office, or it can be very difficult and complex, as in the case of a large hospital that employs a fully computerized billing system.

Some facilities may choose to use a type of *external billing* system, in which the institution hires an outside service to handle all patient accounts with regard to billing and collection procedures. A major advantage of the external billing system is that it cuts out much of the time-consuming tasks involved in billing.

No matter which system of billing is employed by your facility, completeness and accuracy are the keys to a successful billing and collection program. This means that all information pertaining to the patient's name, address, telephone number, health insurance coverage, and medical history must be secured at the time the patient is first seen by your facility, since all of this will be necessary at the time of billing. Most of the data obtained on the patient's registration form can provide you with the facts you will later need for collecting payments.

Collecting Fees for Services Rendered

All fees for medical services rendered by your facility must be in clear view and explained to patients. A typed itemized list of the most common and frequently employed services that the physician or department offers is often used, since it is readily available to the patient. Most states require such a list to be posted in the institution and made available to all patients.

In cases where a patient does not understand the fee schedule or is incapable of making rational decisions regarding his or her care or treatment, you must discuss the disclosure of fees with both the patient and the person responsible for paying the bill. Once it has been determined that the persons involved fully comprehend the process of billing and collection of fees, you must make a determination as to the method of collection of these fees.

Many smaller facilities require payment at the time services are provided. In this instance, the facility would be responsible for explaining the system of payment at the time the patient first calls to make an appointment. In some situations, however, this may not always be practical. If this is the case, the facility may choose to extend credit to the patient. This usually occurs when a patient faces large fees for service, such as in the case of surgery or multiple visits to the facility.

Many health care facilities have opted to use credit card billing as a method of obtaining payments for services rendered. In these cases, your employer will probably require you to carefully check the expiration date on the credit card, as well as the name of the person listed on the card. If you do accept credit cards, you should be prepared for the patient to become defensive if the card is rejected. They may become insistent that you accept the card because the "credit card company has made a mistake." Remember, you are not responsible for dealing with any problems or discrepancies between the credit card company and the patient. Your job is to be polite and not to pass judgment on the patient.

Superbill Billing

Many states have adopted the superbill system, which combines a bill and an insurance claim in one statement. The statement is provided to the patient at the time he or she is seen at the facility. The superbill usually includes the patient's name, date, identification of services received, treatment codes, diagnostic information as it classified in the ICD-9-CM coding system, insurance requirements, assignment of benefits, and the physician's identification number.

A major advantage of using the superbill system is that it eliminates a great deal of the paperwork needed for processing insurance claims, as well as encourages the patient to provide payment immediately after the services have been rendered. The patient can then submit the superbill directly to his or her insurance company, where benefits can either be assigned to the patient, or directly to the health care facility, if credit has been previously granted.

Statements, Cycle Billing, and Ledger Card Billing

Some health care facilities send their patients a monthly itemized statement as a bill for services. Sending out these statements is not always the best method of collecting payments for services rendered, since it can often increase the facility's costs for collection, as well as significantly delay the amount of time in which the payments are received.

Institutions that use statements often use cycle billing to send statements out. Cycle billing involves sending statements according to an alphabetical breakdown. When the facility uses this system, billing goes on throughout the month and therefore can allow for continuous cash flow during the entire month.

Another frequently used method involves billing patients by way of a ledger card. Ledger cards, which generally include all charges, credits, and any adjustments that might be necessary for each patient, are usually copied and then mailed directly to the patient. Bills that remain unpaid are often flagged by using a color strip at the top of the ledger card. When the bill is paid, the color strip can then be removed.

A much more sophisticated method of billing that many larger facilities use involves a billing software application and a computer system. In this method, the computer is searched throughout the billing cycle, and printouts of patients with outstanding balances are identified. Once the system has identified patients who still owe payments to the facility, the software can generally provide you with a standard reminder letter that can be sent to the patient regarding his or her delinquent bill.

Collecting Fees on Overdue Accounts

Unfortunately, patients are not always as prompt as they should be when it comes to paying for their medical costs. Because of this, all health care facilities generally employ a policy regarding the collection of late payments.

There are several ways in which a facility can identify which accounts may be overdue and unpaid. One system is to use a method of *aging accounts*. When a patient's account is aged, it helps to identify both the accounts and the length of time that the account has been delinquent. A color-coding system can be used to identify the length of time the account has been left unpaid.

If your agency uses a computerized billing system, accounts can be aged automatically. The first notation might be a record of a superbill given at the time of the patient's visit. A statement would be sent after 1 month, and after 2 months, a statement with an overdue notice might be sent. Letters would be sent after 3 and 4 months, reminding the patient of the overdue account.

If a patient's account becomes so delinquent that "gentle" reminders are not working, your facility may choose to send out a collection letter in an attempt to collect the overdue bill. However, before you can send out any letters, you must become aware of the *Fair Debt Collections Practice Act*, which is a federal act passed in 1978, established for the protection of people from undue harrassment. The act outlaws any abusive, deceptive, and unfair collection practices by any business, including health care facilities. As long as your agency understands this legislation, after 90 days of delinquency for an account, your facility may begin to write collection letters. The goal of these letters should be to encourage the patient to pay the balance due, which keeps the health care facility from having to pay a collection agency to secure the payment.

Although the length of time may vary as to how long a facility is willing to wait to be paid, most facili-

ties generally wait no longer than 5 or 6 months before they turn the patient's account over to a professional collection agency. During the seventh month, the agency will attempt to collect the payment. If the amount is worth going after, by the eighth month, a lawsuit can be generated by the collection agency on behalf of the facility.

In some cases, you may encounter patients who have a balance due, but who can no longer be reached at the address they provided on their patient record sheet. If this occurs, and no forwarding address has been left, this is called a *skip*.

When a collection letter has been sent by the facility to the patient regarding his or her overdue bill, a skip problem becomes quite evident when the letter is returned with a notation of *Address Correction Requested* or *Address Unknown*. As soon as you realize that a skip has taken place, you should begin the task of locating the patient. This can be done in a number of ways. You may be able to call the patient's employer; however, if you do this, you must be very careful not to disclose the reason for your search. You may also call the person listed on the patient's registration form as his or her nearest relative. You may even attempt to locate the patient's neighbor or landlord to see if they have a forwarding address for the patient. Other ways in which you can attempt to locate a person who has skipped without paying his or her bill include checking the telephone book for last names similar to the patient's; asking the Department of Motor Vehicles if they have a change of address; calling the patient's bank, if you have that information; asking for a transfer address, if one has been provided; and checking with utility companies, such as the telephone or gas and electric company, to see if they have a forwarding address.

Banking Procedures in the Health Care Environment

If you are involved in billing and collection procedures for your health care facility, there is a very good possibility that you will also be in charge of banking procedures. You should understand that banking institutions are involved in many different aspects of financial transactions. They receive deposits for checking and savings accounts, loan money to businesses and individuals, and service loans for savings and loan associations. Your institution may use the bank for many of the services it provides.

The most common type of banking services most health care facilities use is maintaining a checking account, which is a bank account against which checks can be written. A majority of the payments received by the health care facility are generally provided by checks.

There are many different varieties of checking accounts, including some that pay interest, like a savings account. It may be your responsibility to determine which kind of checking account offered in your community will best suit your facility.

When money is not needed to pay for the facility's expenses, it is often deposited into a savings account. Savings accounts earn interest on the amount deposited. Like checking accounts, there are several kinds of savings accounts, such as a simple passbook account that draws interest at the lowest rate offered by the financial institution, and that generally does not require a minimum balance to maintain, and has no check-writing options. Another type of savings account is called a money market account. This type of account usually requires a minimum balance, generally over $1000, and provides the depositor the option of writing a prearranged number of checks per month.

As you carry out your banking responsibilities, you may encounter various types of checks. The most common of these include *cashier's checks*, which are bank checks drawn against itself and signed by a bank official; *certified checks*, which is a customer's own check, with "certified" or "accepted" written across the face of the check; money orders, which can be sold by banks and other businesses; *bank drafts*, which are checks used to pay funds drawn by a bank or its account at another bank; *traveler's checks*, which have been designed for travelers to be used in situations in which a personal check would not be accepted; a *limited check*, which is a check that is limited as to the amount as well as the time during which it can be cashed; *voucher checks*, which usually have a detachable form used to notate the purpose for which the check was written; and *warrants*, which are checks that cannot be cashed but are evidence of a debt due. Warrants are most often used by governmental agencies and insurance companies, who use them to authorize the agency or company to pay for a specific claim.

Accepting Checks and Credit Cards for Payment of Services Rendered

If your facility takes checks from patients to pay for their fees for services rendered, there are certain things you must remember. First of all, you should never accept a check that has been erased or appears to have visible errors. Never accept a check that has been written out to "cash," as opposed to the name of the facility. If you receive a check that has been sent back to your facility marked "account closed" or "account overdrawn," you must contact the

person who wrote the check immediately, to make sure that your facility is not only paid for the services provided, but also is reimbursed for any additional charges incurred for the check being returned.

You must also make sure that any check you receive is properly endorsed. An endorsement is put on the back of a check or money order and is an indication that all rights in the check are transferred to another party. Endorsements must always be made in ink, pen, or rubber stamp, and should be made on the left, or perforated end, of the check.

If your facility also accepts credit cards for payment of services rendered, you must be very careful in checking to be sure that the name on the credit card matches the bearer's name. You should also check the expiration date of the card, and if your employer uses an automatic credit card machine, you may be required to enter the number of the credit card to make sure that the card is not over the company's limit of expenditures. In addition, you must make sure that the information that has been provided on the card is clear on the credit card charge slip and that you give the patient the proper receipt. There are often three parts to a charge slip, with the individual copies clearly marked as to where they should go.

Making Bank Deposits

An important part of banking has to do with making accurate deposits of the daily checks and cash brought into your facility. All deposits should be made as soon as possible in order to avoid losing checks or having them stolen. Delays may cause a check to be returned for insufficient funds, or the check may eventually have a stop-payment placed on it. It is also a courtesy to the patient to cash checks promptly, and insurance checks often have a restricted period for their cashing.

Whenever a deposit is made, it must be accompanied by a deposit slip. The slip contains the name and address of your employer and the date of the deposit, as well as the checking account number. It is always a good idea to make a copy of the deposit slip for your facility.

The total amount of the deposit is immediately entered into the checkbook, and the checks are clipped together or put in bank wrappers, and all coins, currency, and checks should be put in a large bank envelop or bag.

Bank deposits can be made in several ways. Depending upon your employer, he or she may choose to make their deposits by mail, in an after-hours bank depositor, or at an automatic bank teller machine.

Processing Bank Statements

A bank statement is a list that provides an itemized accounting by date and amount of all deposits and withdrawals made from a specific account. Most financial institutions provide these statements at regular intervals, usually on a monthly basis. When the statement is received by your facility, it should be immediately reconciled against the checkbook stubs or check register. You may receive canceled checks, or you may have an account where checks are available upon demand.

Reconciling the bank statement should be done as soon as possible after its arrival. In some cases, the balances in the checkbook and the bank statement differ because some checks have not yet appeared on the bank statement. The reconciliation is therefore necessary.

If, after you have completed the reconciliation, the balances agree, you are finished. If they do not, you must determine the amount of the disagreement. Some of the most common mistakes leading to a disagreement on the reconciliation include forgetting to include an outstanding check, incorrect or inaccurate math, failing to record deposits or recording a deposit more than once, carrying out figures incorrectly, failing to write down a check, and transposing a figure.

Summary

In this chapter, we discussed the role of the cardiovascular technology health care provider who finds him or herself in the position of being responsible for carrying out billing and banking procedures in the health care environment. We talked about how to perform basic bookkeeping procedures, as well as how to bill patients for services rendered. We also explained how to perform specific banking procedures utilized by most health care facilities, including processing payments made by check, making bank deposits, and reconciliating bank statements.

Review Questions

1. Define the following abbreviations:

   a. A/C _____

   b. A/R _____

2. Define the difference between a *debit* and a *credit*.

3. Briefly explain the process of *cycle billing*.

4. Define the difference between *Medicare* and *Medicaid*.

5. What is meant by the term *Medi-Medi*?

6. What does the abbreviation *DRG* mean, and what does it represent?

7. When must a release of information form be signed, and by whom?

8. Briefly explain the differences between the following:

   a. Worker's compensation insurance

   b. Group insurance

   c. Individual insurance

9. What is the purpose of an HMO, and who generally uses its services?

10. Give at least three examples of coding books used for billing:

   a. _____

   b. _____

   c. _____

35

Insurance Coding and Indexing

Performance Objectives

Upon completion of this chapter, you will be able to:

1. Identify and briefly discuss various types of insurance programs available for health care.
2. Discuss reference manuals available for coding medical insurance claims.
3. Describe the importance of accuracy as it relates to coding an insurance claim form.
4. Explain and be able to demonstrate how to produce a rough draft copy of an insurance claim form.

Terms and Abbreviations

Alphanumeric code   a code with both letters and numbers and sometimes other symbols, such as punctuation marks.

CHAMPUS   abbreviation for Civilian Health and Medical Program for the Uniformed Services, a military program responsible for providing medical care for those in military service and their dependents and retired military personnel.

CHAMPVA   abbreviation for Civilian Health and Medical Program for the Veterans Administration, a government insurance program that covers families of veterans with 100% service-connected disability, or the surviving spouse and children of a veteran who died as a result of a service-connected disability.

CPT   abbreviation for Current Procedural Terminology codes, a coding system published by the American Medical Association and used to communicate procedures performed by a physician.

Deductible   the amount of money a patient or responsible party must pay prior to the insurance company starting to pay.

FECA   abbreviation for Federal Employee Compensation Act, which is a program that reimburses federal employees for medical expenses related to accidents or injuries which occurred on-the-job.

HCFA   abbreviation for Health Care Financing Administration, an administrative agency within the United States Department of Health and Human Services that is responsible for handling all issues related to Medicare and Medicaid.

ICD codes   abbreviation for International Classification of Diseases codes, an internationally recognized coding system for all known diseases, originally designed by the World Health Organization of the United Nations.

Medicaid   a state government program designed to help indigent or poor people with medical benefits.

Medicare   a federal government program designed to help elderly and disabled people who have paid into the Social Security system with medical expenses, and whose deductibles and coverage change annually.

Medicare Part A   the part of Medicare that pays a portion of an inpatient's hospital care, daily skilled care received in a skilled nursing facility, home health care, and hospice care.

Medicare Part B   the part of Medicare that pays a portion of a patient's physician and outpatient services.

SNF   abbreviation for skilled nursing facility.

Subscriber   the person who is the insurance policyholder; also called the insured.

Workers' compensation   medical payments made by employers when an employee has a work-related illness or injury.

According to most health insurance providers, approximately 80% of the money paid to a physician's office or to a health care facility comes in the form of insurance payments from private insurance companies or government insurance programs. Since the costs of health care continue to rise, it is mandatory that physicians, hospitals, and clinics be paid on a timely basis. Therefore, as a member of the health care delivery team, if you find yourself responsible for processing health insurance claims for your facility, the first thing you must realize is that you have a very important task in gathering the data necessary to accurately file claims for monies owed, as well as grouping illnesses that allow for indexing.

Careers in Insurance Coding

Although this text deals more specifically with careers in cardiovascular technology, it is important for you to know that with the coming changes in the national health care system, an accurate insurance coding clerk, or someone who possesses the skills and knowledge required to process health insurance claims, will be in great demand. People specializing in health insurance should be able to work with a high degree of accuracy and attention to details. A knowledge of medical terminology is a definite asset, and computer keyboarding skills are a major advantage. If you are really ambitious, you may choose to enroll in any one of a number of vocational schools or colleges throughout the country, and become a Certified Coding Specialist.

Health Insurance Programs

There are two major programs that exist exclusively to pay for health care. These two systems include one that is financed by the individual and one that is financed by state and federal government funds. Approximately 2000 different private health care programs are available, including all types of commercial plans, preferred provider organizations (PPOs), and health maintenance organizations (HMOs).

Comprehensive health care is provided by the federal government for large groups of qualified people. The groups that fall under this category include coverage for members of the uniformed services and retired military personnel and their dependents through CHAMPUS and CHAMPVA; coverage for the elderly through Medicare, which is administered by the Social Security Administration; coverage for disabled and indigent through Medicaid, which is also administered by the Social Security system; and coverage for those with job-related injuries or illnesses, which is administered through FECA/Black Lung or individual workers' compensation insurance companies. All funds for payment through health insurance coverage are financed through general taxation or, in the case of the Social Security system, from a trust fund of contributions paid by employees, employers, and self-employed workers.

When a service or a procedure is performed by a health care provider, that person expects to be paid. In order to obtain insurance compensation, either the patient or the provider must submit a completed form that details the specific services provided. *Codes* are used to standardize and simplify these forms. The code numbers, which are used to identify individual physicians; diseases being treated; and procedures, services, and supplies provided to a patient, are obtained from publications called *manuals*, which provide listings referred to as *coding systems*.

Since payment is made according to the code that has been assigned for a diagnosis and procedure, it is imperative that you be accurate in choosing the correct code. An incorrect code can result in a form being returned to the doctor's office or the health care facility, or, in some cases, a reduced amount being paid.

Understanding and Using Coding Systems

When a doctor examines a patient at his or her office or the hospital, a procedure has been performed for which the physician is expected to be paid, either by the patient, a private insurance company, or a government health care agency. In a regular sequence of events, the physician or health facility will first identify the procedures performed for the patient. For uniformity in reporting procedures and treatments, the American Medical Association has developed and published a coding system called *Current Procedural Terminology* codes, or CPT codes. These procedures and their codes are generally marked on a superbill, charge slip, or the medical record.

The CPT manual is used for determining the correct five-digit code. It is divided into several sections, including *Introduction*, *Medicine*, *Anesthesia*, *Surgery* (by individual body systems), *Radiology*, *Nuclear Medicine*, *Diagnostic Ultrasound*, *Pathology and Laboratory*, and the *Appendix*. When your responsibilities include insurance coding, it is extremely important that you code the procedure accurately because insurance companies and government agencies will only pay according to the correct coding.

Identifying CPT Codes

If you are working with insurance codes, there are three steps you must follow in order to obtain a correct procedure. These include:

- Referring to the alphabetical index at the end of the CPT manual in order to locate the procedure
- Noting the five-digit code that has been provided for the procedure
- Locating the correct numerical code in the manual for the exact description of the procedure

In order for you to be able to gain an understanding of how procedures are assigned a specific code number, let's look at the two examples provided below. In Figure 35-1A the codes being represented are those that would be found under *Medicine*, while the codes shown in Figure 35-1B, are found under *Surgery, Procedures for the Integumentary System*.

Coding Under the International Classification of Diseases

Several years ago, the World Health Organization (WHO) of the United Nations was entrusted with the responsibility of devising a list of all known diseases.

90000	office and other outpatient medical service, NEW PATIENT; *brief service*
90010	*limited* service
90015	*intermediate* service
90017	*extended* service
90020	*comprehensive service*

Figure 35-1A
Codes found under Medicine.

10000	incision and drainage of infection or noninfected sebaceous cyst; *one* lesion
10001	*second* lesion
10002	*more than two* lesions
10003	incision and drainage of infected or noninfected epithelial inclusion cyst (sebaceous cyst) with complete removal of sac and treatment of cavity

Figure 35-1B
Codes found under Surgery, Procedures for the Integumentary System.

Once this list was developed, WHO assigned code numbers to the various diseases. Ultimately, the *International Classification of Diseases*, or *ICD* codes were developed and are now used internationally.

ICD codes are identified in three bound volumes, known as ICD books. Volume I is a tabular list of diseases listed as a three-digit number and, at times, a two-digit extension, such as 003.22 *Salmonella pneumonia*. Volume II of the ICD code book is an alphabetic index of diseases. An insurance clerk would look first in Volume II at the alphabetic name, and then use the number given to refer to Volume I. It is important to remember that you should never code from Volume II alone. It should be used only as a reference. Coding from Volume I will provide you with much more extensive information.

Volume III of the ICD code books is both a tabular and an alphabetic index of procedures used for the purpose of billing hospital patients, and it coordinates with the HCPCS coding used for all government claims.

Coding Under the Health Care Procedural Coding System (HCPCS)

In 1983, HCPCS, which is pronounced "hicpics," was created by Medicare in order to standardize procedural coding for all Medicare and Medicaid claims. It is an alphanumeric coding system that was developed by the federal Health Care Financing Administration (HCFA), defined to be used as a supplement to the CPT codes for filing insurance claims for Medicare, CHAMPUS, and Medicaid. These codes relay information about nonphysician procedures, services, and specific supplies.

There are three levels of coding found in the HCPCS system. *Level I* uses the CPT codes from the CPT manual to code the services and procedures provided by physicians. The five-digit code represents Level I, such as 90040, brief office visit. Level II codes are published and updated on an annual basis by the Health Care Financing Administration, and are used to code nonphysician procedures, services, and supplies. Level II codes are represented by one alphabetic character followed by four numbers, such as A0040, ambulance service, air, helicopter service. Level III codes may be assigned by the Medicare office responsible for a specific geographic region. Local codes will have an alphabetic letter "S" through "Z" and four digits, and are provided by the regional Medicare office as they are updated. Local codes have the highest priority and should always be used first.

Processing Coding Changes and Charges

As a member of the administrative medical services staff, you have a responsibility to stay current with the different coding procedures, government rules and regulations, and newly assigned coding numbers. Updates are printed every year for each of the coding manuals, and if you are assigned to process insurance claims, you must make sure that you are using the very latest edition of your coding manuals. If an update, addendum, or appendix is printed, it should be placed immediately in the appropriate manual so that you are using the current codes.

Each year, Medicare changes the amounts for deductible charges and pricing for procedures that can be charged by the physician who is a Medicare provider. Medicaid also changes its rules and regulations very often. Medical office workers who are responsible for handling Medicare and Medicaid are also responsible for noting any changes and charging the patients for their deductible part accordingly. In addition, you must also bill the government for the Medicare or Medicaid approved amount.

Processing Insurance Claim Forms

In order for the physician's office or the health care facility to receive payment from an insurance company or government insurance system, an insurance claim form must be properly filled out. The common form most widely used by private insurance companies and government insurance agencies is FORM HCFA-1500 (Figure 35-2). It is commonly referred to as the "universal insurance claim form," because it can easily be adopted for almost every private and government insurance agency. If you are responsible for filling out this form, you must remember that there are two types of information required. The first includes all routine information regarding the patient, his or her subscriber, and the insurance company. The second type of information required involves all the medical information and health-related issues that is provided by the patient's physician.

The most accurate way to obtain information regarding health insurance is to ask the patient or the person insured for his or her insurance identification card and then make a copy of both the front and the back of the card. This card contains information that is required for processing the claim, and usually includes the person's social security number and group number. In addition, the insurance company's name, address, telephone number, and service representa-tive are usually printed on the back of the identification card.

If you are responsible for processing Medicare claims, you should also make a copy of the patient's or subscriber's identification card, so that verification can be made concerning coverage under Parts A and B. Part B is currently optional for all patient's receiving Medicare benefits.

Filling Out the Insurance Claim Form

If you plan on receiving payment for your physician or the health care facility, especially in a timely manner, it is extremely important that the claim form be accurately filled out, since any errors can result in either not receiving the payment or in waiting an undue amount of time to be paid. Therefore, when processing the HCFA-1500 insurance claim form, there is a specific way you must respond to each and every section of the form.

At the top of the form, you must first check the applicable program block. If the patient has private or employer's group insurance, check *Other* and write the name of the insurance company in the top right hand corner. After you have checked the appropriate box or written in the name of the company, complete the form by following the information provided in Appendix C.

Upon completion of the insurance claim form, make sure you double-check it for accuracy and completness. Check for any omissions of information and for any math errors. Once you have made copies for your billing records, send the completed form to the appropriate insurance company.

Summary

In this chapter, we discussed the process and skills involved in coding procedures and treatments performed by the physician or health care provider. We talked about how to use the *Current Procedural Terminology* manual for coding descriptions of procedures, the International Classification of Diseases, for coding a diagnosis or disease, and the Health Care Procedural Coding System (HCPCS), when coding non-physician procedures, services, and supplies for Medicare and Medicaid. Finally, we discussed the purpose of health insurance claim forms, including how to code and fill out properly the HCFA-1500, which is a universal health insurance claim form used by most private and government insurance agencies.

PLEASE
DO NOT
STAPLE
IN THIS
AREA

| | PICA | | | HEALTH INSURANCE CLAIM FORM | PICA | | |

1. MEDICARE   MEDICAID   CHAMPUS   CHAMPVA   GROUP HEALTH PLAN   FECA BLK LUNG   OTHER

(Medicare #) (Medicaid #) (Sponsor's SSN) (VA File #) (SSN or ID) (SSN) (ID)

1a. INSURED'S I.D. NUMBER (FOR PROGRAM IN ITEM 1)

2. PATIENT'S NAME (Last Name, First Name, Middle Initial)

3. PATIENT'S BIRTH DATE MM DD YY   SEX M   F

4. INSURED'S NAME (Last Name, First Name, Middle Initial)

5. PATIENT'S ADDRESS (No., Street)

6. PATIENT RELATIONSHIP TO INSURED Self   Spouse   Child   Other

7. INSURED'S ADDRESS (No., Street)

CITY   STATE

8. PATIENT STATUS Single   Married   Other

CITY   STATE

ZIP CODE   TELEPHONE (Include Area Code) (   )

Employed   Full-Time Student   Part-Time Student

ZIP CODE   TELEPHONE (INCLUDE AREA CODE) (   )

9. OTHER INSURED'S NAME (Last Name, First Name, Middle Initial)

10. IS PATIENT'S CONDITION RELATED TO:

11. INSURED'S POLICY GROUP OR FECA NUMBER

a. OTHER INSURED'S POLICY OR GROUP NUMBER

a. EMPLOYMENT? (CURRENT OR PREVIOUS) YES   NO

a. INSURED'S DATE OF BIRTH MM DD YY   SEX M   F

b. OTHER INSURED'S DATE OF BIRTH MM DD YY   SEX M   F

b. AUTO ACCIDENT? YES   NO   PLACE (State)

b. EMPLOYER'S NAME OR SCHOOL NAME

c. EMPLOYER'S NAME OR SCHOOL NAME

c. OTHER ACCIDENT? YES   NO

c. INSURANCE PLAN NAME OR PROGRAM NAME

d. INSURANCE PLAN NAME OR PROGRAM NAME

10d. RESERVED FOR LOCAL USE

d. IS THERE ANOTHER HEALTH BENEFIT PLAN? YES   NO   *If yes*, return to and complete item 9 a-d.

READ BACK OF FORM BEFORE COMPLETING & SIGNING THIS FORM.

12. PATIENT'S OR AUTHORIZED PERSON'S SIGNATURE I authorize the release of any medical or other information necessary to process this claim. I also request payment of government benefits either to myself or to the party who accepts assignment below.

SIGNED _____   DATE _____

13. INSURED'S OR AUTHORIZED PERSON'S SIGNATURE I authorize payment of medical benefits to the undersigned physician or supplier for services described below.

SIGNED _____

14. DATE OF CURRENT: MM DD YY   ILLNESS (First symptom) OR INJURY (Accident) OR PREGNANCY(LMP)

15. IF PATIENT HAS HAD SAME OR SIMILAR ILLNESS. GIVE FIRST DATE MM DD YY

16. DATES PATIENT UNABLE TO WORK IN CURRENT OCCUPATION MM DD YY FROM TO MM DD YY

17. NAME OF REFERRING PHYSICIAN OR OTHER SOURCE

17a. I.D. NUMBER OF REFERRING PHYSICIAN

18. HOSPITALIZATION DATES RELATED TO CURRENT SERVICES MM DD YY FROM TO MM DD YY

19. RESERVED FOR LOCAL USE

20. OUTSIDE LAB? YES   NO $ CHARGES

21. DIAGNOSIS OR NATURE OF ILLNESS OR INJURY. (RELATE ITEMS 1,2,3 OR 4 TO ITEM 24E BY LINE)

1. ⌊___.__⌋   3. ⌊___.__⌋

2. ⌊___.__⌋   4. ⌊___.__⌋

22. MEDICAID RESUBMISSION CODE   ORIGINAL REF. NO.

23. PRIOR AUTHORIZATION NUMBER

24. A DATE(S) OF SERVICE			B Place of Service	C Type of Service	D PROCEDURES, SERVICES, OR SUPPLIES (Explain Unusual Circumstances) CPT/HCPCS | MODIFIER	E DIAGNOSIS CODE	F $ CHARGES	G DAYS OR UNITS	H EPSDT Family Plan	I EMG	J COB	K RESERVED FOR LOCAL USE
From MM DD YY	To MM DD YY											
1												
2												
3												
4												
5												
6												

25. FEDERAL TAX I.D. NUMBER SSN EIN

26. PATIENT'S ACCOUNT NO.

27. ACCEPT ASSIGNMENT? (For govt. claims, see back) YES   NO

28. TOTAL CHARGE $

29. AMOUNT PAID $

30. BALANCE DUE $

31. SIGNATURE OF PHYSICIAN OR SUPPLIER INCLUDING DEGREES OR CREDENTIALS (I certify that the statements on the reverse apply to this bill and are made a part thereof.)

SIGNED _____   DATE _____

32. NAME AND ADDRESS OF FACILITY WHERE SERVICES WERE RENDERED (If other than home or office)

33. PHYSICIAN'S, SUPPLIER'S BILLING NAME, ADDRESS, ZIP CODE & PHONE #

PIN#   GRP#

(APPROVED BY AMA COUNCIL ON MEDICAL SERVICE 8/88)   **PLEASE PRINT OR TYPE**   APPROVED OMB-0938-0008 FORM HCFA-1500 (12-90),   FORM RRB-1500,
APPROVED OMB-1215-0055 FORM OWCP-1500,   APPROVED OMB-0720-0001 (CHAMPUS)

CARRIER   PATIENT AND INSURED INFORMATION   PHYSICIAN OR SUPPLIER INFORMATION

FOLD HERE / USE ENVELOPE NO. 1500E

Figure 35-2
HCFA-1500 insurance claim form.

Review Questions

1. Briefly explain the following types of insurance programs:

   a. CHAMPUS _____

   b. CHAMPVA _____

   c. Workers' compensation _____

   d. Medicare _____

   e. Medicaid _____

2. Define the following abbreviations:

   a. HMO _____

   b. ICD codes _____

   c. CPT _____

   d. SNF _____

   e. HCFA _____

   f. FECA _____

3. What does the term *subscriber* mean?

4. Briefly explain what an *alphanumeric code* is.

36

Job-Seeking Skills and Employment Opportunities

Performance Objectives

Upon completion of this chapter, you will be able to:

1. Identify where most jobs will occur by the year 2000.
2. Describe the steps and process involved in beginning a job search.
3. Explain how to fill out a job application form.
4. Discuss the purpose of a cover letter.
5. Define the function of a resume and identify its basic components.
6. Identify the three types of resumes most often used in securing a position in the field of cardiovascular technology and briefly explain when each should be used.
7. List the proper guidelines for preparing a resume.
8. Discuss the steps involved in preparing for a job interview.
9. Discuss the process involved in conducting oneself in a professional manner during the job interview process.
10. Briefly explain the follow-up process that should occur after an interview has taken place.

Terms and Abbreviations

Chronological resume   a type of resume that provides an employer with specific dates and employers listed in chronological order.

Combination resume   a type of resume that emphasizes the applicant's work skills and at the same time lists previous employers with dates of employment.

Cover letter   a personal introduction to a perspective employer; always enclosed with a resume.

DNA   abbreviation for *does not apply.*

Employment agency   an organization whose sole purpose is to assist applicants and employers in attaining employment for the prospective worker and filling a position for the employer.

Functional resume   a type of resume that highlights an applicant's qualifications and marketable skills.

Interview   the process by which an applicant speaks with a potential employer regarding employment.

N/A   abbreviation for *not applicable.*

Resume   a one- to two-page document that is used to provide prospective employers with information regarding a future employee's educational and employment history.

According to the U.S. Bureau of Labor Statistics, by the year 2000, over half of the jobs available in the United States will occur in professional, clerical, and service-oriented occupations. All information generated from these statistics point to health care being the industry offering the highest number of jobs and the brightest prospects. Physicians, nurses, ECG technicians, echocardiographic technicians, respiratory therapy and pulmonary function assistants, and laboratory assistants and phlebotomists will all be in great demand throughout rural and urban communities. Key factors contributing to increased employment opportunities for cardiovascular workers and other allied health care professionals include the need to staff medical offices for the increasing numbers of medical doctors being graduated from medical schools, public awareness for the need to provide quality health care, and an increase in the volume of paperwork emanating from insurance companies and from state and government regulatory agencies.

Research studies seem to bear out the fact that although the job-seeking person has all the clinical skills and theoretical knowledge to do a job, he or she often lacks the basic skills required to *get* the job. Therefore, before you begin actively seeking employment in a health care facility, there are specific steps you should take in order to prepare to find and *obtain* the best position possible. The first question you should consider, however, is why do employers reject job applicants?

There are many reasons why an employer rejects a job applicant. Some of the most frequent responses employers give include applicants showing little interest or poor reasons for desiring a position. Also, showing a past history of "job hopping" and an inability to verify previous employment and/or educational background tends to make a perspective employer hesitant to hire an individual. Demonstrating a lack of maturity or an inability to communicate effectively during the interview process are two additional reasons employers sometimes give for not being interested in an applicant. Dressing unacceptably or showing a lack of professionalism and manners during the interview are other reasons. Finally, providing the employer with a poorly completed job application form or resume, or demonstrating a lack of job-related skills are good reasons why employers would not hire someone for a position.

Initiating the Job Hunt

When you are ready to begin your search for a position, you should try to follow through on all possible job leads. An individual who recently completed his or her education might contact the school placement office and place his or her name on file. You might also attend meetings, seminars, and workshops that are run by professional organizations in the cardiovascular occupations but are open to the public. Those announcements are usually placed in a special section of your local newspaper. Because many jobs are never formally advertised, you should try to spread the word that you are "looking" to classmates,

teachers, family, and acquaintances who work for cardiovascular medical practices, outpatient centers, individual physicians, or health care facilities. If you own a computer, you may also want to go "online" or hook up with an E-mail listing, since many online services, such as America OnLine and Prodigy offer users bulletin boards of job listings and classified ads.

You should understand that hiring, especially in the field of health care, is often most effective when it is completed through a network or grapevine of contacts, called a *hidden job market*. This process involves an employer passing the word of a specific job opening to his or her friends and colleagues, who in turn spread the word and refer qualified persons they know. Approximately 75% of all health-related jobs are secured through personal contacts, the hidden job market, and the greatest and most abundant source, through acquaintances.

As you conduct your search for employment, try to visit public and private employment agencies, fill out application forms, and take the required skills tests that may be required of a specific position. Many of the employment and personnel agencies work as referral services and make their money by placing applicants in jobs. Often when a job applicant calls an employment agency about an advertised job opportunity, chances are that it may have already been filled. Even though the position may have already been filled by someone else, you can expect the agency to suggest that you still visit the office so that you can talk about other openings.

Before agreeing to any appointment at an employment or personnel agency, it is always in your best interests to first find out as much as possible about other job listings, since you may already have learned about them from another source or agency. That is because many positions are listed with more than one agency. Some agencies may require you to sign a written binding contract before they can assist you in your job search. Before you agree to this, make sure you read it very carefully to determine whether you or the employer is required to pay the agency a fee for finding you the job.

Another good source of leads is the help wanted section of your local newspaper. The advertisement explains how to make the initial contact, usually by telephone or written communication. Help wanted advertisements appearing in newspapers generally cannot mention the age, sex, and race requirements of the job; however, some ads, such as situation want ads, do allow this.

Another good way to begin your job search is to visit the personnel or human resources departments of local hospitals, clinics, and health care facilities. Many of these facilities also keep questionnaires and application forms on hand for potential employees to review. If you do read through these forms, it is important to study each question carefully before indicating an answer. This is because in some agencies and facilities, the object of the question may be to see if you can follow directions rather than just answer the question. If you do fill out one of the application forms, always try to furnish as much information as possible, but if an item does not apply or cannot be answered, you should indicate that the question has not been overlooked by inserting *no, none, NA (not applicable),* or *DNA (does not apply).*

Filling Out the Job Application Form

When filling out a job application form, you should always read the entire form before beginning to fill it out, since some instructions may be on the last line of the page. Make sure you read the fine print and take note of any special instructions, such as *please print* or *put last name first,* since doing so shows the employer your ability to follow instructions. Also, unless you are told to do otherwise, always make sure you fill the application out in ink, and if your handwriting is illegible, you should block print, and never abbreviate words when there is ample space to write them out. Try to keep a completed application form on hand with you that has been checked for accuracy. You may use it as a "guide" to copy information onto each master application form. If the form asks for your experience using equipment, make sure you list each specific type of equipment. And when listing your previous employment, make sure you are exact when listing the dates. This is very important, since most employers will require a verification of your employment history. If the form asks the reason why you left a position, this may be left blank for discussion during the interview. And finally, make sure you sign the application upon its completion.

Occasionally a blind letter to an office where a possible job opportunity is discovered through a friend or where you would especially like to work may result in a positive response.

Seeking Employment in Another Location

If you are planning to seek employment in a geographical area that may be unfamiliar to you, advance planning is highly desirable. Nothing is more discouraging to an unemployed person than a prolonged job search in unfamiliar surroundings. Dun and Bradstreet, Inc.'s *Million Dollar Directory* and the *Middle Market Directory* are two national publications that can provide you with information on potential employers in many cities throughout the United States. Your local *Yellow Pages* directory, which is provided by most telephone companies, can also provide you with a comprehensive listing of professional offices and hospitals. Chambers of Commerce publications also include membership directories, names of major professional employers in specific areas, and brochures describing regional facts. It is even a good idea to subscribe to the principal newspaper of a city where employment is desired, since this is one way of *tuning in* to the local job market of that area and responding to their advertisements.

The Cover Letter

A *cover letter* is like a personal introduction to a prospective employer (Figure 36-1). It should be typed and addressed to the name of a person. If you are applying for a position that you saw advertised in the newspaper, and that ad listed only a telephone number or a post office box, you should call and ask for the name of the personnel supervisor or who the person is that is most likely to be doing the interviewing. This is done so that the cover letter can include that person's name. If you are unable to ascertain the name of the person to whom the letter is to be addressed, it is acceptable to use the salutation "Dear Sir or Madam," or "To Whom It May Concern." In some cases, you may even use a less formal salutation, such as "Hello" or "Good Morning."

If your intention is to attract the reader's interest, you should use the first 20 words of the letter to state the reason you are applying for the position. This part of the letter should also provide the reader with a summary of your qualifications and a statement as to how you learned about the position. If you choose, you may even provide a short accounting of your career objectives. The concluding sentence of your cover letter should pave the way for an interview appointment by calling attention to a telephone number. Remember, too, that the cover letter should be a preview of your writing skill and should therefore be free of any errors in spelling, punctuation, and grammar. A personal touch can also be added to make the letter stand out.

Preparing the Resume

Most human resources supervisors agree that the sole purpose of providing a prospective employer with a resume is to sell your job qualifications in a format that is as brief and as attractive as possible in order to obtain an interview. A well-written resume should be able to summarize your educational and vocational history, with an analysis of problems effectively con-

Personnel Dept.
Free Memorial Hospital
601 Graceland Avenue
Anywhere, USA 55555

Dear Sir or Madam:

Please allow me a few moments from what I am sure is a very busy schedule, to respond to the ad you are currently running in the <u>Anywhere Times</u>, in which your company is seeking to fill the position of Manager of the ECG Department for your facility.

As you will note from my enclosed resume, I have an extensive background both as an ECG Technician and as a manager and supervisor. In addition to being highly skilled in these areas, my expertise has also afforded me with a strong background in public relations and clinical, both of which are disciplines that I believe to be of great benefit to the position you are seeking to fill.

Figure 36-1
Cover letter.

If you believe, as I do, that my background and expertise may be what you are looking for in order to fill the very challenging position of Manager of your ECG department, my hope is that you will consider me for this very rewarding position. I eagerly look forward to hearing from you so that we may further discuss the benefits I could bring to your very prestigious hospital.

Sincerely,

Susie Jones

fronted and solved, emphasizing organizational, administrative, and clinical skills.

The ideal resume is a one-page document, written in language similar to a telegram. It should contain as many action words as possible and should avoid the personal pronoun. If it is impossible to confine the resume to one page, it can be typed on a 10 by 14 inch page for reduction to standard letter size. Brevity is also important as long as it is possible to include all relevant information.

All data on the resume should be originally typed or printed on high-quality, wrinkle-free bond paper, single spaced internally with double spacing between unrelated items, and with balanced spacing on all four margins. Headings should stand out, and can be typed using a different style of type from the rest of the resume.

Types of Resumes

There are three formats that are generally accepted for future employees seeking a position in the health care industry. These include the *chronological resume*, the *functional resume,* and the *combination resume.*

The chronological resume (Figure 36-2), is the most widely used because of its familiarity to employers. It provides the employer with an interview script and is the easiest for the applicant to prepare. Specific dates and employers are listed in chronological order, with either experience or education first, depending on the area of background to be empha-

sized. The major advantage of using a chronological format is that it stresses a steady employment record. However, the two greatest disadvantages of this resume are that any lack of experience is quickly revealed and, although a steady working history may be exposed, absence of job skills also seem to stand out. To counteract these weaknesses, you may want to enclose photocopies of any certificates or licenses that emphasize specific skills.

For most applicants who have recently graduated from high school or college, the functional resume (Figure 36-3) is the best choice for highlighting the person's qualifications and marketable skills. It does not list specific job titles or descriptions with dates, but rather, emphasizes growth and development in skills.

The combination resume emphasizes the applicant's work skills and identifies specific employers and dates in which the employee worked. A major advantage of this format is that it shows at a glance an applicant's entire working and educational history, particularly stressing the most relevant skills and employment experience, while at the same time minimizing less significant experience. A major weakness, however, of this format, is that it tends to run on and on.

Whether you select the chronological format, the functional format, or the combination format for your resume, personal data such as your name, address, and telephone number should be stated in as brief a manner as possible. According to a decision made by the Civil Rights Act of 1964 and enforced by the Equal

SUSIE SMITH
12345 Green Street
Youknow, CA 11111
(213) 555–5555

EMPLOYMENT HISTORY

1981 to Present: **Outpatient Cardiovascular Services, Inc.,** Van Nuys, PA

As the owner of my own *outpatient cardiovascular services* company, I have been involved in all aspects of providing outpatient cardiovascular services to patients. These areas have included performing ECGs, echocardiograms, holtor monitoring, and obtaining laboratory specimens. I have also been involved in basic billing and collection procedures involved in HMOs, Medicare and Medicaid, private insurance companies, and workers' compensation, as each of these have related to performing cardiovascular procedures for patients on an as needed and outpatient basis.

1979 to 1981:   **Doctor's Medical Group,** Los Angeles, California

As a part-time *ECG Technician and Medical Lab Assistant* for a large physicians-operated medical group, I was responsible for recording and monitoring ECGs, as well as performing basic laboratory tests on patients. My responsibilities in this role also included performing and teaching others how to perform basic administrative tasks required of my position, such as coding insurance forms for billing cardiology procedures.

1976 to 1979:   **Concorde Cardiology Medical Group,** Kansas City, Missouri

As an *ECG Technician and Office Manager,* I was responsible for both administrative and clinical procedures, such as greeting patients and other people coming into the office, answering telephones, scheduling appointments, completing correspondence for executives, and performing other clerical tasks required of my position. As a clinician, my responsibilities included recording both 12-lead and 3-channel electrocardiograms, monitoring out-patient cardiology patients for the physicians, and overseeing all in-office procedures related to cardiology and clinical laboratory monitoring.

EDUCATION

Cardiovascular Technician   Here and There Vocational School, Philadelphia, PA 1975
B.A.   Health Sciences Management, Anywhere University, Jonesville, CA 1974
A.A.   Business Management, Los Angeles Valley College, Greenville, CA 1971

References Furnished Upon Request

Figure 36-2
The chronological resume.

Employment Opportunity Commission, no employer is allowed to ask you about information regarding your height, weight, date of birth, marital status, Social Security number, or presence of any physical disability; therefore, you may omit any information related to these topics from your resume.

Guidelines for Preparing the Resume

When preparing your resume, you will be much more successful in obtaining the position you desire if you follow some very simple guidelines. These include:

- Being as brief as possible; get to the purpose of your resume, and remember, you will always get better results if you do not "bore" your prospective employer with all the details of your skills on your resume; save something for your interview!
- Explaining previous job titles and duties, mentioning awards, special interests, credentials, certifications, and licenses.
- Emphasizing the positive points about your employment history, while at the same time being very careful not to identify your weaknesses.
- Only enclosing photocopies of certificates, licenses, or diplomas if they will be of value to the interviewer for recall purposes and indication of skills.
- Indicating that references are available on request.
- Always typing your resume, the cover letter, and the envelope.

JANE DOE
5311 Corteen Place, #28
No. Hollywood, CA 91607
(818) 761–2345

7/90–5/95   DR. JOHN SMITH, M.D.
Los Angeles, California
Office Manager

Overall responsibility for management of high-volume medical cardiology office. In addition to performing cardiology tasks, such as recording ECGs and monitoring laboratory tests, duties also included answering the telephone and scheduling appointments, billing, banking and collections, insurance claim processing, maintenance and management of all medical and financial records, correspondence, generation of new patients into practice, public and patient relations, and administration of all clerical and office tasks as required for practice.

4/87–5/90   TWIN-TOWERS CARDIOLOGY GROUP
Los Angeles, California
ECG Technician

Responsibilities included recording, interpreting, and mounting ECGs, monitoring out-patient cardiology patients, and performing basic laboratory tests. Additional clerical responsibilities often included billing, insurance claim processing, financial record-keeping, answering the telephone and appointment scheduling, banking and collections, and maintenance and management of patients medical records for high volume cardiology medical group.

1/78–12/86   CARDIOVASCULAR MEDICAL SERVICES
Philadelphia, PA
Cardiovascular Specialist

Responsibilities included performing basic cardiology and laboratory procedures for large out-patient medical services agency specializing in out-patient procedures.

References Furnished Upon Request

Figure 36-3
The functional resume.

- Never mentioning salary requirements, unless you are requested to do so.
- Only listing volunteer activities if they are related to the health care industry or the position for which you are seeking employment.

If the bulk of your resume is devoted to educational qualifications and skills, you should provide details of courses that relate to clinical and organizational skills. Awards may also be mentioned, as well as grade averages. The names of high schools and any colleges attended can also be included. Any diplomas from vocational schools or degrees achieved, with the most recent listed first, should also be identified.

Work experience should include the name and address of the employer, the job title, the length of time employed, and a brief description of duties. Most recent employment is always listed first. Remember, prospective employers usually verify the applicant's employment history, so it is important that you are able to state the exact employment dates of any of your previous employers. Also, unless required, past salaries should never be included in the resume or cover letter. Miscellaneous information, selectively chosen, belongs at the end of the resume. This information might include volunteer work, honors, awards, certificates, special language skills, and leadership positions in the health care industry or professional health care organizations and associations.

Because prospective employers usually ask for names of people who can provide references, you should contact friends and former employers *before* an interview in order to ask them if they will serve as references. This courtesy allows the person time to prepare a response before receiving an unexpected telephone call or communication from the prospective employer.

Taking Part in the Interview Process

The interview process is perhaps the most important aspect in securing a position, chiefly because it often determines whether an applicant will be offered employment. Research studies have shown that when two applicants have similar skills and education, the choice of which candidate to hire is based almost entirely on the physical appearance and attitude of the person at the time of the interview. The importance of good grooming in projecting a favorable first impression cannot be overemphasized. Your clothing should always be immaculate. Wear conservative clothing that fits the image of the job. You may choose to use coordinated accessories, but only if they show good taste. Remember, a picture's worth a thousand words and looks often speak much louder, and may reveal inner feelings. When you know you look your best, you will be more confident and relaxed at the time of your interview.

What Should You Bring?

A portfolio of information related to the current job opening, carried to the interview, suggests that you are serious about obtaining the position and are well organized. Such information often includes letters of recommendation, school diplomas or degrees, transcripts, certificates, names and addresses of references, a copy of your resume, your Social Security card, and items related to your prior education and training.

It is important to find out as much as possible about the position you are applying for before the interview. Because the interview appointment is the only time you may have with the interviewer or prospective employer, this is the time to show that person firsthand your ability to be a professional. Remember, during the interview process, it is the employer who desires a firsthand evaluation of your maturity, manners, personality, and verbal skills. You will find that being knowledgeable about the requirements of the position and only responding to questions that are asked of you, will help you to feel much more relaxed during the interview process.

The Actual Interview

If you are contacted by the employer to be interviewed, you should always arrive on time, usually at least 15 minutes before your scheduled appointment time. Once the interviewer comes to greet you, always allow the first handshake to be initiated by interviewer, and remember to address him or her by name. It is also a good idea to wait to be seated until the interviewer sits down or directs you to be seated. Listen attentively to each question and ask for clarification if there can be more than one interpretation. Always use your common sense, and think before answering a question. There is no need to hurry through your responses.

Never answer questions about your personal life unless the answer demonstrates a reflection of your ability to perform the job, and always be discreet in your references to former employers. Make sure your responses are short, but avoid one-word answers, such as "yes" or "no." And never, never, use slang or swear words!

A confident prospective employee always demonstrates a genuine interest in the position for which he or she is applying, by asking questions about job specifications, continuing education policies, medical benefits, and to whom he or she will be responsible. You should also be prepared to respond to a question concerning salary expectations, and if you are unable to answer a question, be honest and state that you are unable to respond. Most important, always speak confidently to the interviewer without letting your eyes wander. You must appear relaxed, yet interested in the position.

There may be some questions that may be asked by the interviewer that legally do not have to be answered unless the information is job related. Jobs are to be offered on the basis of qualifications, so any questions related to your marital status, religious preference, club memberships, height, weight, dependents, or age do not have to be answered. Inquiries dealing with credit ratings, home and automobile ownership, family planning, and pregnancy are also illegal.

The way in which the interview process ends is as important as how it begins. Most prospective employers usually terminate the interview by standing. This should be your cue to stand and prepare to leave. As you did in the beginning, allow the interviewer to initiate the shaking of hands at the conclusion of the interview process. Before departing, you may want to ask the interviewer when you might expect to hear if the job is to be offered, so that you will not miss the call. The interview process is completed by saying a simple "thank you" to both the interviewer and the receptionist.

After the Interview, What's Next?

In today's employment market, an offer of employment is seldom initiated during the interview process. Therefore, if there has been no contact from the employer within a day or two, it is time for you to write a follow-up note of thanks (Figure 36-4). If the inter-

JANE DOE
5311 Corteen Place, Apt. #28
No. Hollywood, CA 91607
(818) 761-2345

May 15, 1995

Dr. John Smith
9001 Green St., Suite 306
Anywhere, USA 12345

Dear Dr. Smith:

Please allow me to take this opportunity to personally thank you for the time you gave me during my recent interview.

As I am sure you are aware, I am most interested in working for you and would consider it a privilege if you were to select me for a position in your practice. If I am fortunate enough to be offered a job, I can promise you someone that is a hard worker, and who is extremely dedicated to working "above and beyond the call of duty" for her employer.

Once again, I would like to thank you for your consideration. I eagerly look forward to hearing from you, so that we may further discuss the possibility of me working as a member of your team.

Most sincerely,

Jane Doe

Figure 36-4
The thank you note.

viewer has provided you with a telephone number, you may also choose to place a call in order to express your continued interest in the position and to keep from being forgotten. The object of these "gentle reminders" is to briefly restate your assets, emphasizing your strong feelings toward obtaining the position, while at the same time reinforcing the time you may be reached by telephone. Even if the position is not offered, you will learn from each interview until you are able to secure the right job.

Once you have secured a position, it will be well for you to remember that no matter what level you are hired at, you are still a beginner in that position, with much to learn. It is a good idea to borrow the office or department's procedure manual to preview the facility's routines. Arriving for work the first day with a notebook to take notes saves the subsequent embarrassment of having to ask how to carry out tasks after they have been explained, and taking notes also reinforces procedures and demonstrates your genuine desire to do the best job possible.

Summary

During this chapter, we discussed the basic skills involved in obtaining a position in the health care industry. We discussed the various steps and process involved in beginning the job search, how to fill out a job application form properly, and how to create a cover letter, resume, and thank you note. We also explained how to prepare for and take part in the actual interview process. Finally, we discussed the follow-up process required of the prospective employee once the interview has taken place.

Review Questions

1. Identify at least three reasons an employer might reject a job applicant:

   a. _____

   b. _____

   c. _____

2. Differentiate between a chronological resume, a functional resume, and a combination resume.

3. Give at least one example an applicant may demonstrate to show interest in a job interview.

4. Why is it important to read the "fine print" on an employment agency contract before signing it?

5. Identify at least one disadvantage of using a chronological resume.

6. What steps can be taken by the cardiovascular worker to help him or her in securing a position of employement?

7. List three personal items that legally do not have to be included on a resume or answered during an interview:

a. _____

b. _____

c. _____

8. What follow-up steps can be taken after a resume has been sent and an interview has been completed?

9. What does the abbreviation *DNA* mean?

10. What does the abbreviation *N/A* mean?

Medical Abbreviations and Symbols

a	before	AKA	above-the-knee amputation
@	at	ALS	amyotrophic lateral sclerosis
aa	of each	alt	alternate
AAA	abdominal aortic aneurysm	a.m.	morning
AB	abortion	AMA	against medical advice
abd	abdomen	amp	ampule
ABG	arterial blood gases	amt	amount
abn	abnormal	A&O	alert and oriented
ac	before meals	AODM	adult onset diabetes mellitus
accom	accommodation	A&P	auscultation and percussion; anterior and posterior
ACH	adrenocortical hormone		
ACTH	adrenocorticotropic hormone	AP	anterior-posterior
AD	right ear	AP&Lat	anterior-posterior and lateral
ADA	American Dietetic Association	ART	accredited records technician
ADH	antidiuretic hormone	AS	left ear
ADL	activities of daily living	ASA	aspirin
ad lib	as desired	ASAP	as soon as possible
adm	admission	ASCVD	arteriosclerotic cardiovascular disease
AF	acid fast	ASCVRD	arteriosclerotic cardiovascular renal disease
AFB	acid-fast bacillus ratio		
AgNo2	silver nitrate	ASHD	arteriosclerotic heart disease
A/G ratio	albumin globulin ratio	as tol	as tolerated
AK	above knee	astig	astigmatism

at fib	atrial fibrillation		**conv**	convalescent
AU	both ears		**COPD**	chronic obstructive pulmonary disease
aud	auditory		**CORT**	certified operating room technician
aux	auxillary		**CPT**	chest physical therapy
AV	atrioventricular		**CRNA**	certified registered nurse anesthetist
Ax	axillary		**CRP**	C-reactive protein
Bact	bacteria		**C&S**	culture and sensitivity
BacT	bacteriology		**C-sect**	cesarean section
BBB	bundle branch block		**CSD**	central supply room
BE	barium enema		**CSF**	cerebrospinal fluid
bet	between		**CT**	computerized tomography
bid	twice a day		**CVA**	cerebrovascular accident (stroke)
bilat	bilateral		**CVP**	central venous pressure
BKA	below-the-knee amputation		**CXR**	chest x-ray
bld	blood		**cysto**	cystoscopy
BM	bowel movement		**D**	dorsal
BP	blood pressure		**DAT**	diet as tolerated
BPH	benign prostatic hypertrophy		**D&C**	dilatation and curretage
BR	bathroom		**DC**	discontinue
BRP	bathroom privileges		**DDS**	doctor of dental surgery
BS	blood sugar		**decub**	decubitus
BSC	bedside commode		**del**	delivery
BUN	blood urea nitrogen		**dept**	department
Bx	biopsy		**dict**	dictation
c̄	with		**diff**	differential
C	centigrade		**Dig**	digoxin; digitalis
C1, C2, C3	cervical vertebrae		**dil**	dilute
Ca	cancer; calcium		**Dir**	director
cal	calorie		**disc**	discontinue
Cap	capsule		**disch**	discharge
cardio	cardiology		**DJD**	degenerative joint disease
CAT	computerized axial tomography		**SM**	diabetes mellitus
Cath	Catholic		**DO**	doctor of osteopathy
cath	catheter		**DOA**	dead on arrival
cauc	caucasian		**DON**	director of nursing
caut	cauterization		**doz**	dozen
CBC	complete blood count		**DP**	discharge plan
CBI	continuous bladder irrigation		**DPM**	doctor of podiatric medicine
CBR	complete bed rest		**DPT**	diptheria, pertussis, tetanus
cc	cubic centimeter		**dr**	dram
CC	chief complaint		**Dr**	doctor
CCU	coronary care unit		**DRGs**	diagnosis related groups
CHF	congestive heart failure		**D/S**	dextrose in saline
CHO	cholesterol		**dsg**	dressing
CHUC	certified health unit coordinator		**DT**	delirium tremens
Cl	chloride		**DUB**	dysfunctional uterine bleeding
CL	chlorine		**D/W**	dextrose in water
clysis	hypodermoclysis		**Dx**	diagnosis
cm	centimeter		**dysp**	dyspnea
CNA	certified nurse assistant		**EBL**	estimated blood loss
CNS	central nervous system		**ECF**	extended care facility
c/o	complains of		**ECG or EKG**	electrocardiogram
CO₂	carbon dioxide		**Echo**	echocardiogram
coag	coagulation		**Echo EG**	echoencephalogram
compd	compound		***E. coli***	*escherichia coli*
cond	condition		**ECT**	electroconvulsive therapy

EDC	expected day of confinement		**GTT**	glucose tolerance test
EEG	electroencephalogram		**gtts**	drops
EENT	eyes, ears, nose, and throat		**GU**	genitourinary
e.g.	for example		**Gyn**	gynecology
elix	elixir		**HB**	heart block
EMG	electromyogram		**HCG**	human chorionic gonadotropin
EMS	electrical muscle stimulation		**Hct**	hematocrit
EMT	emergency medical technician		**Hgb**	hemoglobin
ENT	ears, nose, and throat		**H&H**	hemoglobin and hematocrit
eq	equivalent		**HHC**	home health care
equip	equipment		**H&P**	history and physical
ER	emergency room		**H₂O**	water
ERCP	endoscopic retrograde cholangio-pancreatography		**hosp**	hospital
ESR	erythrocyte sedimentation rate		**hr**	hour
est	estimate		**hs**	bedtime
et	and		**hyper**	above
etiol	etiology		**hypo**	under or below
ETOH	ethanol		**hyst**	hysterectomy
EUA	examination under anesthesia		**Hx**	history
evac	evacuate		**ICF**	intermediate care facility
ex	example		**ICU**	intensive care unit
exam	examination		**I&D**	incision and drainage
exp lap	exploratory laparotomy		**ID**	identification
ext	external		**i.e.**	that is
F	Fahrenheit		**IM**	intramuscular
FB	foreign body		**IMC**	intensive medical care
FBS	fasting blood sugar		**in**	inch
Fe	iron		**inf**	infusion
FeSO₄	ferrous sulfate		**ing**	inguinal
FHT	fetal heart tones		**inj**	injection
fib	fibrillation		**insuff**	insufficiency
fl	fluid		**int**	internal
fl dr	fluid dram		**invol**	involuntary
fl oz	fluid ounce		**I&O**	intake and output
FP	flat plate		**IOP**	interoccular pressure
FS	frozen section		**IPPB**	intermittent positive pressure breathing
FSH	follicle stimulating hormone		**irrig**	irrigat
ft	foot		**ISC**	intensive surgical care
FTI	free thyroxin index		**IU**	International Units
FUO	fever of unknown origin		**IUD**	intrauterine device
FWB	full weight bearing		**IV**	intravenous
Fx	fracture		**IVC**	intravenous cholangiogram
g	gram		**IVP**	intravenous pyelogram
gal	gallon		**JCAHO**	Joint Commission for Accreditation Health Care Organizations
GB	gallbladder		**K**	potassium
GC	gonorrhea		**KCl**	potassium chloride
G&E	gastroscopy and esophagoscopy		**Kg**	kilogram
GED	gastroscopy, esophagascopy, duodenoscopy		**KJ**	knee jerk
			KUB	kidneys, ureters, bladder
GH	growth hormone		**KVO**	keep vein open
GI	gastrointestinal		**l**	liter
glauc	glaucoma		**L**	left
gr	grain		**lab**	laboratory
grav	gravida		**lac**	laceration
GSW	gunshot wound		**lact**	lactation

lam	laminectomy		**MSW**	master of science in social work
lap	laparotomy		**myop**	myopia
lat	lateral		**Na**	sodium
LBBB	left bundle branch block		**NaCl**	sodium chloride
LBP	low back pain		**NaHCo₃**	sodium bicarbonate
LDH	lactic dehydrogenase		**NAHUC**	National Association of Health Unit Co-ordinators
LE	lower extremity		**N/C**	no complaints
lg	large		**neg**	necessary
LH	luetenizing hormone		**neuro**	neurology
lig	ligament		**NF**	*National Formulary*
liq	liquid		**NG**	nasogastric
LLE	left lower extremity		**NG-tube**	nasogastric tube
LLL	left lower leg		**NH**	nursing home
LLQ	left lower quadrant		**NICU**	neonatal intensive care unit
l/M	liters per minute		**NKA**	no known allergies
LMP	last menstrual period		**no**	number
LOA	leave of absence		**N₂O**	nitrous oxide
LOC	level of consciousness		**noct**	night
LPN	licensed practical nurse		**norm**	normal
L-S	lumbosacral		**NPO**	nothing by mouth
lt	left		**NS**	normal saline
LUE	left upper quadrant		**Nsg**	nursing
LV	left ventricle		**NSR**	normal sinus rhythm
LVH	left ventricular hypertrophy		**NTG**	nitroglycerin
LVN	licensed vocational nurse		**N/V; N&V**	nausea and vomiting
L&W	living and well		**NWB**	non-weight bearing
lymphs	lymphocytes		**o**	oral
lytes	electrolytes		**O₂**	oxygen
M	male		**Ob**	obstetrics
macro	macrocytic		**Ob-Gyn**	obstetrics and gynecology
MAO	manoaminooxidase		**OBS**	organic brain syndrome
MAR	medication administration record		**OD**	right eye; overdose
mcg	microgram		**off**	office
MCH	mean cell hemoglobin		**oint**	ointment
MCL	midclavicular line		**OJ**	orange juice
MCV	mean cell volume		**OOB**	out of bed
MD	doctor of medicine		**op**	operation
MDR	minimum daily requirement		**OPD**	outpatient department
med	medical		**ophth**	ophthalmology
meds	medications		**OR**	operating room; open reduction
mEq	milliequivalents		**ORIF**	open reduction with internal fixation
Met Ca	metastatic cancer		**ORT**	operating room technician
mg	milligram		**ortho**	orthopedic
MgSo₄	magnesium sulfate		**os**	mouth
MI	myocardial infarction		**OS**	left eye
min	minute		**OT**	occupational therapy
misc	miscellaneous		**OU**	both eyes
mL	milliliter		**oz**	ounce
mm	millimeter		**p**	pulse
mn	midnight		**p̄**	after
mod	moderate		**P&A**	percussion and auscultation
MOM	Milk of Magnesia		**PA**	posterior-anterior
MRA	medical records administrator		**PAC**	premature atrial contraction
MRI	magnetic resonance imaging		**PA & Lat**	posterior-anterior and lateral
MS	morphine sulfate		**palp**	palpitation
MSN	master of science in nursing			

Pap	Papanicolaou (smear)		**qhs**	every hour of sleep
PAT	paroxysmal atrial tachycardia		**qid**	four times a day
path	pathology		**QNS**	quantity not sufficient
PBI	protein bound iodine		**qod**	every other day
pc	after meals		**qs**	quantity sufficient
PE	physical examination		**qt**	quart
Ped	pediatric		**quad**	quadrant
PEEP	positive end expiratory pressure		**quant**	quantity
per	by		**R**	right
PERRLA	pupils equal, round, reactive to light and accommodation		**Ra**	radium
			RA	rheumatoid arthritis
PFT	pulmonary function test		**RBBB**	right bundle branch block
PG	pregnant		**RBS**	random blood sugar
PH	past history		**re**	regarding
Pharm	pharmacy		**rec**	record
phys	physician		**ref**	reference
Physio	physiotherapy		**ref phys**	referring physician
PID	pelvic inflammatory disease		**reg**	registered
PKU	phenolketonuria		**rehab**	rehabilitation
p.m.	afternoon		**resp**	respiration
PMH	past medical history		**ret cath**	retention catheter
PMS	premenstrual syndrome		**retro**	retrograde
pneu	pneumonia		**RFR**	refraction
po	by mouth		**Rh**	rhesus blood factor
PO	phone order		**RHD**	rheumatic heart disease
postop	postoperative		**RHF**	right heart failure
PPBS	postprandial blood sugar		**R/L**	Ringer's lactate
PPN	partial parenteral nutrition		**RLE**	right lower extremity
PRBC	packed red blood cells		**RLL**	right lower lobe
preop	preoperative		**RLQ**	right lower quadrant
prep	prepare		**RN**	registered nurse
PRN	as needed		**R/O**	rule out
Proct(o)	proctology		**Roent**	roentgenology
prog	prognosis		**ROM**	range of motion
Prot	Prostestant		**RPh**	registered pharmacist
pro-time	prothrombin time		**R&R**	rate and rhythm
PSRO	Professional Standards Review Organization		**RR**	recovery room
			RRA	registered records administrator
psych	psychiatric		**Rt**	right
pt	patient		**RT**	respiratory therapy
PT	physical therapy		**RUE**	right upper extremity
PTA	physical therapy assistant		**RUL**	right upper lobe
PTT	partial thromboplastin time		**RUQ**	right upper quadrant
PVC	premature ventricular contraction		**Rx**	prescription
PVD	peripheral vascular disease		**s̄**	without
PWB	partial weight bearing		**S&A**	sugar and acetone
Px	prognosis		**SA**	sinoatrial
PZI	protamin zinc insulin		**SB**	stillborn
q	every		**SC**	subcutaneous
qd	every day		**sec**	second
qh	every hour		**sed rate**	sedimentation rate
q2h	every 2 hours		**SGOT**	serum glutamic pyruvic transaminase
q4h	every 4 hours		**sib**	siblings
q6h	every 6 hours		**sig**	instructions
q8h	every 8 hours		**SL**	sublingual
q12h	every 12 hours		**SNF**	skilled nursing facility

SO	significant other	**TP**	total protein
SOB	short of breath	**TPN**	total parenteral nutrition
Soc Sec	social security	**TPR**	temperature, pulse, respiration
Soc Serv	social services	**tr**	tincture
sol	solution	**T/R**	timed release
SOP	standard operating procedure	**trach**	trachea
SOS	once only, if necessary	**TSH**	thyroid stimulating hormone
sp	specific	**tsp**	teaspoon
spans	spansule	**TURP**	transurethral resection of prostate
spec	specimen	**TV**	tidal volume
Sp Gr	specific gravity	**TWB**	total weight bearing
ss	one half	**TWE**	tap water enema
S&S	signs and symptoms	**Tx**	traction
SSE	soap suds enema	**U**	units
Staph	staphylococcus	**UA**	urinalysis
STAT	immediately	**UCD**	usual childhood diseases
STD	sexually transmitted disease	**UCG**	urinary chorionic gonadotropin
Strep	streptococcus		pregnancy test
Sub Q	subcutaneous	**UGI**	upper gastrointestinal
suff	sufficient	**ULQ**	upper left quadrant
supp	suppository	**umb**	umbilical
surg	surgical	**UMS**	urethral meatal stricture
susp	suspension	**ung**	ointment
SW	social worker	**UO**	undetermined origin
Sx	symptom(s)	**U/O**	urinary output
syph	syphilis	**URI**	upper respiratory infection
syr	syrup	**urol**	urology
T	temperature	**URQ**	upper right quadrant
T1; T12	thoracic vertebrae or nerves	**USP**	*United States Pharmacopeia*
T3	triiodothyronine	**Ut Dict**	as directed
T4	thryroxine	**UTI**	urinary tract infection
T&A	tonsillectomy and adenoidectomy	**VA**	Veterans Administration; visual acuity
tab	tablet	**vag**	vaginal
tach	tachycardia	**vasc**	vascular
TAH	total abdominal hysterectomy	**VD**	venereal disease
TB	tuberculosis	**VDRL**	Venereal Disease Research Laboratory
tbsp	tablespoon	**vent**	ventricular
TCDB	turn, cough, deep breath	**vent fib**	ventricular fibrillation
TCI	transient cerebral ischemia	**VER**	visual evoked response
TDP	tentative discharge plan	**vert**	vertical
tech	technician	**VF**	visual fields
TENS	transcutaneous electrical nerve stimulator	**V fib**	ventricular fibrillation
THR	total hip replacement	**vib**	vibration
TIA	transient ischemic attack	**Vit**	vitamin
tid	three times a day	**VNA**	Visiting Nurse Association
tinct	tincture	**VO**	verbal order
TJR	total joint replacement	**vol**	volume
TKO	to keep open	**VP**	venous pressure
TL	team leader	**VS**	vital signs
TLC	tender loving care	**WBC**	white blood count
TMJ	temperomandibular joint	**WBTT**	weight bearing to tolerance
TO	telephone order	**Wt**	weight
		ZSR	zeta sedimentation rate

Root Words, Prefixes, and Suffixes

_____
_____
_____

_____

_____

Root Words

abdomin/o	abdominal
acro/o	extremity
aden/o	gland
adip/o	fat
aer/o	air
alveol/o	air sac
an/o	anus
angi/o	vessel
aort/o	aorta
append/o	appendix
aqua	water
arteri/o	artery
arthr/o	joint
articul/o	joint
atri/o	atrium
audi/o	to hear
axill/o	armpit
blephar/o	eyelid
brachi/o	arm
bronch/o	bronchial tube
bucc/o	cheek
calcul/o	stone
cardi/o	heart
caud/o	tail
cephal/o	head
cerebell/o	cerebellum
cerebr/o	cerebrum
cerumin/o	wax
cervic/o	cervix, neck
cheil/o	lip
chole	bile, gall
chondr/o	cartilage
clavic/o	clavicle
col/o	colon
colp/o	vagina
corona	crown
cost/o	rib
crani/o	skull
crypt/o	hidden
cutis	skin
cyan/o	blue
cyst/o	bladder
cyt/o	cell
dacry/o	tear
dent/o	tooth
derm/o	skin

duct	tube	**or/o**	mouth
dura	hard	**orchi/o**	testicle
dyps/o	thirst; drink	**oste/o**	bone
encephal/o	brain	**ot/o**	ear
endocrin/o	endocrine glands	**ovari/o**	ovary
enter/o	intestines	**para**	to give birth
episi/o	perineum	**patell/o**	patella
erythr/o	red	**path**	disease
esophag/o	esophagus	**perine/o**	perineum
femor/o	femur	**phag/o**	swallow
fib/o	fibrous	**pharyng/o**	pharynx
gastr/o	stomach	**phil**	like
gingiv/o	gum	**phleb/o**	vein
gluc/o	glucose	**pneum/o**	lung; air
glyc/o	glycogen	**poly**	many
gravid/o	pregnant	**primi**	first
gynec/o	female reproductive system; woman	**proct/o**	rectum
hepat/o	liver	**pseud/o**	false
herni/o	hernia	**psych/o**	mind
hist/o	tissue	**pty/o**	saliva
hydr/o	water	**pulm/o**	lung
hyster/o	uterus	**pyel/o**	kidney pelvis
ile/o	ilium; part of the small intestine	**py/o**	pus
immun/o	immune system	**ren/o**	kidney
inguin/o	groin	**reticul/o**	network
intestin/o	intestine	**rhin/o**	nose
irid/o	iris	**rubr/i**	red
jejun/o	jejunem	**salping/o**	fallopian tube
kal/o	potassium	**sarc/o**	flesh
lact/o	milk	**scapul/o**	scapula
lapar/o	abdomen	**scler/o**	hard
larynx/o	larynx	**sepsis**	decay
leuk/o	white	**sept/o**	wall
lingu/o	tongue	**sphygmos**	pulse
lith/o	stone	**spir/o**	breathe
lumbar	lower back	**splen/o**	spleen
lymph/o	lymphatic system	**spondyl/o**	spine; vertebra
mast/o	breast	**stern/o**	sternum
maxillo/o	upper jaw	**steth/o**	chest
meat/o	meatus	**tend/o**	tend
melano	black	**thorac/o**	chest
men/o	month flow, menses	**thrombo/o**	clot
mening/o	meninges	**thyr/o**	thyroid
multi	many	**toxic/o**	toxis
my/o	muscle	**trache/o**	trachea
myel/o	bone marrow; spinal cord	**trich**	hair
nas/o	nose	**tympan/o**	drum
nat/o	birth	**ur/o**	urine
nephr/o	kidney	**ureter/o**	ureter
neur/o	nerve	**urethr/o**	urethra
noct	night	**uter/o**	uterus
ocul/o	eye	**valv/o**	valve
odont/o	teeth	**varic/o**	enlarged and twisted vein
onc/o	cancer; tumor	**vas/o**	vessel
oophor/o	ovary	**ven/o**	vein
ophthalm/o	eye	**ventriculo/o**	ventricle

venul/o	venule
vertebr/o	vertebrae
vesic/o	bladder
viscer/o	large internal organ; intestine
vitre/o	glassy

Prefixes

a	without
ab	away from
ad	toward
aero	air
ambi	both
an	without
andro	male
ante	before
anti	against
auto	self
bi	two
brady	slow
circum	around
con	together
contra	against
cryo	cold
de	down
di	two
dia	through
dis	apart
dys	painful; difficult
ecto	outer
en	in
endo	within
epi	upon
eu	good
ex	away from
exo	outside
extra	outside
hemato	blood
hemi	half
hemo	blood
hydro	water
hyper	above
hypo	below
in	in
infra	beneath; below
inter	between
intra	within
intro	into
macro	large
mal	bad
mega	large
meso	middle
meta	change
micro	small
mono	one

multi	many
neo	new
noct	night
null	none
oligo	few
pan	all
para	beside
per	through
peri	around
poly	many
post	after
pre	before
primi	first
pro	before
pseudo	false
pyo	pus
quadri	four
re	again
retro	backward; behind
semi	half
sub	under
super	above
supra	above
syn	together
tachy	fast
tetra	four
trans	across
tri	three
ultra	excessive or beyond

Suffixes

ac	pertaining to
al	pertaining to; of
alg	pain
ar	pertaining to
asis	condition
cele	protrusion
centesis	puncture
cise	to cut out
cyte	cell
dyn	pain
eal	pertaining to
ectomy	to cut out
emia	blood
er	one who
esthesia	pain
genesis	beginning
genic	producing
graph	instrument used to record
graphy	recording
ia	condition; pathological state
ism	condition
itis	inflammation
ive	performs

logist	one who studies and practices
logy	study of
lysis	breakdown
malacia	softening
megaly	enlargment
metry	measurement
oid	resembling
ole	small
oma	tumor
opsy	to view
osis	condition of
path	disease
penia	abnormal reduction
pexy	surgical fixation
phagia	swallowing
phasia	speaking
phobia	exaggerated fear
phone	voice
plasty	surgical repair
plegia	paralysis
pnea	breathing
poiesis	formation

ptosis	downward displacement
ptysis	to spit
rrhage	excessive flow
rrhaphy	surgical repair
rrhea	discharge or flow
rrhexis	rupture
sclerosis	hardening
scope	instrument for viewing
scopy	examination of
sis	condition
stasis	stopping or controlling
stat	stopping or controlling
stomy	to make an opening
thermy	heat
tic	pertaining to
tion	state of; result
tome	instrument to cut
tomy	incision
trophy	development; nourishment
ule	very small
uria	urine
y	condition

Billing Forms

―――――
―――――
―――――
―――――
―――――

HCFA 1500

Field No.	Description
1	Medicare, Medicaid, CHAMPUS, CHAMPVA, Feca Black Lung or Other. Check the appropriate box for which you are submitting this claim for payment
1A	Insured's ID number. Social security number of the insured
2	Patient's name. Same
3	Patient's birth date and sex. Write all dates as month/day/year; check box of appropriate sex
4	Insured's name. Subscriber's name
5	Patient's address and phone number. Same
6	Patient's relationship to insured. Same
7	Insured's address and phone number. Same
8	Patient's status. Check the appropriate boxes
9	Other insured's name. Other insured whose coverage may be responsible, in whole or in part, for the payment of this claim
9A	Other insured's policy or group number. Same
9B	Other insured's date of birth and sex. Same
9C	Employer's name or school name. Employer or school name of other insured party
9D	Insurance plan name of program name. Name of the insurance company and/or the group plan for the other insured
10A	Was condition related to employment? If yes, then there is workers' compensation involved. If no, then no workers' compensation was involved. Circle whether employment is current or previous

Field No.	Description
10B	Was condition related to an auto accident? If yes, check for an injury date (block 14) and an injury diagnosis (block 23). The state in which the accident occurred should also be indicated. If no, then the claim may not be for an injury
10C	Was condition related to other accident? If yes, check for an injury date (block 14) and an injury diagnosis (block 23). If no, then the claim may not be for an injury
10D	Reserved for local use. Same
11	Insured's policy group of FECA number. Subscriber's group number. This information refers to primary insured listed in 1A above
11A	Insured's date of birth. Same
11B	Employer's name or school name. Refers to employer or school name of insured party
11C	Insurance plan name or program name. Refers to the name of insurance company and/or the group plan
11D	Is there another health benefit plan? Check the appropriate box. If yes, then items 9A through 9D must be completed
12	Patient's or authorized person's signature. Patient's release of information for medical services
13	Assignment of benefits. This box should be signed by the patient in order to allow the insurer to pay provider for services rendered directly instead of paying the patient and waiting for patient to pay provider
14	Date of illness, injury, accident, or pregnancy. All claims for injury must have an injury or accident date. If the patient's condition is pregnancy, then put down the date of the last menstrual period
15	If patient has had same or similar illness, give first date. Same
16	Dates patient unable to work in current occupation. Same
17	Name of referring physician or other source. Fill in if patient was referred to current physician by another physician, a hospital, or a clinic. Also list the name of the referring party
17A	I.D. number of referring physician. Same
18	Hospitalization dates relating to current services. Same
19	Reserved for local use
20	Outside lab. Was laboratory work performed outside of your office? If it was, check box yes and show total amount of charges
21	Diagnosis or nature of illness or injury. The diagnosis states why the patient went to see the provider. Use both an ICD-9 code and a description
22	Medicaid resubmission code. Leave this blank
23	Prior authorization number. Refers to authorization number for services that were approved prior to being provided
24A	Date of service. This is the date service was rendered by the provider. Use complete date
24B	Place of service. This is the location where the services were performed
24C	Type of service. Leave blank
24D	Procedure code. Use the 5-digit procedure code found in the CPT or HCPC manuals
24D	Modifier code. Use the 2-digit modifier from the CPT
24E	Diagnosis code. This is used in conjunction with field 21. The number placed in field 24E refers to diagnosis 1, 2, 3, and 4 in block 21
24F	Charges. This is the charge per line of service
24G	Days or units. This is the number of times a service was performed
24H	EPSDT family plan. Leave this blank
24I	EMG. If service was performed in the hospital emergency room, this should match the service code listed in item 24B
24J	COB. This is the coordination of benefits. List any other insurance policies or plans which may be responsible for payment on this claim. Indicate by a Y for yes or an N or no
24K	Reserved for local use. Leave this blank
25	Federal tax ID number. If the provider is a physician or an individual, his or

Field No.	Description
	her social security number should be used. If provider is a facility, use employer identification number
26	Patient's account number. Same
27	Accept assignment for government claims. This refers to medicare or CHAMPUS. Do not use to assign payment on this claim to the provider. Instead, use item 13 only for your assignment of payment
28	Total charge. This is the total charge of the claim
29	Amount paid. This is the amount paid by the patient or the subscriber
30	Balance due. This is the difference between the total charge and the amount paid by the patient or subscriber, if any
31	Signature of physician or supplier of service. Must be signed by the provider requesting the payment
32	Name and address of facility where services rendered. If the same as item number 33, leave blank
33	Physician's/supplier's billing name, address, zip code, and phone number. This is the name, address, and phone number of the provider of service. This is the address that payments will be addressed and sent to if assignment of benefits has been signed in field 13

HCFA 1500 ITEM 24B: PLACE OF SERVICE

This is a numerical code that is used to indicate the place where the service was rendered.

00–10	Unassigned
11	Office (location other than a hospital, SNF, military treatment facility, community health center, state or local public health clinic, or ICF, where the health professional routinely provides health care services, diagnosis and treatment of illness or injury on a walk-in or ambulatory basis)
12	Home (location other than a hospital or other health care facility where the patient receives care in a private residence
13–20	Unassigned
21	Inpatient hospital, other than

	psychiatric, which provides diagnostic, therapeutic, and rehabilitative services by or under the supervision of a licensed physician to patients admitted for a number and variety of medical conditions
22	Outpatient hospital, provides diagnostic, therapeutic, and rehabilitation services to sick and injured persons not requiring hospitalization; a patient who is not admitted to a hospital is defined as an outpatient
23	Emergency room, hospital. Patients in the emergency room are considered to be facility outpatients, therefore, remember to complete box number 24
24	Ambulatory surgical center, free-standing facility, other than a doctor's office, where surgical and diagnostic procedures are performed on an ambulatory basis
25	Birthing center, a facility other than a doctor's office or hospital's maternity department that provides a setting for labor, delivery, and immediate postpartum care and immediate care of the newborn
26	Military treatment facility, a facility operated by one or more of the uniformed services
27–30	Unassigned
31	Skilled nursing facility, a facility that primarily provides inpatient skilled nursing care and related services to patients who require medical, nursing, or rehabilitative care
32	Nursing facility, a facility providing skilled nursing care and related services for the rehabilitation of injured, disabled, or sick persons or, on a regular basis, health-related care services above the level of custodial care to mentally retarded persons
33	Custodial care facility, a facility providing room, board, and personal assistance services, usually on a long-term basis
34	Hospice, a facility other than a patient's home, which provides palliative and supportive care for terminally ill patients and their families
35–40	Unassigned
41	Ambulance (land), a vehicle designed,

Field No.	Description
	equipped, and staffed for lifesaving and transporting the sick or injured
42	Ambulance (air or water), a vehicle specifically designed, equipped, and staffed for life-saving and transporting the sick or injured
43–50	Unassigned
51	Inpatient psychiatric facility, a facility providing inpatient psychiatric services for the diagnosis and treatment of mental illness
52	Psychiatric facility partial hospitalization, a facility for the diagnosis and treatment of mental illness providing a planned therapeutic program for patients who do not require inpatient or full-time hospitalization
53	Community mental health center, a facility providing comprehensive mental health care and services on an ambulatory basis
54	Intermediate care facility/mentally retarded, a facility providing care and other health-related services for persons above the level of custodial care of mentally retarded persons
55	Residential substance abuse treatment facility, a facility providing treatment for substance (alcohol and drug) abuse to live-in residents who do not require acute medical care
56	Psychiatric residential treatment center, a facility or part of a facility in which psychiatric care is provided on a 24-hour basis
57–60	Unassigned
61	Comprehensive inpatient rehabilitation facility, a facility providing comprehensive rehabilitation services under the supervision of a physician to inpatients with physical disabilities
62	Comprehensive outpatient rehabilitation facility, a facility providing comprehensive rehabilitation services under the supervision of a physician to inpatients with physical disabilities
63–64	Unassigned
65	End-stage renal disease treatment facility, a facility other than a hospital that provides dialysis treatment, mainte-

Field No.	Description
	nance, and/or training to patients or care-givers on an ambulatory or home-care basis
66–70	Unassigned
71	State or local public health clinic, a facility maintained by either state or local health departments that provides ambulatory primary medical care under the direction of a physician
72	Rural health clinic, a certified facility located in a rural medically undeserved area that provides ambulatory primary medical care under the direction of a physician
73–80	Unassigned
81	Independent laboratory, a laboratory that has been certified to perform diagnostic and/or clinical tests independent of an institution or a physician's office
82–98	Unassigned
99	Other unlisted facility, a facility other than those listed and identified

UB-92 BILLING FORM

Field No.	Description
1	Provider name, address, and telephone number. This is the name, address and telephone number of the hospital or clinic where the services were provided
2	Reserved (untitled). This is where all the unlabeled fields are reserved for state or national use
3	Patient control number. This refers to the patient's account number
4	Type of bill. This is a 3-digit code that is used to provide information regarding the type of bill being submitted
5	Federal tax number. This is the provider's identification or social security number
6	Statement covers period. These are the dates of services this billing statement represents
7	Covered days. These are the number of days services were covered by the primary payer
8	Non-covered days (inpatient only). These are the days services were not covered by the primary payer

Field No.	Description
9	Coinsurance days. These are the number of days for which the patient is responsible for paying a portion of the costs of services
10	Lifetime reserve days. Under medicare, each beneficiary has a lifetime reserve of 60 additional days of inpatient hospital services after using 90 days of inpatient services during a particular period of an illness
11	Reserved for state assignment
12	Patient's name. Same
13	Patient's address. Same
14	Birthdate. This is the patient's date of birth
15	Sex. This is the patient's sex
16	Marital status. This represents the patient's marital status. Mark as S (single), M (married), X (legally separated), D (divorced), W (widowed), or U (unknown)
17	Date of admission. This represents the date in which the patient was admitted to the hospital
18	Hour of admission. This is the hour in which the patient was admitted to the hospital based on a 24-hour clock
19	Type of admission. This is the numerical code which denotes the priority of the admission
20	Source of admission. This is the numerical code denoting the source of this admission
21	Discharge hour. This is the hour in which the patient was discharged from the hospital, based upon a 24-hour clock
22	Patient status. This is the numerical code used to denote the status of the patient as of the time of the statement through date
23	Medical record number. This is the number that has been assigned by the provider by the medical record
24–30	Condition codes. These are codes that are used to identify conditions relative to the claim that may affect the payer processing
31	Reserved for national assignment
32–35	Occurrence codes. These are the codes and the associated dates that de-
	fine a significant event relative to this bill that might effect the payer processing
36	Occurrence span. These are the codes and the related dates that identify a specific event that relates to the payment of the claim
37	Internal control number. This is the control number that has been assigned to the original bill by the payer or the payer's intermediary
38	Responsible party name and address. This is the name and address of a person who is ultimately responsible for insuring payment of the bill
39–41	Value codes and amounts. These are codes and related dollar amounts that identify specific data regarding the monetary nature that is necessary for the processing of this claim
42	Revenue code. This is a code that is referenced as the type of services that were provided
43	Revenue description. This is a description of the type of services that were provided
44	HCPCS/Rates. This is the accommodation rate for inpatient bills, or the CPT or HCPCS code for ancillary or outpatient services
45	Service date. This is the date in which services were provided if this is a series bill in which the date of service differs from the from/through date on the bill
46	Units of service. This is the quantitative measure of services, days, miles, pints of blood, units, or treatments
47	Total charges. This is the amount of the total charges for that line of services
48	Non-covered charges. This is the amount per line of service that was not covered by the primary payer
49	Reserved for national assignment
50	Payer identification. This is the name of the insurer(s) covered by the patient who may be ultimately responsible for payment on this bill.
51	Provider name. This is the number that has been assigned to the provider by the listed payer
52	Release information. Y for yes and N

Field No.	Description
	for no as to whether the patient signed a release of information form
53	Assignment of benefits. Y for yes and N for no as to whether the patient signed an assignment of benefits form
54	Prior payments. This is the amount that has been paid toward this bill prior to the current billing date
55	Estimated amount due. This is the amount that has been estimated by the provider to be due from the indicated payer
56	Reserved for state assignment
57	Reserved for national assignment
58	Insured's name. This is the name of the person listed on the insurance forms (subscriber's name)
59	Patient's relationship to insured. This is a numerical code designation that indicates the relationship between the patient and the insured
60	Subscriber's certificate number. This is the policy number under which the insured is covered if it is an individual policy
61	Insured group name. This is the name of the group or company that holds the insured's policy
62	Insurance group number. This is the group number that denotes the group policy or plan under which the insured is covered
63	Treatment authorization code. This is a number that indicates that the treatment described by this bill has been authorized by the payer
64	Employment status code. This is a code that denotes whether the employee is currently working part or full-time, retired, or is in active military service
65	Employer name. This is the name of the insured person's employer
66	Employer location. This is the address of the employer of the insured or responsible party
67	Principal diagnosis code. This is the ICD-9-CM code used for the diagnosis of the patient's condition
68–75	Other diagnosis codes. These are the ICD-9-CM, V, and E codes that may be

	used for additional diagnosis of the patient's condition
76	Admitting diagnosis. This is the ICD-9 code used at the time of the admission to the hospital
77	External cause of injury code (E code). This is the ICD-9 code used for an external cause of injury, poisoning, or adverse effect
78	Reserved for state assignment
79	Procedure coding method used. This is an indicator code used to identify the coding method used for procedure coding on the claim (1-3 reserved for state assignment, 4 - CPT-4, 5 HCPCS, 6-8 reserved for national assignment, and 9 ICD-9-CM)
80	Principal procedure codes and date. This is the CPT code for the principal procedure that was rendered. For medicare, the ICD-9-CM codes must be entered here and on item number 81
81	Other procedure codes and dates. These are the CPT codes used for additional procedures that were provided and the dates those procedures were performed
82	Attending physician ID. This is the name and license number of the physician who was primarily responsible for the patient during this hospitalization
83	Other physician ID. This is the name and license number of the secondary physician, the assistant surgeon, and any other physician who provided services to the patient during this hospitalization
84	Remarks. This is used for any pertinent data for which there is no other specific place on the form
85	Provider representative signature. This is the signature of the provider's representative
86	Date bill submitted. This is the date on which this bill was signed and submitted for payment

UB-92 ITEM NO. 4

Type of Bill

The following code structure should be used to classify the type of bill used for this hospitalization. Each individual claim should have its own 3-digit code entered in the space provided that corresponds with the following information.

First Digit	Type of Facility
1	Hospital
2	Skilled nursing facility
3	Home health
4	Christian Science (hospital)
5	Christian Science (extended care facility)
6	Intermediate care facility
7	*Clinic
8	*Special facility
9	Reserved for national use

*If the type of facility is a clinic, then the "Bill classifications for clinics only" must be used; if the type of facility is a special facility, then the "Bill classifications for special facilities only" must be used.

Second Digit	Bill Classification (used for all except clinics)
1	Inpatient, including Medicare Part A only
2	Inpatient, including Medicare Part B only
3	Outpatient
4	Other (for hospital referenced diagnostic procedures or home health under the plan of treatment)
5–7	Reserved for national use only
8	Swing beds
9	Reserved for national use only
	Bill Classification (used for clinics only)
1	Rural health
2	Hospital based or independent renal dialysis center
3	Free standing
4	Outpatient rehabilitation facility
5	Comprehensive outpatient rehabilitation facility
6–8	Reserved for national use only
9	Other
	Bill Classification (used for special facilities only)
1	Hospice (non-hospital based only)
2	Hospice (hospital based only)
3	Ambulatory surgical center
4	Free standing birthing center
5–8	Reserved for national use only
9	Other

Third Digit	Frequency of Billing
0	Non-payment/zero claim
1	Admit through discharge claim
2	Interim first claim. Pertains to the first claim in a series for the same course of action
3	Interim continuing claim. Pertains to a prior claim has been submitted for this course of treatment or for hospital confinement and a subsequent bill is also expected to be issued
4	Interim last claim. Pertains to prior claims having already been submitted for this course of treatment or for hospital confinement and this is expected to be the last bill issued
5	Late charge(s). Pertains to a prior claim or complete set of claims having already been submitted to the provider and late charge(s) being added to the prior billing(s)
6	Adjustment of prior claim. This is an adjustment(s) being made that ultimately alters the prior claim with the addition of an explanation and a credit or additional charge(s) added to the claim
7	Replacement of prior claim. This pertains to a claim replacing a prior claim and the prior claim then being considered null and void
8	Void/Cancel prior claim. This pertains to the prior bill being voided, and subsequently cancelled
9	Reserved for national assignment

UB-92 ITEM 19

Type of Admission

These pertain to 1-digit codes which are used to indicate the priority of this admission according to the following structure.

Code No.	Priority
1	Emergency. Used when the patient requires immediate medical intervention as a result of a severe, life-threatening, or potentially disabling medical condition, in which the

Code No.	Priority
	patient must be admitted through the hospital emergency room
2	Urgent. Used when the patient requires immediate attention for the care and/or treatment of a physical or mental disorder in which the patient is admitted to the first available and suitable accommodation
3	Elective. Used when the patient's medical condition permits adequate time to schedule the availability of a suitable accommodation
4	Newborn. Used in conjunction with a special Source of Admission Code (item 20), when a baby is born within the healthcare facility
5–8	Reserved for national assignment
9	Information not available

UB-92 ITEM 20

Source of Admission

These pertain to 1-digit codes used to indicate the source of this admission according to the following structure.

Code No.	Emergency, Elective, or Other Types of Admission
1	Physician referral
2	Clinic referral
3	HMO referral
4	Transfer from a hospital
5	Transfer from a skilled nursing facility
6	Transfer from another health care facility
7	Emergency room
8	Court or law enforcement
9	Information not available
A–Z	Reserved for national assignment

Code No.	Newborn Admission
1	Normal delivery. Delivery with no complications
2	Premature delivery. Baby delivered with time and/or weight factors qualifying it for premature status
3	Sick baby. Baby delivered with medical complications, other than those related to prematurity

Code No.	
4	Extramural birth. Baby born in a non-sterile environment
5–8	Reserved for national assignment
9	Information not available

UB-92 ITEM 92

Patient Status

These are 2-digit codes that refer to the status of the patient at the time of the last date that was covered by this billing statement.

Code No.	Status
01	Discharged to home or self care
02	Discharged or transferred to another short-term general inpatient hospital
03	Discharged or transferred to a skilled nursing facility
04	Discharged or transferred to an intermediate care facility
05	Discharged or transferred to another type of inpatient or outpatient institution
06	Discharged or transferred to home under the care of an organized home health care service agency
07	Left or discontinued care against medical advice
08	Discharged or transferred to home under the care of a home IV provider
09	Admitted as an inpatient to this hospital
10–19	Discharged to be defined at the state level
20	Expired
21–29	Expiration to be defined at the state level
30	Patient is still expected to return for outpatient services
31–39	Patient is still defined at the state level
40*	Expired at home
41*	Expired in a health care facility such as a hospital, free-standing clinic, or hospice
42*	Expired, location unknown

*These codes are for use only on Medicare claims for hospice care.

UB-92 ITEMS 24 through 30

Condition Codes

These are 2-digit codes that are used to identify specific conditions relating to this bill that may affect the payer processing. There are no specific dates associated with these codes as there are in items 32 through 36.

Code No.	Insurance Code
01	Military service related
02	Condition is employment related
03	Patient is covered by insurance not reflected here
04	Patient is enrolled in an HMO
05	Lien has been filed on this claim
06	Patient is in end-stage renal disease (ESRD) and the first 18 months of the entitlement has been covered by the employer group health insurance
07	Treatment of nonterminal condition for hospital patient
08	Beneficiary would not provide information regarding other insurance coverage
09	Neither the patient nor his/her spouse is employed
10	Patient and his/her spouse is employed but no employer group plan exists
11	Disabled beneficiary but no large group health plan
12–16	Payer codes

Special Condition

17	Reserved for national assignment
18	Maiden name has been retained
19	Child retains the mother's name
20	Beneficiary has requested billing
21	Billing for denial notice
22–25	Reserved for national assignment
26	VA-eligible patient chooses to receive services in a Medicare-certified facility
27	Patient has been referred to a sole community hospital for a diagnostic laboratory test
28	Patient and/or his/her spouse's employee health plan is secondary to Medicare
29	Disabled beneficiary and/or his/her family member's large group health plan is secondary to Medicare
30	Reserved for national assignment

Student Status

(Used only when the patient is a dependent child over the age of 18)

31	Patient is a full-time day student
32	Patient is a cooperative or work-study student
33	Patient is a full-time night student
34	Patient is a part-time student
35	Reserved for national assignment

Accommodation

36	General care patient in a special unit
37	Ward accommodation at the patient's request
38	Semi-private room is not available
39	Private room is medically necessary
40	Same-day transfer
41	Partial hospitalization services are necessary
42–45	Reserved for national assignment

CHAMPUS and SNF

46	Non-availability certificate on file
47	Reserved for CHAMPUS
48	Psychiatric residential treatment centers for children and adolescents
49–54	Reserved for national assignment
55	SNF bed is not available
56	Medical appropriateness. Patient's SNF admission was delayed more than 30 days after discharge from hospital because condition made it inappropriate to begin active care within that period
57	SNF readmission
58–59	Reserved for national assignment

Prospective Payment

60	Day outlier
61	Cost outlier
62	Payer code indicating that the claim was paid under a DRG
63–65	Payer codes set aside for payer use
66	Provider does not wish cost outlier payment

Renal Dialysis Setting

70	Self-administered erythropoietin (EPO)
71	Full care in the dialysis unit
72	Self-care in the dialysis unit

Code No.	Renal Dialysis Setting
73	Self-care training
74	Home
75	Home 100 percent reimbursement for dialysis
76	Back-up in facility dialysis
77	Provider accepts or is obligated to accept payment by a primary payer as payment in full
78	New coverage has not been implemented by the HMO
79	CORF services (physical therapy, occupational therapy, or speech pathology) have been provided offsite

Code No.	PPO Approval Indicator Service
C0	Reserved for national assignment
C1	Approved as billed
C2	Automatic approval as billed based on a focused review
C3	Partial approval
C4	Admission and services have been denied
C5	Postponement review applicable
C6	Admission has been pre-authorized
C7	Extended authorization has been approved
C8–C9	Reserved for national assignment

UB-92 ITEMS 32 through 35

Occurrence Codes

These codes and their associated date define a significant event that relates to this bill and that may affect the payer's processing.

Code No.	Occurrence (relating to accidents)
01	Auto accident
02	No fault insurance involved
03	Accident involving a tort liability
04	Accident that was employment related
05	Other accident
06	Crime victim involved
07–08	Reserved for national assignment

	Occurrence (arising from medical condition)
09	Start of infertility treatment cycle
10	Last menstrual period
11	Onset of symptoms and/or illness

12	Date of onset for a chronically dependent person
13–16	Reserved for national assignment

	Occurrence (related to insurance)
17	Date outpatient occupational therapy plan established or was last reviewed
18	Date of patient's or beneficiary's retirement
19	Date of spouse's retirement
20	Guarantee in which payment began
21	Utilization review (U/R) notice was received
22	Date in which active care ended
23	Reserved for national assignment
24	Date insurance was denied
25	Date benefits were terminated by primary payer
26	Date skilled nursing facility bed become available
27	Date home health plan was established or was last reviewed
28	Date CORF (outpatient plan) was established or last reviewed
29	Date outpatient physical therapy plan was established or last reviewed
30	Date outpatient speech pathology plan was established or last reviewed
31	Date beneficiary was notified of intent to bill accommodations
32	Date beneficiary was notified of intent to bill for procedures or treatment
33	First day in which Medicare coordination of benefits for ESRD beneficiaries were instituted by the employee's group health plan
34	Date of election of extended care facilities
35	Date treatment began for physical therapy
36	Date patient was discharged as an inpatient for covered transplant procedure
37	Date patient was discharged as an inpatient for noncovered transplant procedure
38–39	Reserved for national assignment
40	Schedule date of admission as an inpatient in the hospital
41	Date of first test for a pre-admission into the hospital

Code No.	Service-Related
42	Date of discharge
43	Scheduled date of canceled surgery
44	Date occupational therapy treatment began
45	Date speech therapy treatment began
46	Date cardiac rehabilitative treatment began
47–49	Payer codes. These are reserved for use by the payer
50–69	Reserved for state assignment
70–99	These are occurrence span codes and dates and include the following:

	A1	Birth date-insured A. This is the birth date of the insured person who is covered by the insurance and who is considered as the primary payor
	A2	Effective date-insured A policy. This is the date the insurance coverage under the primary payer first began
	A3	Benefits exhausted-payer A. This is the last date for which benefits are available
	A4–A9	Reserved for national assignment
	B0	Reserved for national assignment
	B1	Birth date-insured B. This is the date of birth of the insured person who is covered by the insurance and who is considered to be the secondary payor
	B2	Effective date-insured B policy. This is the date the insurance coverage under the secondary payer first began
	B3	Benefits exhausted-payer B. This is the last date for which benefits became available.
	B4–B9	Reserved for national assignment
	C0	Reserved for national assignment
	C1	Birth date-insured C. This is the birth date of the insured person who is covered by the insurance and who is considered to be the tertiary payor

	C2	Effective date-insured C policy. This is the date the insurance coverage for the tertiary payer first began
	C3	Benefits exhausted-payer C. This is the last date for which the benefits were available
	C4–I9	Reserved for national assignment
	J0–L9	Reserved for state assignment
	M0–Z9	Occurence span codes and dates

Occurrence Span

These are codes and their related dates that identify a specific event that relates to the payment of the claim.

70	Qualifying stay dates
70	Payer code-nonutilization dates
71	Prior stay dates
72	First/last visit
73	Benefit eligibility period for primary payer
74	Noncovered level of care
75	SNF level of care
76	Patient liability
77	Provider liability period
78	SNF prior stay dates
79	Payer code
80–99	Reserved for state assignment
M0	PRO/UR approved stay dates
M1–W9	Reserved for national assignment
Z0–Z9	Reserved for state assignment

UB-92 ITEMS 39 through 41

Value Codes and Amounts

These are codes and their related dollar amounts that are used to identify specific data of a monetary nature that is necessary to process the claim.

Code No.	Value and Amount
01	Most common semi-private rate
02	Hospital has no semi-private rooms
03	Reserved for national assignment
04	Inpatient professional component
05	Outpatient professional component included in charges and is also billed separately to the carrier
06	Medicare blood deductible

Code No.	Value and Amount
07	Reserved for national assignment
08	Medicare lifetime reserve amount
09	Medicare co-insurance amount
10	Lifetime reserve amount during the second calendar year
11	Co-insurance amount during the second calendar year
12	Working aged beneficiary/spouse with employer group health plan
13	ESRD beneficiary in a medicare coordination period with an employer group health plan
14	No fault auto/other
15	Workers' compensation
16	PHS or other federal agency
17–20	Payer codes. These are used for payer only

Medicaid-Specific Codes

21–24	Reserved for state assignment
25–29	Reserved for national assignment for Medicaid

Code Structure

30	Pre-admission testing
31	Patient liability amount
32–36	Reserved for national assignment
37	Pints of blood that have been furnished
38	Blood deductible pints
39	Pints of blood that have been replaced
40	New coverage that has not been implemented by an HMO
41	Black Lung
42	VA
43	Disabled beneficiary under the age of 65 with a large group health plan
44	Amount provider agreed to accept from primary payer, which amount is less than charges but higher than payment received for which a Medicare secondary payment is due
45	Accident hour
46	Number of grace days
47	Amount of liability insurance
48	Amount for hemoglobin reading
49	Amount for hematocrit reading
50	Amount for physical therapy visits

51	Amount for occupational therapy visits
52	Amount for speech therapy visits
53	Amount for cardiac rehabilitation visits
54–55	Reserved for national assignment
56	Skilled nursing-home visit hours
57	Home health aide-home visit hours
58	Amount for arterial blood gas (PO_2/PA_2)
59	Amount for oxygen saturation (O_2 SAT/Oximetry)
60	HHA branch MSA. This is the branch location of the Metropolitan Statistical Area
61–67	Reserved for national assignment
68	EPO-drug. This is the number of units of erythropoietin administered and/or supplied during the billing period. Amount is reported in whole units
69	Reserved for national assignment
70–72	Payer codes
73	Reserved for national assignment
75–79	Payer codes
80	Most common ward rate
81–99	Reserved for state assignment
A0	Reserved for national assignment
A1	Deductible payer A
A2	Coinsurance payer A
A3	Estimated responsibility for payer A
A4–A9	Reserved for national assignment
B0	Reserved for national assignment
B1	Deductible for payer B
B2	Coinsurance payer B
B3	Estimated responsibility for payer B
B4–B9	Reserved for national assignment
C0	Reserved for national assignment
C1	Deductible for payer C
C2	Coinsurance for payer C
C3	Estimated responsibility for payer C
C4–C9	Reserved for national assignment

Code Structure

D0–D2	Reserved for national assignment
D3	Estimated responsibility for patient
D4–W9	Reserved for national assignment
X0–Z9	Reserved for state assignment

UB-92 ITEM 42

Hospital Revenue Codes

These codes are used to identify a specific accommodation, ancillary service, or billing calculation.

Code No.	Revenue
001	Total Charges: used to reflect the total of all charges on this bill
01X	Reserved for internal payer use
02X–06X	Reserved for national assignment
07X–09X	Reserved for state use
10X	All inclusive rate

    0   All inclusive room and board plus ancillary (ALL INCL R&B/ANC)

    1   All inclusive room and board (ALL INCL R&B)

11X   Room and board private medical or general: routine service charges for single-bed rooms

    0   General classification (ROOM-BOARD/PVT)

    1   Medical/surgical/gyn (MED-SUR-GYN/PVT)

    2   OB (OB/PVT)

    3   Pediatric (PEDS/PVT)

    4   Psychiatric (PSYCH/PVT)

    5   Hospice (HOSPICE/PVT)

    6   Detoxification (DETOX/PVT)

    7   Oncology (ONCOLOGY/PVT)

    8   Rehabilitation (REHAB/PVT)

    9   Other (OTHER/PVT)

12X   Room and board semi-private two-bed medical or general: Routine service charges that have been incurred for accommodations with two beds

    0   General classification (ROOM-BOARD/SEMI)

    1   Medical/surgical/gyn (MED-SUR-GYN/2 BED)

    2   OB (OB/2 Bed)

    3   Pediatric (PEDS/2 Bed)

    4   Psychiatric (PSYCH/2 Bed)

    5   Hospice (HOSPICE/2 Bed)

    6   Detoxification (DETOX/2 Bed)

    7   Oncology (ONCOLOGY/2 Bed)

    8   Rehabilitation (REHAB/2 Bed)

    9   Other (OTHER/2 Bed)

13X   Semi-private, three, and four beds: Routine service charges incurred for accommodations with three or four beds

    0   General classification (ROOM-BOARD/3&4 Bed)

    1   Medical/surgical/gyn (MED-SUR-GYN/3&4 Bed)

    2   OB (OB/3&4 Bed)

    3   Pediatric (PEDS/3&4 Bed)

    4   Psychiatric (PSYCH/3&4 Bed)

    5   Hospice (HOSPICE/3&4 Bed)

    6   Detoxification (DETOX/3&4 Bed)

    7   Oncology (ONCOLOGY/3&4 Bed)

    8   Rehabilitation (REHAB/3&4 Bed)

    9   Other (OTHER/3&4 Bed)

14X   Private or deluxe: Deluxe rooms are accommodations with special amenities substantially in excess of those that have been provided to other patients

    0   General classification (ROOM-BOARD/PVT/DLX)

    1   Medical/surgical/gyn (MED-SUR-GYN/DLX)

    2   OB (OB/DLX)

    3   Pediatric (PEDS/DLX)

    4   Psychiatric (PSYCH/DLX)

    5   Hospice (HOSPICE/DLX)

    6   Detoxification (DETOX/DLX)

    7   Oncology (ONCOLOGY/DLX)

    8   Rehabilitation (REHAB/DLX)

    9   Other (OTHER/DLX)

15X   Room and board, ward (medical or general): Routine service charge for accommodations with five or more beds

    0   General classification (ROOM-BOARD/WARD)

    1   Medical/surgical/gyn (MED-SUR-GYN/WARD)

    2   OB (OB/WARD)

Code No.   Revenue

      3   Pediatric (PEDS/WARD)

      4   Psychiatric (PSYCH/WARD)

      5   Hospice (HOSPICE/WARD)

      6   Detoxification (DETOX/WARD)

      7   Oncology (ONCOLOGY/WARD)

      8   Rehabilitation (REHAB/WARD)

      9   Other (OTHER/WARD)

16X   Other room and board: Any routine service charges for accommodations that cannot be included in the more specific revenue codes

      0   General classification (R&B)

      4   Sterile environment (R&B/STERILE)

      7   Self care (R&B/SELF)

      9   Other (R&B/Other)

17X   Nursery: Charges for nursing care to the newborn and premature infants in the nurseries

      0   General classification (NURSERY)

      1   Newborn (NURSERY/NEWBORN)

      2   Premature (NURSERY/PREMIE)

      5   Neonatal ICU (NURSERY/ICU)

      9   Other (NURSERY/OTHER)

18X   Leave of absence: Charges that are made to hold a room while the patient is temporarily away from the provider

      0   General classification (LEAVE OF ABSENCE OR LOA)

      1   Reserved (RESERVED)

      2   Patient convenience (LOA/PT CONV)

      3   Therapeutic leave (LOA THERAPEUTIC)

      4   ICF/MR-any reason (LOA/ICF/MR)

      5   Nursing home (for hospitalization (LOA/NURS HOME)

19X   Not assigned

20X   Intensive care: Routine service charges for medical or surgical care that is provided to patients who require a more intensive level of care than that which is rendered within the general medical or surgical unit

      0   General classification (INTENSIVE CARE or ICU)

      1   Surgical (ICU/SURGICAL)

      2   Medical (ICU/MEDICAL)

      3   Pediatric (ICU/PEDS)

      4   Psychiatric (ICU/PSYCH)

      6   Post ICU (POST ICU)

      7   Burn care (ICU/BURN CARE)

      8   Trauma (ICU/TRAUMA)

      9   Other intensive care (ICU/OTHER)

21X   Coronary care: Routine service charges for medical or surgical care that has been provided to patients with a coronary illness and who require a more intensive level of care than care which is rendered within the general medical care unit

      0   General classification (CORONARY CARE or CCU)

      1   Myocardial infarction (CCU/MYO INFARC)

      2   Pulmonary care (CCU/PULMONARY)

      3   Heart transplant (CCU/TRANSPLANT)

      4   Post CCU (POST CCU)

      9   Other coronary care (CCU/OTHER)

22X   Special charges: Charges that have been incurred on a daily basis during a patient's stay in the hospital

      0   General classification (SPECIAL CHARGES)

      1   Admission charge (ADMIT CHARGE)

      2   Technical support charge (TECH SUPPT CHG)

      3   U.R. service charge (UR CHARGE)

      4   Late discharge, medically necessary (LATE DISCH/MED NEC)

      9   Other special charges (OTHER SPEC CHG)

23X   Incremental nursing charge rate: The charge for nursing services that are assessed in addition to those for room and board

      0   General classification (NURSING INCREM)

      1   Nursery (NUR INCR/NURSERY)

      2   OB (NUR INCR/OB)

      3   ICU (NUR INCR/ICU)

      4   CCU (NUR INCR/CCU)

      5   Hospice (NUR INCR/HOSPICE)

      9   Other (NUR INCR/OTHER)

Code No.   **Revenue**

24X   All inclusive ancillary: This is a flat rate charge for incurred services on either a daily or total-stay basis for ancillary services only

    0   General classification (ALL INCL ANCIL)

    9   Other inclusive ancillary (ALL INCL ANCIL/OTHER)

25X   Pharmacy: Charges for medications produced, manufactured, packaged, controlled, assayed, dispensed, and distributed to the patient under the direction of a licensed pharmacist. Also includes blood plasma and other components of blood and IV solutions

    0   General classification (PHARMACY)

    1   Generic drugs (DRUGS/GENERIC)

    2   Non-generic drugs (DRUGS/NONGENERIC)

    3   Take home drugs (DRUGS/TAKEHOME)

    4   Drugs incident to other diagnostic services (DRUGS/INCIDENT OTHER DX)

    5   Drugs incident to radiology (DRUGS/INCIDENT RAD)

    6   Experimental drugs (DRUGS/EXPERIMT)

    7   Nonprescription (DRUGS/NONPSCRPT)

    8   IV solution (IV SOLUTIONS)

    9   Other pharmacy (DRUGS/OTHER)

26X   IV therapy: Includes administration of intravenous solution by specially trained personnel to patients requiring such treatment

    0   General classification (IV THERAPY)

    2   Infusion pump (IV THER/INFSN PUMP)

    3   IV therapy-pharmacy services (IV THER/PHARM/SVC)

    4   IV therapy/drug/supply delivery (IV THER/DRUG/SUPPLY DELV)

    9   Other IV therapy (IV THERP/OTHER)

27X   Medical-surgical supplies and devices: These are charges for supply items required for the patient's care

    0   General classification (MED-SUR SUPPLIES)

    1   Nonsterile supply (NON-STER SUPPLY)

    2   Sterile supply (STERILE SUPPLY)

    3   Take home supplies (TAKE HOME SUPPLY)

    4   Prosthetic/orthotic devices (PROSTH/ORTH DEV)

    5   Pacemaker (PACEMAKER)

    6   Intraocular lens (INTRA OC LENS)

    7   Oxygen-take home (O$_2$/TAKEHOME)

    8   Other implants (SUPPLY/IMPLANTS)

    9   Other supplies (SUPPLY/OTHER)

28X   Oncology: These are charges for the treatment of tumors and related diseases

    0   General classification (ONCOLOGY)

    9   Other Oncology (ONCOLOGY/OTHER)

29X   Durable medical equipment other than renal: These are charges for medical equipment, other than for renal equipment, that can withstand use repeated use

    0   General classification (MED EQUIP/DURAB)

    1   Rental (MED EQUIP/RENT)

    2   Purchase of new DME (MED EQUIP/NEW)

    3   Purchase of used DME (MED EQUIP/USED)

    4   Supplies/drugs for DME effectiveness (MED EQUIP/SUPPLIES/DRUGS)

    9   Other equipment (MED EQUIP/OTHER)

30X   Laboratory: These are charges for the performance of diagnostic and routine clinical laboratory tests

    0   General classification (LABORATORY or LAB)

    1   Chemistry (LAB/CHEMISTRY)

    2   Immmunology (LAB/IMMUNOLOGY)

    3   Renal patient (home) (LAB/RENAL HOME)

Code No.   **Revenue**

4   Nonroutine dialysis (LAB/NR DIALYSIS)

5   Hematology (LAB/HEMATOLOGY)

6   Bacteriology and microbiology (LAB/BACT-MICRO)

7   Urology (LAB/UROLOGY)

9   Other laboratory (LAB/OTHER)

31X   Laboratory pathological: These are charges for diagnostic and routine laboratory tests on tissues and cultures

0   General classification (PATHOLOGY LAB or PATH LAB)

1   Cytology (PATHOL/CYTOLOGY)

2   Histology (PATHOL/HYSTOL)

4   Biopsy (PATHOL/BIOPSY)

9   Other (PATHOL/OTHER)

32X   Radiology-diagnostic: These are charges for diagnostic radiology services that are provided for the purpose of examination and care of patients, and include taking, processing, examining, and interpreting radiographs and fluorographs

0   General classification (DX X-RAY)

1   Angiocardiography (DX X-RAY/ANGIO)

2   Arthrography (DX X-RAY/ARTH)

3   Arteriography (DX X-RAY/ARTER)

4   Chest x-ray (DX X-RAY/CHEST)

9   Other (DX X-RAY/OTHER)

33X   Radiology-therapeutic: These are charges for therapeutic radiology services and chemotherapy that are required for the patient's care and treatment, and include therapy for injection or ingestion of radioactive substances

0   General classification (RX X-RAY)

1   Chemotherapy-injected (CHEMOTHER/INJ)

2   Chemotherapy-oral (CHEMOTHER/ORAL)

3   Radiation therapy (RADIATION RX)

5   Chemotherapy-IV (CHEMOTHERAP-IV)

9   Other (RX X-RAY/OTHER)

34X   Nuclear medicine: These are charges for procedures and tests performed by a radioisotope laboratory that utilizes radioactive materials required for diagnosis and treatment of patients

0   General classification (NUCLEAR MEDICINE or NUC MED)

1   Diagnostic (NUC MED/DX)

2   Therapeutic (NUC MED/RX)

9   Other (NUC MED/OTHER)

35X   CT scan: These are charges for computerized tomography scans of the head and other parts of the body

0   General classification (CT SCAN)

1   Head scan (CT SCAN/HEAD)

2   Body scan (CT SCAN/BODY)

9   Other scan (CT SCAN/OTHER)

36X   Operating room services: These are charges for services provided to patients during the performance of surgical and related procedures during and immediately following surgery

0   General classification (OR SERVICES)

1   Minor surgery (OR/MINOR)

2   Organ transplant-other than (OR/ORGAN TRANS) kidney

7   Kidney transplant (OR/KIDNEY TRANS)

9   Other operating services (OR/OTHER)

37X   Anesthesia: These are charges for anesthesia services in the hospital

0   General classification (ANESTHESIA)

1   Anesthesia incident to radiology (ANESTHE/INCIDENT RAD)

2   Anesthesia incident to other diagnostic services (ANESTHE/INCDNT OTHER DX)

4   Acupuncture (ANESTHE/ACUPUNC)

9   Other anesthesia (ANESTHE/OTHER)

38X   Blood

0   General classification (BLOOD)

1   Packed red cells (BLOOD/PKD RED)

2   Whole blood (BLOOD/WHOLE)

3   Plasma (BLOOD/PLASMA)

4   Platelets (BLOOD/PLATELETS)

Code No.   **Revenue**

5   Leukocytes (BLOOD/LEUKOCYTES)

6   Other components (BLOOD/OTHER)

7   Other derivatives (BLOOD/DERIVA-TIVES)

9   Other blood (BLOOD/OTHER)

39X   Blood storage and processing

0   General classification (BLOOD/STOR-PROC)

1   Blood administration (BLOOD/ADMIN)

9   Other blood storage and processing (BLOOD/OTHER STOR)

40X   Other imaging services

0   General classification (IMAGE SERVICES)

1   Diagnostic mammography (DIAG MAMMOGRAPHY)

2   Ultrasound (ULTRASOUND)

3   Screening mammography (SCRN MAMMOGRAPHY)

4   Positron emission tomography (PET SCAN)

9   Other imaging services (OTHER IMAGE SVS)

41X   Respiratory therapy services: These are charges for the administration of oxygen and certain potent drugs through inhalation or positive pressure and other forms of rehabilitative therapy through the exchange of oxygen and other gases

0   General classification (RESPIRATORY SVC)

2   Inhalation services (INHALATION SVC)

3   Hyperbaric oxygen therapy (HYPERBARIC O_2)

9   Other respiratory therapy services (OTHER RESPIR SVS)

42X   Physical therapy: These are charges for therapeutic exercises, massage, and utilization of effective properties of light, heat, cold, water, electricity, and assistive devices used in the diagnosis and rehabilitation of patients who have neuromuscular, orthopedic, and other physical disabilities

0   General classification (PHYSICAL THERP)

1   Visit charge (PHYS THERP/VISIT)

2   Hourly charge (PHYS THERP/HOUR)

3   Group rate (PHYS THERP/GROUP)

4   Evaluation or re-evaluation (PHYS THER/EVAL)

9   Other physical therapy (OTHER PHYS THERP)

43X   Occupational therapy: These are charges for teaching manual skills and independence in activities of daily living and personal care that are necessary to stimulate mental and emotional activity on the part of the patient

0   General classification (OCCUPATION THERP)

1   Visit charge (OCCUP THERP/VISIT)

2   Hourly charge (OCCUP THERP/HOUR)

3   Group rate (OCCUP THERP/GROUP)

4   Evaluation or re-evaluation (OCCUP THERP/EVAL)

9   Other occupational therapy (OTHER OCCUP THERP)

44X   Speech-language pathology: These are charges for services provided to patients with impaired functional communication skills

0   General classification (SPEECH PATHOL)

1   Visit charge (SPEECH PATH/VISIT)

2   Hourly charge (SPEECH PATH/HOUR)

3   Group rate (SPEECH PATH/GROUP)

4   Evaluation or re-evaluation (SPEECH PATH/EVAL)

9   Other speech-language pathology (OTHER SPEECH PATH)

45X   Emergency room: These are charges for emergency treatment to those persons who are ill or injured and who require immediate and unscheduled medical or surgical care or treatment

0   General classification (EMERG ROOM)

9   Other emergency room (OTHER EMER ROOM)

46X   Pulmonary function: These are charges for test that measure inhaled and

Code No.	Revenue

exhaled gases and the analysis of blood and for tests that are used to evaluate the patient's ability to exchange oxygen and other gases

   0   General classification (PULMONARY FUNC)

   9   Other pulmonary function (OTHER PULMON FUNC)

47X   Audiology: These are charges for the detection and management of communication disabilities centering in whole or in part on the function of hearing

   0   General classification (AUDIOLOGY)

   1   Diagnostic (AUDIOLOGY/DX)

   2   Treatment (AUDIOLOGY/RX)

   9   Other (OTHER AUDIOL)

48X   Cardiology: These are charges for cardiac procedures that are rendered in a separate unit within the hospital, and include, but are not limited to, cardiac catheterization, Swan-Ganz catheterization, coronary angiography, and exercise stress testing

   0   General classification (CARDIOLOGY)

   1   Cardiac cath lab (CARDIAC CATH LAB)

   2   Stress test (STRESS TEST)

   9   Other cardiology (OTHER CARDIOL)

49X   Ambulatory surgical care

   0   General classification (AMBUL SURG)

   9   Other ambulatory surgical care (OTHER AMBL SURG)

50X   Outpatient services: These are charges for services that have been rendered to the patient who is admitted as an inpatient before midnight of the day following the date of service

   0   General classification (OUTPATIENT SVS)

   9   Other outpatient services (OUTPATIENT/OTHER)

51X   Clinic: These are charges for providing diagnostic, preventive, curative, rehabilitative, and educational services on a scheduled basis to ambulatory patients

   0   General classification (CLINIC)

   1   Chronic pain center (CHRONIC PAIN CL)

   2   Dental clinic (DENTAL CLINIC)

   3   Psychiatric clinic (PSYCH CLINIC)

   4   OB-GYN clinic (OB-GYN CLINIC)

   5   Pediatric clinic (PEDS CLINIC)

   9   Other clinic (OTHER CLINIC)

52X   Free-standing clinic

   0   General classification (FREESTAND CLINIC)

   1   Rural health-clinic (RURAL/CLINIC)

   2   Rural health-home (RURAL/HOME)

   3   Family practice (FAMILY PRACTICE)

   9   Other freestanding clinic (OTHER FR/STD CLINIC)

53X   Osteopathic services: These are charges for a structural evaluation of the cranium and the entire cervical, dorsal, and lumbar spine by a doctor of osteopathy

   0   General classification (OSTEOPATH SVS)

   1   Osteopathic therapy (OSTEOPATH RX)

   9   Other osteopathic services (OTHER OSTEOPATH)

54X   Ambulance: These are charges for ambulance service, usually on an unscheduled basis to the ill or injured person who requires immediate medical attention

   0   General classification (AMBULANCE)

   1   Supplies (AMBUL/SUPPLY)

   2   Medical transport (AMBUL/MED TRANS)

   3   Heart mobile (AMBUL/HEART MOBL)

   4   Oxygen (AMBUL/OXY)

   5   Air ambulance (AIR AMBULANCE)

   6   Neonatal ambulance services (AMBUL/NEONAT)

   7   Pharmacy (AMBUL/PHARMACY)

   8   Telephone transmission ECG (AMBUL/TELEPHONIC ECG)

   9   Other ambulance (OTHER AMBULANCE)

Code No.　**Revenue**

55X　Skilled nursing: These are charges for nursing services that must be provided under the direct supervision of a licensed nurse to assure the safety of the patient and to achieve the medically desired results

　0　General classification (SKILLED NURSING)

　1　Visit charge (SKILLED NURS/VISIT)

　2　Hourly charge (SKILLED NURS/HOUR)

　9　Other skilled nursing (SKILLED NURS/OTHER)

56X　Medical social services: These are charges for services such as counseling and interviewing patients and interpreting problems of social situations that are rendered to patients on any basis

　0　General classification (MED SOCIAL SVS)

　1　Visit charge (MED SOC SERVS/VISIT)

　2　Hourly charge (MED SOC SERVS/HOUR)

　9　Other medical social services (MED SOCIAL SERVS/OTHER)

57X　Home health aide: These are charges made by a home health agency for personnel that are primarily responsible for the personal care of the patient

　0　General classification (AIDE/HOME HEALTH)

　1　Visit charge (AIDE/HOME HLTH/VISIT)

　2　Hourly charge (AIDE/HOME HLTH/HOUR)

　9　Other home health aide (AIDE/HOME HLTH/OTHER)

58X　Other visits (home health): These are charges by a home health agency for visits other than for physical therapy, occupational therapy, or speech therapy, and must be specifically identified

　0　General classification (VISIT/HOME HEALTH)

　1　Visit charge (VISIT/HOME HLTH/VISIT)

　2　Hourly charge (VISIT/HOME HLTH/HOUR)

　9　Other home health (VISIT/HOME HLTH/OTHER)

59X　Units of service (home health): These are revenue codes used by home health agencies that bill on the basis of units of service

　0　General classification (UNIT/HOME HEALTH)

　9　Home health other units (UNIT/HOME HLTH/OTHER)

60X　Oxygen home health: These are charges by a home health agency for oxygen equipment, supplies, or contents, excluding purchased equipment

　0　General classification (O_2/HOME HEALTH)

　1　Oxygen-stationary equipment, supplies or contents (O_2/STAT EQUIP/SUPPL/CONT)

　2　Oxygen-stationary equipment or supplies under 1 LPM (O_2/STAT EQUIP/UNDER 1 LPM)

　3　Oxygen-stationary equipment or supplies over 4 LPM (O_2/STAT EQUIP/OVER 4 LPM)

　4　Oxygen-portable add-on (O_2/PORTABLE ADD-ON)

61X　MRI: These are charges for magnetic resonance imaging of the brain and other parts of the body

　0　General classification (MRI)

　1　Brain (including brain stem) (MRI-BRAIN)

　2　Spinal cord (including spine) (MRI-SPINE)

　9　Other MRI (MRI-OTHER)

62X　Medical-surgical supplies: These are charges for supplies required for patient care

　1　Supplies incident to radiology (MED-SUR SUPP/INCDNT RAD)

　2　Supplies incident to other diagnostic services (MED-SUR SUPP/INCDNT ODX)

63X　Drugs requiring specific identification

　0　General classification (DRUGS)

　1　Single source drug (DRUG/SNGLE)

　2　Multiple source drug (DRUG/MULT)

　3　Restrictive prescription (DRUG/RSTR)

Code No.	Revenue

4   Erythropoietin (EPO) less than 10,000 units (DRUG/EPO<10,000 Units)

5   Erythropoietin (EPO) more than 10,000 units (DRUG/EPO>10,000 Units)

6   Drugs requiring detailed coding (DRUGS/DETAIL CODE)

64X   Home IV therapy services

0   General classification (IV THERAPY SVC)

1   Non-routine nursing, central line (NON RT NURSING/CENTRAL)

2   IV site care, central line (IV SITE CARE/CENTRAL)

3   IV start-change peripheral line (IV STRT/CHNG/PERIPHRL)

4   Non-routine nursing peripheral line (NON RT NURSING/PERIPHRL)

5   Training patient/caregiver, central line (TRNG PT/CAREGVR/CENTRAL)

6   Training disabled patient, central line (TRNG DSBLPT/CENTRAL)

7   Training patient/caregiver, peripheral line (TRNG PT/CAREGVR/PERIPHRL)

8   Training disabled patient, peripheral line (TRNG DSBLPT/PERIPHRL)

9   Other IV therapy services (OTHER IV THERAPY SVC)

65X   Hospice service: These are charges for hospice care services for a terminally ill patient

0   General classification (HOSPICE)

1   Routine home care (HOSPICE/RTN HOME)

2   Continuous home care (HOSPICE/CTNS HOME)

3   Reserved

4   Reserved

5   Inpatient respite care (HOSPICE/IP RESPITE)

6   General inpatient care (HOSPICE/IP NON-RESPITE)

7   Physician services (HOSPICE/PHYSICIAN)

9   Other hospice (HOSPICE/OTHER)

66X   Respite care: These are charges for hours of service under the Respite Care Benefit for homemaker or home health aide, personal care services, and nursing care provided by a licensed professional nurse

0   General classification (RESPITE CARE)

1   Hourly charge/skilled nursing (RESPITE/SKILLED NURSE)

2   Hourly charge/home health aide/homemaker (RESPITE/HMEAID/HMEMKR)

67X   Not assigned

68X   Not assigned

69X   Not assigned

70X   Cast room: These are charges for services related to the application, maintenance, and removal of casts

0   General classification (CAST ROOM)

9   Other cast room (OTHER CAST ROOM)

71X   Recovery room

0   General classification (RECOVERY ROOM)

9   Other recovery room (OTHER RECOV RM)

72X   Labor and delivery

0   General classification (DELIVROOM/LABOR)

1   Labor (LABOR)

2   Delivery (DELIVERY RM)

3   Circumcision (CIRCUMCISION)

4   Birthing center (BIRTHING CENTER)

9   Other labor room/delivery (OTHER/DELIV-LABOR)

73X   ECG services

0   General classification (EKG/ECG)

1   Holter monitor (HOLTER MON)

2   Telemetry (TELEMETRY)

9   Other EKG/ECG (OTHER EKG-ECG)

74X   EEG services

0   General classification (EEG)

9   Other EEG services (OTHER EEG)

75X   Gastrointestinal services

0   General classification (GASTR-INTS SVS)

Code No.   **Revenue**

     9   Other gastrointestinal services (OTHER GASTRO-INTS)

76X   Treatment and observation room: These are charges for the use of a treatment room or other observation room for outpatient observation services

     0   General classification (TREATMENT-OBSERVATION RM)

     1   Treatment room (TREATMENT RM)

     2   Observation room (OBSERVATION RM)

     9   Other treatment/observation room (OTHER TREAT/OBSERV RM)

77X   Not assigned

78X   Not assigned

79X   Not assigned

80X   Inpatient renal dialysis

     0   General classification (RENAL DIALYSIS)

     1   Inpatient hemodialysis (DIALY/INPT)

     2   Inpatient peritoneal (DIALY/INPT/PER)

     3   Inpatient continuous ambulatory peritoneal dialysis (DIALY/INPT/CAPD)

     4   Inpatient continuous cycling peritoneal dialysis (DIALY/INPT/CCPD)

     9   Other inpatient dialysis (DIALY/INPT/OTHER)

81X   Organ acquisition: These are charges for the acquisition of a kidney, liver, or heart for use in transplantation. Other organs are included in category 89X

     0   General classification (ORGAN ACQUISIT)

     1   Living donor-kidney (KIDNEY/LIVE)

     2   Cadaver donor-kidney (KIDNEY/CADAVER)

     3   Unknown donor-kidney (KIDNEY/UNKNOWN)

     4   Other kidney acquisition (KIDNEY/OTHER)

     5   Cadaver donor-heart (HEART/CADAVER)

     6   Other heart acquisition (HEART/OTHER)

     7   Donor-liver (LIVER ACQUISIT)

     9   Other organ acquisition (ORGAN/OTHER)

82X   Hemodialysis-outpatient or home

     0   General classification (HEMO/OP OR HOME)

     1   Hemodialysis/composite or other rate (HEMO/COMPOSITE)

     2   Home supplies (HEMO/HOME/SUPPL)

     3   Home equipment (HEMO/HOME/EQUIP)

     4   Maintenance 100% (HEMO/HOME/100%)

     5   Support services (HEMO/HOME/SUPSERV)

     9   Other outpatient hemodialysis (HEMO/HOME/OTHER)

83X   Peritoneal dialysis-outpatient or home

     0   General classification (PERITONEAL/OP OR HOME)

     1   Peritoneal/composite or other rate (PERTNL/COMPOSITE)

     2   Home supplies (PERTNL/HOME/SUPPL)

     3   Home equipment (PERTNL/HOME/EQUIP)

     4   Maintenance 100% (PERTNL/HOME/100%)

     5   Support services (PERTNL/HOME/SUPSERV)

     9   Other outpatient peritoneal (PERTNL/HOME/OTHER)

84X   Continuous ambulatory peritoneal dialysis (CAPD)-outpatient or home

     0   General classification (CAPD/OP OR HOME)

     1   CAPD/composite or other rate (CAPD/COMPOSITE)

     2   Home supplies (CAPD/HOME/SUPPL)

     3   Home equipment (CAPD/HOME/EQUIP)

     4   Maintenance 100% (CAPD/HOME/100%)

     5   Support services (CAPD/HOME/SUPSERV)

     9   Other outpatient CAPD (CAPD/HOME/OTHER)

Code No.	Revenue

85X — Continuous cycling peritoneal dialysis (CCPD)-outpatient or home

  0 General classification (CCPD/OP OR HOME)

  1 CCPD/composite or other rate (CCPD/COMPOSITE)

  2 Home supplies (CCPD/HOME/SUPPL)

  3 Home equipment (CCPD/HOME/EQUIP)

  4 Maintenance 100% (CCPD/HOME/100%)

  5 Support services (CCPD/HOME/SUPSERV)

  9 Other outpatient CCPD (CCPD/HOME/OTHER)

86X — Reserved for dialysis (national assignment)

87X — Reserved for dialysis (national assignment)

88X — Miscellaneous dialysis: These are charges for dialysis services not identified anywhere else

  0 General classification (DAILY/MISC)

  1 Ultrafiltration (DIALY/ULTRAFILT)

  2 Home dialysis aid visit (HOME DIALYSIS AID VISIT)

  9 Miscellaneous dialysis other (DIALY/MISC/OTHER)

89X — Other donor bank: These are charges for the acquisition, storage, and preservation of all human organs except kidneys

  0 General classification (DONOR BANK)

  1 Bone (DONOR BANK/BONE)

  2 Organ (other than kidney) (DONOR BANK/ORGN)

  3 Skin (DONOR BANK/SKIN)

  9 Other donor bank (OTHER DONOR BANK)

90X — Psychiatric and psychological treatments: These are charges for treatment for emotionally disturbed patients, including those admitted for diagnosis and for treatment

  0 General classification (PSYCH TREATMENT)

  1 Electroshock treatment (ELECTRO SHOCK)

  2 Milieu therapy (MILIEU THERAPY)

  3 Play therapy (PLAY THERAPY)

  9 Other (OTHER PSYCH RX)

91X — Psychiatric and psychological services: These are charges for providing nursing care and employee, professional services for emotionally disturbed patients, including those admitted for diagnosis and treatment

  0 General classification (PSYCH SERVICES)

  1 Rehabilitation (PSYCH/REHAB)

  2 Day care (PSYCH/DAYCARE)

  3 Night care (PSYCH/NIGHTCARE)

  4 Individual therapy (PSYCH/INDIV RX)

  5 Group therapy (PSYCH/GROUP RX)

  6 Family therapy (PSYCH/FAMILY RX)

  7 Bio feedback (PSYCH/BIOFEED)

  8 Testing (PSYCH/TESTING)

  9 Other (PSYCH/OTHER)

92X — Other diagnostic services: These are charges for other diagnostic services not otherwise categorized

  0 General classification (OTHER DX SVS)

  1 Peripheral vascular lab (PERI VASCUL LAB)

  2 Electromyogram (EMG)

  3 Pap smear (PAP SMEAR)

  4 Allergy testing (ALLERGY TEST)

  5 Pregnancy testing (PREG TEST)

  9 Other diagnostic service (ADDL DX SVS)

93X — Not assigned

94X — Other therapeutic services: These are charges for other therapeutic services not otherwise categorized

  0 General classification (OTHER RX SVS)

  1 Recreational therapy (RECREATION RX)

  2 Education and training (EDUC/TRAINING)

  3 Cardiac rehabilitation (CARDIAC REHAB)

Code No.	Revenue
	4 Drug rehabilitation (DRUG REHAB)
	5 Alcohol rehabilitation (ALCOHOL REHAB)
	6 Complex medical equipment-routine (CMPLX MED EQUIP-ROUT)
	7 Complex medical equipment-ancillary (CMPLX MED EQUIP-ANC)
	9 Other therapeutic services (ADDITIONAL RX SVS)
95X	Not assigned
96X	Professional fees: These are charges for medical professionals that the hospitals or third-party payers require to be separately identified
	0 General classification (PRO FEE)
	1 Psychiatric (PRO FEE/PSYCH)
	2 Ophthalmology (PRO FEE/EYE)
	3 Anesthesiologist (MD) (PRO FEE/ANES MD)
	4 Anesthetist (CRNA) (PRO FEE/ANES CRNA)
	9 Other professional fees (OTHER PRO FEE)
97X	Professional fees (continued)
	1 Laboratory (PRO FEE/LAB)
	2 Radiology-diagnostic (PRO FEE/RAD/DX)
	3 Radiology-therapeutic (PRO FEE/RAD/RX)
	4 Radiology-nuclear medicine (PRO FEE/NUC MED)
	5 Operating room (PRO FEE/OR)
	6 Respiratory therapy (PRO FEE/RESPIR)
	7 Physical therapy (PRO FEE/PHYSI)
	8 Occupational therapy (PRO FEE/OCUPA)
	9 Speech pathology (PRO FEE/SPEECH)
98X	Professional fees (continued)
	1 Emergency room (PRO FEE/ER)
	2 Outpatient services (PRO FEE/OUTPT)
	3 Clinic (PRO FEE/CLINIC)
	4 Medical social services (PRO FEE/SOC SVC)
	5 ECG (PRO FEE/ECG)
	6 EEG (PRO FEE/EEG)

	7 Hospital visit (PRO FEE/HOS VIS)
	8 Consultation (PRO FEE/CONSULT)
	9 Private duty nurse (PRO FEE/NURSE)
99X	Patient convenience items: These are charges for items that are generally considered by the third-party payers to be strictly convenience items and, therefore, are not generally covered
	0 General classification (PT CONVENIENCE)
	1 Cafeteria-guest tray (CAFETERIA)
	2 Private linen service (LINEN)
	3 Telephone-telegraph (TELEPHONE)
	4 TV-radio (TV/RADIO)
	5 Nonpatient room rentals (NONPT ROOM)
	6 Late discharge charge (LATE DISCHARGE)
	7 Admission kits (ADMIT KITS)
	8 Beauty shop-barber (BARBER/BEAUTY)
	9 Other patient convenience items (PT CONVENCE/OTH)

UB-92 ITEM 59

Relationship Codes

These are numerical codes that provide the designation of the patient to the insured.

Code No.	Relationship
01	Insured party
02	Spouse of insured
03	Child of insured
04	Natural child of the insured who does not have financial responsibility of the child
05	Step-child of the insured
06	Foster child
07	Ward of the court
08	Employee, who is employed by the insured
09	Unknown
10	Handicapped dependent
11	Organ donor
12	Cadaver donor
13	Grandchild

Code No.	Relationship
14	Niece or nephew
15	Injured plaintiff
16	Sponsored dependent
17	Minor dependent of a minor dependent
18	Parent
19	Grandparent
20–99	Reserved

UB-92 ITEM 64

Employment Status Codes

These are codes that are used to define the employment status of the person identified in Item 63.

Code No.	Employment Status
1	Employed full time
2	Employed part time
3	Not employed
4	Self-employed
5	Retired
6	On active military duty
7–8	Reserved for national assignment
9	Employment status unknown

MEDICAID CODES

Field No.	Description
1	Leave blank
1A	Type providers name and address
2	Type in the provider's 9-digit medicaid provider number
3	Leave blank
4	Enter an "X" in the medicaid box
5	For patients that have medicare and medicaid, enter an "X" in boxes 4 and 5
6	Enter the 5-digit zip code number
7A	Enter the provider's telephone number
7B	Attach a medicaid sticker for the month of services
8	Enter the patient's last name, first name, and middle initial and full address as it appears on the medicaid card
9	Leave blank on medicaid forms. For medi-medi, enter the medicare number as it appears on the medicare ID card
10	Enter the patient's sex. M for male, F for female
11	Complete this field only for services associated with an accident by entering an "X" in the yes or no box in order to show if the patient's condition is related to his or her employment
12	Enter the date of onset of the patient's illness or the date of the last menstrual period
13	Enter the complete 11-digit TAR control number; if a TAR is not required, leave blank
14	Enter the patient's medicaid ID number exactly as it appears on the eligibility label
15	Enter the patient's date of birth in six digits
16	Enter the patient's last name, account number, or record number
17–18	Enter the hospital admission and discharge dates if the services were related to a hospitalization
19	Leave this field blank unless billing for emergency services
20	Enter an "X" if the patient has other insurance coverage; enter the name and address of the carrier
21	Claims must be submitted within two months of the month the services are rendered. Exceptions to this include the following:

Code No.	Description
1	Proof of eligibility was unknown or unavailable
2	Other coverage
3	Delays in obtaining authorization
4	Delay by department or fiscal intermediary in providing certification or in supplying billing
5	Do not use
6	Substantial damage to provider's records was caused by fire, flood, or other natural disaster
7	Employee committed theft, sabotage, or other willful acts

Code No.	Description
8	Court decisions, fair hearing decisions, provider appeals, or other circumstances in which the provider had no control
22	Enter an "X" if attachments are included; if not, leave space blank
23	Leave blank
24	Leave blank if patient is receiving medicare benefits; if not, enter one of the codes listed below:

Code No.	Description
0	Under the age of 65, and does not qualify for medicare benefits
1	Benefits are exhausted
2	Utilization committee has denied or physician noncertification
3	No prior hospitalization
4	Facility has denied claim
5	Provider is not eligible
6	Recipient is not eligible
7	Medicare benefits have been denied or cut short by a medicare intermediary
8	Services are not covered
9	PSRO denial

25	Optional
26	Optional
27	Enter the full 9-digit medicaid provider number of the facility where the services were provided
28	If a claim submitted to a health insurer has not been paid within 90 days, the provider may then bill medicaid using the Billing Limit Exception reason (code 2)
29	Leave blank
30	Leave blank
31	Optional
32	Enter the medicaid number of the referring or prescribing doctor
33	Optional if an entry is made in field number 34
34	Enter all the letters and numbers of the ICD-9 code
35	Optional if an entry is made in field number 36
36	Enter all the letters and numbers of the ICD-9 code, if applicable
37	Optional, except if billing for procedures not listed
38	Leave blank
39	If a mistake was made, delete the entire line by typing an "X" in this space; then enter correct information on next line
40	Enter date of service in 6-digit format
41	Enter the location where the services were rendered, using the codes listed below:

Code No.	Location of Services Rendered
1	Office
2	Home
3	Inpatient hospital
4	Skilled nursing facility
5	Out-patient hospital
6	Independent laboratory
7	Other (describe in section identified as "Remarks")
8	Independent kidney treatment center
9	Clinic
A	Surgery clinic
B	Emergency room
C	Intermediate-care facility
D	Extended-care facility

42	Enter code 1 or 2 if the services are related to family planning
43	Enter the medicaid provider number or state license number of the provider only if it is different from the billing provider number
44	Enter the applicable code and modifiers from the CPT
45	Enter the number of medical visits or surgical lesions
46	Enter the usual and customary fee for services provided
47–116	Follow the same instructions for each claim line
117	Leave blank
118	Leave blank
119	Leave blank

Code No.	Description
120	Leave blank
121	Leave blank
122	Leave blank
123	Leave blank
124	Leave blank
125	Enter amount of payment received from third-party payer identified in field number 28
126	Enter amount paid by other insurance coverage (the amount in field 127); leave blank unless medicare denies or this is a noncovered service
128	Using a 6-digit format, enter date the claim is being submitted to medicaid
129	Enter the difference between the total charges and deductions (field 119 minus field 126 equals field 129)
130–134	Leave blank
135	Leave blank
136	Leave blank
137A	Leave blank
137B	Use this space to identify any services that required additional explanation or for entering the "emergency certification statement"
138	Leave blank
139	The claim form must be signed and dated by the provider of services. Do not use a stamped signature or initials
140	Leave blank
141	Leave blank

Index

Page numbers followed by *t* indicate tables; page numbers in italics indicate figures.

fibroma(s), echocardiography in, 136
FICA deduction(s), 273
fire blanket(s), 140
fire extinguisher(s), 140–141
fire safety, in laboratory, 140–141
first-degree heart block, on electrocardiogram, 106, *106*
fixative(s), 207
flammable liquid(s), in laboratory, 141
flask(s), 150, *151*
flexion, 37
floppy valve syndrome, echocardiography in, 128–129
flora, normal, 184, 189
Florence flask(s), 150, *151*
flowmeter(s), on respiratory therapy equipment, 220, 222–223, *223*
foreign body(ies), on echocardiography, 135
frangible disc(s), on cylinders for gases, 222
frontal plane, 36, *36*
frozen section, 207
functional resume(s), 284, 287, *289*
fusible plug(s), on cylinders for gases, 222

gas(es), administration of, 221–224
  color-coding system for, 221–222
  cylinders for, 221–224, *223*
  movement of, 55–56
gas sterilization, 217, 218
glassware, in laboratory, use of, 150–151, *150–151*
glove(s), protective, 142, *144*
glucose, testing for, 197–198
Good Samaritan Act, 18, 20–21
graduated cylinder(s), 149
Gram staining, 194
granular cast(s), in urine, 169
granulocyte(s), 174
Guedel airway, 241, 242, *242*
Guillain-Barré syndrome, 236

handwashing, 26, *27*
  aseptic, 143
HbS (hemoglobin S), 174
HCFA (Health Care Financing Administration), 278
HCG (human chorionic gonadotropin), 184
HCPCS (Health Care Procedural Coding System), 270, 280
health, and illness or disease, 12–13, *12–13*
  beliefs about, 13–14
  definition of, 10
  factors affecting, 13–14
  holistic, 13, *13*
  personal definition of, development of, 11–12
  trends in, 16
health behaviors, 13–14
health care, legal aspects of, 85
health care delivery, models of, *11*, 11–12
Health Care Financing Administration (HCFA), 278
Health Care Procedural Coding System (HCPCS), 280
health care worker(s), licensing of, 20
health insurance program(s), 279
health maintenance organization(s) (HMOs), 3, 270
Healthdyne ventilator, 249
heart. See also entries under *Cardiac.*
  anatomy of, 48–50, *49*, 74, *75*
  blood flow to, 79
  electrical activity of, *80*, 80–81
  innervation of, 79
  physiology of, 74, *75*
heart block, electrocardiography in, 106, *106*
heart disease(s), 59–60
  congenital, 59–60, 237–238
  ischemic, echocardiography in, 133
heart failure, 60
  congestive, 236
heart rate, on electrocardiogram, 100
heart valve(s), anatomy of, 75
heating block(s), 156, *157*

Heimlich maneuver, 54–55, *55*
hematocrit, 174, 175, 178
hematologic study(ies), 174–182. See also specific study(ies).
hematology, 44–48, *45–47*, 47t
hematoxylin, 208
hemocytometer, 174
hemodynamics, in Doppler echocardiography, 118, *119*, 120
hemoglobin, 174, 175, 177–178
hemoglobin electrophoresis, 199
hemolysis, during venipuncture, prevention of, 161
hemolytic disease, of newborn, 204
hemoptysis, 58, 59
hemothorax, 235
heterophil antibody(ies), in infectious mononucleosis, testing for, 186–187
high-pulsed repetition frequency Doppler echocardiography, 118, 118t
histology, 207–210
histology laboratory(ies), safety precautions in, 210
histology specimen(s), clearing of, 208–209
  mounting of, 208–209
  processing of, 207–208
  records of, 208
  slides for, storage of, *209*, 209–210
  staining of, 208, *209*
histotechnologist(s), role of, 144–145
HMO(s) (health maintenance organizations), 3, 270
holistic health, 13, *13*
Holter monitor, 89–90, *89–90*
hospital(s), organization of, 5–7, 7t, 8t
hospitalization, effects of, 15–16
hot air oven(s), 156
human chorionic gonadotropin (HCG), 184
human need(s), of cardiac patients, 90–92
humidifier(s), types of, 226, *226*
humidity, absolute, 220, 226
  potential, 221, 226
  relative, 226
hyaline cast(s), in urine, 169
hydatiform mole, 184
hydrosphere nebulizer, 227
hydrostatic testing, 221
hypercapnia, 233
hypercarbia, 233
hyperinflation, 241
hypertension, 58, 61
  pulmonary, echocardiography in, 131
hypotension, 58
hypoxemia, 241

ICD code(s), 270, 278, 280
idiopathic hypertrophic subaortic stenosis (IHSS), echocardiography in, 127, 129
I:E ratio, 241
illness, and families, 15
  and wellness, 12–13, *12–13*
  definition of, 10
  stages of, 14–15
  trends in, 16
immunization(s), for laboratory personnel, 143
IMV/SIMV, 241
incentive spirometry, 228, 229–230
income tax, payroll deductions for, 273
incoming payment(s), processing of, 268
infant(s), cardiopulmonary resuscitation in, 253–254
  echocardiography in, 124
  ventilators for, 247, 249, *249*
infarction, 73
infection(s), definition of, 24
  nosocomial, 24
  susceptibility to, 25
infection control, 25–28
infection cycle, 25–26, *26*
infectious mononucleosis, testing for, 186–187